Kalil

A Manual for Histologic Technicians

A *Manual for*

HISTOLOGIC

TECHNICIANS

THIRD EDITION

ANN PREECE, H.T. (ASCP)
SCRIPPS MEMORIAL HOSPITAL, LA JOLLA, CALIFORNIA

LITTLE, BROWN AND COMPANY
BOSTON

TO *Sheldon C. Sommers, M.D.*

Preface

Like its previous editions, A *Manual for Histologic Technicians* is published with a twofold purpose: (1) to convey a practical working knowledge of histologic techniques and (2) to fill a need for fundamental and standard material for the student. Because the course in histologic techniques requires coverage of much material in an abbreviated time, it is expedient to omit all nonessentials in order to facilitate the learning process. Although the *Manual* is primarily a teaching book, advanced and special staining techniques are included in an appendix in order to extend its usefulness.

The third edition continues to offer a condensation of basic essentials presented in a simple style and a compilation of standard accepted methods in the field of histologic technology. Only enough theory and background relevant to promoting greater understanding and satisfactory results are included. More coverage is given to what may be encountered daily in a diagnostic histopathology laboratory than to specialized procedures.

With modifications and additions for the third edition, the *Manual* is evolving into an all-purpose textbook. An effort has been made to retain the desirable features of previous editions and at the same time to keep abreast of current trends. Material new to the third edition includes Nuclepore filter membrane techniques and also an introduction to fluorescent microscopy and histochemistry. The sections dealing with laboratory equipment and histology and the glossary have been expanded for this revision, and a large portion of the material in the previous edition has been updated or reworked. Review quizzes are included at the ends of most chapters — some testing memory and some testing understanding — so that the student can challenge her knowledge.

I am aware that there are almost as many variations of techniques as there are technicians, and I have made an effort to standardize the material as much as possible. The trade names referred to in the text are products or equipment recommended by the originator of a technique, or they represent material with which the author is most familiar.

With affectionate regard this book is dedicated to Sheldon C. Sommers, M.D., Professor of Pathology, Columbia University College of Physicians and Surgeons, and Director of Laboratories, Lenox Hill Hospital, New York, in appreciation of his guidance and continuing support.

I am particularly indebted to the following members of the staff of Lenox Hill Hospital: Miss Barbro Andersson and Dr. John Terzakis of the electron microscopy department for editing and contributing new material for the section Electron Microscopy in Chapter 9; Dr. Margaret E. Long for her careful editing and helpful suggestions for the section Histochemistry in Appendix I; and Dr. Harry J. Ioachim for reviewing the material on fluorescent microscopy.

I would also express my appreciation to Dr. Phillips L. Gausewitz, Dr. George E. Meador, Dr. Kai Kristensen, and Dr. Edward L. Ellsworth of Scripps Memorial Hospital for their patience, interest, and help. I am grateful to Mr. Dan Groskruger for his work on the drawings.

For their encouragement I thank my colleagues Evelyn Bonvillain, Irma Chilcote, and Mary K. Griffin and my husband Charles O. Preece who monitored my split infinitives and helped with the proofreading.

In the preparation of the first, second, and third editions, I am heavily indebted to the authors of the following reference books:

Baker, J. R. *Cytological Technique*. New York: Wiley, 1960.

Barka, T., and Anderson, P. J. *Histochemistry*. New York: Harper & Row, 1965.

Carleton, C. M., and Drury, R. A. B. *Histological Technique*. New York: Oxford University Press, 1957.

Conn, H. J. *Biological Stains* (7th ed.). Baltimore: Williams & Wilkins, 1961.

Davenport, H. A. *Histological and Histochemical Technics*. Philadelphia: Saunders, 1960.

Lee, A. B. *Microtomist's Vade-Mecum* (11th ed.). Edited by J. B. Gatenby and H. W. Beams. Philadelphia: Blakiston, 1950.

Lillie, R. D. *Histopathologic Technic and Practical Histochemistry* (2d ed.). New York: Blakiston, 1954.

Lillie, R. D. *Histopathologic Technic and Practical Histochemistry* (3d ed.). New York: Blakiston Div., McGraw-Hill, 1965.

Luna, L. G. (Ed.) *Manual of Histologic Staining Methods of the Armed Forces Institute of Pathology* (3d ed.). New York: Blakiston Div., McGraw-Hill, 1968.

Mallory, F. B. *Pathological Technique.* Philadelphia: Saunders, 1938.

McManus, J. F. A., and Mowry, R. W. *Staining Methods, Histologic and Histochemical.* New York: Hoeber, 1960.

Pearse, A. G. E. *Histochemistry, Theoretical and Applied* (2d ed.). Boston: Little, Brown, 1960.

It is my hope that this third edition will continue to be of value to students of histologic technique, histologic workers, teaching technicians, and residents in pathology.

A. P.

Contents

A Manual for Histologic Technicians

1

What Goes On in a Pathology Laboratory

Pathology is the study of disease, particularly the structural and functional changes in cells, tissues, and organs of the body which lead to or are caused by disease. A pathologist is a physician highly trained in the recognition and diagnosis of both normal and diseased tissues. A pathologist has multiple functions. As the Director of Laboratories in a hospital he makes diagnoses in the operating room, interprets and reports findings of all laboratory tests to the attending physician, presents educational programs to the medical staff, and at the autopsy table determines the cause of death. This multifunctional responsibility requires extensive knowledge, proficiency, and judgment.

The anatomic pathologist works primarily with cells and tissues. We define cells as the building blocks of all living things. When groups of these cells unite to perform a specific function we call these cell aggregates *tissue.* Normal cells have definite characteristics and reproduce themselves in an orderly fashion. Diseases, caused by infections or tumors, cause changes in tissue and disrupt this order. Mutation of cells, bizarre forms, or unregulated abnormal growth of cells make up tumors, both benign and malignant.

When the individual cell (as in a smear or cell block) is studied microscopically, the general term for this is *cytology.* When specialized cells aggregate to form a definite structure with a specific function, the study of these tissues or systems is called *histology.*

The pathology department maintains both diagnostic and research histopathology laboratories where technical procedures play a vital role in both the practical and theoretical applications of this branch of medicine. In the research area of the pathology laboratory, experiments on animals and on human tissue specimens together with findings at postmortem examinations provide knowledge that will produce the diagnostic procedures, types of therapy, and disease-prevention measures of the future.

In the hospital routine pathology laboratory, the daily surgical and autopsy tissue is processed for microscopic study and interpretation by the pathologist. It is the pathologist who either confirms or makes the final diagnosis of the patient's disease, a decision that in turn determines or affects the mode of therapy.

The histologic technician is concerned with the preparation and staining of tissue sections from surgical or autopsy material for microscopic study and interpretation by the pathologist. In addition to the knowledge and technical ability required, the technician must have a strong sense of responsibility toward the patient. Conscientious handling of tissue and care in producing the best possible slides can substantially affect and improve the accuracy of the diagnosis. In the field of histologic techniques, what you accomplish as an individual is limited only by your developed skills, knowledge of your subject, and your interest.

The story of the routine pathology laboratory really begins in the operating room and in the autopsy room. Both surgical and postmortem specimens are delivered to the laboratory as soon as possible after removal. Upon arrival at the laboratory, the tissue is given an identifying accession number and is carefully examined by the pathologist (grossing). A complete description of the general findings is recorded. The specimen is dissected and representative tissue blocks (pieces) are taken from it, put in perforated capsules, and immediately placed in a solution (fixative) that will prevent decomposition and preserve the tissue. After several hours in this fixative the tissue blocks are processed through a series of solutions that wash, dehydrate, and clear the tissue. The tissues are then infiltrated with a substance (usually melted paraffin) which, when allowed to solidify, will support the cells and make it possible to cut very thin sections of the material.

Tissue Processing

In almost all routine laboratories the tissue washing, dehydration, clearing, and infiltration are automatically accomplished by a tissue-processing machine. Generally speaking, complete processing, including fixation, takes approximately 18 to 24 hours. Early in the morning the technician detaches from the machine the paraffin-infiltrated material which must be processed further. The tissues are then embedded, i.e., the specimens are cast in a small mold containing melted paraffin and allowed to solidify into blocks. Each block is attached to a machine (microtome) designed to cut sections of tissue-paper thinness. Ribbons of paraffin-encased tissue are placed on glass slides and dried. Once the tissue is secured to the slide, the paraffin is removed and the tissue is stained with dye solutions. The stains facilitate recognition of the various tissue elements by their different color reactions.

After staining, the tissue sections are sealed under a glass coverslip for preservation. The process is now complete, and the tissue is ready for microscopic examination. Identified with the appropriate number on each glass slide, the finished sections are delivered to the pathologist in a special folder or box, accompanied by the laboratory record (protocol) containing information about the patient and the data recorded about the specimen on its arrival at the laboratory.

In the smaller community hospitals, the histologic technician also prepares body fluids and exudates for cell blocks, and processes cytology slides with the Papanicolaou technique. It is not uncommon for the histologic technician to be responsible for the preparation and processing of a wide variety of cytologic material, e.g., Papanicolaou smears, chromosome studies, cell blocks, and membrane filters.

Subsequent chapters in this book take up in detail each phase of those processes in which the technician must be well versed. For a clearer understanding of the material, an early familiarity with the terminology in the Glossary and Chapter 13, Histology, is beneficial.

2

Laboratory Equipment and Care

MICROSCOPES

The *microscope* is a very important instrument in the pathology laboratory. It enlarges minute details of the object under study. A histology laboratory without a microscope is a laboratory without quality control. The microscope not only makes it possible to regulate the results of staining procedures, but also provides the technician with daily opportunity to familiarize herself with the microscopic structure and staining characteristics of the different types of tissue. Concerning tissue, automation will never replace the adaptability and judgment of the individual.

A binocular microscope is to be preferred to the monocular model. A *lens* is used to magnify (increase the apparent size of) the object. Most microscopes are equipped with three or more *power objectives* mounted on a revolving head.

Both low (8× or 10×) and high (40×) power objectives are necessary for differentiation. Always use low power first. Focus by means of the fine adjustment. It is more difficult to find a microscopic field on high power; consequently, orientation is usually accomplished with the low-power lens. The higher magnifications give a sharp focus and provide greater detail on smaller areas. When using a monocular microscope, keep both eyes open. The eye which is not being used will soon become adjusted to ignoring objects in the field of vision.

Daylight, which was formerly used for illumination, seldom gives adequate lighting because the weather is too variable. For this reason, electric lamps are used to provide a controlled, concentrated light

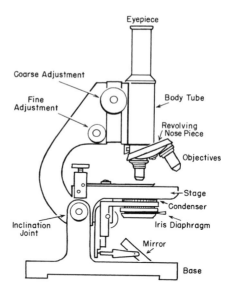

Figure 2-1. Light microscope

source. The objectionable yellowness of artificial illumination can be eliminated with the use of blue glass **filters.**

The **condenser** is located just beneath the stage of the microscope. Its purpose is to concentrate light upon the object to be examined. It consists of a lens or series of lenses mounted in a substage. The condenser should be accurately centered, with the object to be examined placed at the apex of the cone of light formed by it.

The **diaphragm** consists of a series of overlapping opaque plates with an opening of variable size for regulating the illumination of the object to be examined.

The microscope is provided with both a concave and a plane **mirror,** which may be rotated. Use the concave side of the mirror with artificial illumination and the plane side only if using daylight. Adjust the mirror until a flood of light shines up through the center of the stage (Fig. 2-1).

Dark-Field Microscopy

This type of illumination is particularly useful in the examination of *Treponema pallidum,* too small to be seen by light microscopy, and for the study of other **living unstained** microorganisms in motion. Dark-field microscopy is also useful in fluorescent microscopy.

To produce this type of illumination a special dark-field apparatus is installed on an ordinary light microscope. The attachment excludes all direct light by the presence of a disc beneath the condenser (or use of a special condenser) which diffracts the light from the center of the condenser to the periphery so that illumination emanates from the sides only. An opaque ring in the objective cuts out all directly transmitted light. Because the objective lies in the hollow dark portion of the cone of light, it picks up only scattered light so that the minute objects under study glow brightly against a dark field.

Electron Microscopy

The practical magnification possible with an ordinary microscope that uses light rays is limited because objects much smaller than a wave length of light (magnifications of up to a few thousand diameters) cannot be seen clearly, and so the limits of magnification of the microscope are about 2000 times the size of the object. When a beam of electrons is used to "illuminate" the specimen, much greater magnifications are possible, some as high as 500,000 times. The instrument has the disadvantage, however, of producing a silhouette picture (like an x-ray picture), now being improved upon with newer techniques, such as scanning electron microscopy. Personnel must be specially trained in the preparation of materials and in the use of equipment.

The instrument consists of a source of electrons coupled with a series of magnetic lenses which bend and focus the electron beam. The image produced by the electron microscope, invisible to the human eye, is recorded on photographic film by a camera installation within the apparatus. These electron micrographs are used instead of slides for interpretation of the fine structural components of the cell. The electron microscope has made possible many new discoveries and modified or changed our concepts about the structure of cells and tissues (page 111).

Phase Contrast Microscopy

The light microscope relies on differences either in color or in light absorption to provide the contrast that makes it possible for us to identify the object under the microscope. The phase contrast microscope makes it possible for us to see moving, living, and **unstained** cells and intracellular detail. The picture seen in phase contrast is very like that seen with stained sections in the light microscope, except that the image is visualized by contrasting light and dark areas.

The phase contrast microscope is a microscope with a special attachment that changes or alters the phase relationships of the light passing through and around the object. A device installed in the objective and condenser of the microscope reduces and intensifies light while simultaneously introducing a phase shift of one-quarter of a wavelength. It is the phase shifting of the light that produces dark (positive) contrast and bright (negative) contrast, so that some components of the tissue appear bright against a dark background. It is this shifting that allows objects otherwise invisible to become visible.

Polarizing Microscopy

Polarized light is used in histology primarily for the identification of crystals, such as talc, silica, alum, hematein, and urates. To achieve polarized light, a polarizing device is interposed between the material to be studied and the light source. The polarized light then passes through the material and into the objective of the microscope. Between the specimen and the observer's eyes a second polarizing filter (often mica) is inserted, and this may be rotated manually to eliminate most light except that which is altered by doubly refractile materials in the specimen, making these stand out clearly.

Fluorescent Microscope

The fluorescent microscope is basically a light microscope integrated with special filters so that organisms stained with fluorescent dyes are made visible by ultraviolet light. The type of illumination or energy source must have an extremely high intensity, rich in ultraviolet radiation, and for this purpose high-pressure mercury vapor lamps are used. The microscope must be equipped with an **exciter** filter which selectively passes the optimum exciting wavelengths through the microscope condenser into the object under study to stimulate (excite) the fluorochrome in the specimen. In addition, the microscope must have a **barrier** filter interposed between the microscopic objective and the observer to absorb or bar effectively the transmission of undesired wavelengths and pass only the fluorescing wavelengths emitted by the specimen. The barrier filters protect the eyes of the viewer from the damage that would be caused by the ultraviolet radiation. The microscope is usually equipped with interchangeable condensers for both dark-field and bright-field observation. (See additional information on page 130.)

Care of the Microscope

The microscope should be handled carefully and kept covered when not in use. If no other cover is available, an ordinary plastic bag will provide adequate protection.

Condensers, eyepieces, and objectives should be cleaned by breathing on the lens and wiping dry with lens paper made for that purpose. For a sticky lens, and after the use of immersion oil, lens paper moistened with xylene or benzene may be used for cleaning. These must be wiped dry immediately with lens paper. Cleansing or facial tissue is no proper substitute for lens paper. The microscope should be professionally cleaned and adjusted once a year.

MICROTOMES

A *microtome* is a machine specifically designed to cut very thin sections of tissue. There are four major types of microtomes including: (1) the *rotary* microtome for cutting paraffin-embedded sections; (2) the *sliding* microtome for cutting celloidin-embedded sections; (3) the *freezing* microtome, that is used exclusively to cut unembedded tissues that have been frozen with carbon dioxide, freon, or other refrigerants; and (4) the *cold* microtome (cryostat) which is a rotary microtome, mounted within a refrigerated chamber, for cutting uniformly thin frozen sections of unembedded fresh or fixed tissue.

Since the prevailing routine method is paraffin embedding, the rotary microtome is the one most regularly found in pathology laboratories (Fig. 2-2).

All microtomes consist of three major parts:

1. The *block holder,* in which the tissue is held in position.
2. The *knife carrier* and the *knife.*
3. The *adjustment screws* and *rachet* device that line up the tissue

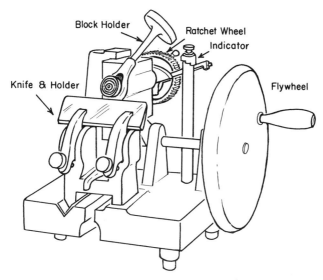

Figure 2-2.   International rotary microtome

in proper relation to the knife and feed the proper thickness of tissue for successive sections. The microtome feeding mechanism is graduated in microns. A micron (μ) is one-millionth of a meter, $\frac{1}{1000}$ of a milli-meter, or about $\frac{1}{25,000}$ of an inch.

Care of the Rotary Microtome

After cutting sections on the microtome, all accumulated paraffin and tissue should be brushed away with a soft brush.

All metal parts may be wiped clean with xylene. Avoid continuous application of xylene to the rest of the machine, as xylene will remove the painted finish. The machine must be dried carefully, with particular attention to the area under the stage (knife holder). Keep this area well oiled to prevent rust formation, which would interfere with the performance of the microtome.

Moving parts of the microtome must be kept oiled with a light oil such as 3-in-One machine oil.

The microtome should be covered when not in use.

A regular maintenance program for all laboratory equipment is recommended.

MICROTOME KNIVES

It is essential that anyone who does much work in a pathology laboratory should learn to care for and sharpen knives. A sharp knife in good condition is indispensable to the histologic technician, and *is the most important requirement for satisfactory cutting.* Poorly prepared material can sometimes be sectioned with a good knife, but a poor knife may fail to cut or may even ruin the best material.

The modern microtome knife is made of a high grade steel, tempered to a specific hardness for its purpose. It is either wedge-shaped with slightly hollow-ground sides or is planoconcave. The latter is used primarily for celloidin sectioning. Microtome knives are provided with a fitted back to ensure the proper angle of the bevel when hand sharpening, and a handle that is screwed into the base of the knife to facilitate handling while honing and stropping manually (Fig. 2-3).

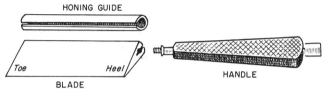

Figure 2-3.　Microtome knife

Every laboratory should have a "bone knife." This merely means that you set aside one regular microtome knife for the exclusive purpose of cutting calcified tissue, in order to protect the edge of the knives used for cutting the other sections. Even when tissue has been decalcified, it is a wise precaution to cut it first on the bone knife, since there is a possibility that not all the calcium has been removed.

A common failing of histologic technicians is to do most of the cutting in the center of the knife. This will cause the knife to wear unevenly and sacrifice the potential usefulness of the rest of the blade.

Although razor blades may be used in conjunction with a special holder to cut paraffin sections, the writer believes that the very best work is obtained with a standard microtome knife. *Advantages of razor blades:* Time is saved since honing and sharpening are unnecessary; the blade is used as long as it has a keen edge, then is discarded. The use of blades has been recommended by some workers for cutting bone sections. ***Disadvantages:*** The blade is not as rigid as a standard microtome knife. The cutting edge is short. If both razor blades and a standard microtome knife are used interchangeably on the same machine, readjustment of angle setting usually is necessary.

Care of the Microtome Knives

Whatever time is invested in the care of the knife will be repaid many times over by the ease of obtaining sections and the quality of the sections produced. Since the knives are subject to corrosion by water and blood, they should be wiped dry and oiled lightly after using. Great care must be taken to protect the edge of the knife at all times. When it is not in use, keep the knife suspended in the box in which it is received. There is no one universally accepted procedure for taking care of the microtome knife. For ***manual*** honing of the knife, some workers prefer a Blue-Green or Belgian Yellow hone, whereas others obtain best results with a glass plate and appropriate abrasives. Many authorities deny the value of stropping, whereas others recommend it. In my own experience a ***light*** stropping (even after honing with a mechanical sharpener) has prolonged the keenness of the cutting edge of the knife.

To keep the knife in good working order it is ***honed*** to remove nicks and ***stropped*** to sharpen it. Honing removes small amounts of the metal first from one side of the edge and then the other. Excellent power knife sharpeners are available in most hospitals. These machines grind the knife more evenly than hand honing and save innumerable technician hours, a factor to be considered in amortizing the cost of such equipment. Each knife sharpener has complete instructions supplied by the manufacturer. It requires only a brief time to learn to use the machine.

Some types of electric sharpeners are low-speed, light-pressure lapping machines which employ glass plates and abrasives. There is the disadvantage that the glass honing plates must be carefully monitored and dressed frequently, either manually or with a special machine, if they are to perform satisfactorily. Some such sharpeners require as long as 1 to 3 hours or more to produce a fine edge. Other electrical knife sharpeners employ high-speed grinding and stropping wheels which both sharpen and polish the knife in as little as 3 to 5 minutes.

Although the electrical sharpeners are excellent for normal maintenance, badly worn or deeply nicked knives should be returned to the factory or sent to a professional grinder for reconditioning.

When a sharpener is not available or is in need of repair, it is necessary to know how to hone by hand. Detachable backs are provided with knives for use during sharpening. Since the purpose of the back supplied with the knife is to ensure the proper bevel for the edge of the knife, a few precautions must be observed. A knife should be honed and stropped only with its *own* back. Knife backs should never be interchanged. The back must fit the blade properly. When backs become flattened or show excessive wear, they should be replaced. They may be ordered from the company that supplied the knife. When ordering a new back, either send out the knife to be fitted or order a new back by the number etched on the back or blade of the knife, or by the number on the box in which it was received.

After hand honing a knife, it cannot be sharpened on the American Optical lapping machine without first returning the knife to this company for grinding to their specific angle setting.

Before any sharpening technique, carefully examine the condition of the knife edge with a microscope. Use a wooden inspection block to hold the knife at the proper angle under the microscope. Periodic reexamination during sharpening is equally important.

HONING.   *The purpose of honing is to remove nicks and irregularities from the knife edge.* Jagged edges on the knife will produce tears or striations in the tissue sections that will be greatly magnified under the microscope. The knife should be carefully examined under the microscope before, during, and after sharpening at a magnification of about 50×. You can anticipate the following steps: (1) Before sharpening, a ragged edge is seen on the knife. (2) Preliminary honing will remove rough spots and nicks. (3) When honing is complete a fine burr edge will be noted on the knife, which is removed by stropping. (4) After the blade has been stropped, the microscope should reveal a cutting edge that is even over the entire length of the knife, represented by a thin, bright, straight line. When the cutting edge is reflected as a broad beam of light, the knife has been improperly sharpened.

Honing Technique.   For hand honing, use a fine yellow Belgian water stone with a coarse and a smooth side. The coarse side of the stone should be used only when the knife edge is badly nicked. The fine side is used when the knife has only minor irregularities or is merely dull. Keep the hone clean by scrubbing with a nailbrush as necessary before, during, and after use. Be sure the knife is free of paraffin and tissue by cleaning it with a soft cloth moistened with xylene, wiping from the back toward and away from the edge. Secure the proper back and handle to the knife.

The author's experience with the use of oil stones for honing coincides fully with the sentiments of Dr. Lorimer Rutty (Krajian and Gradwohl. *Histopathological Technic.* St. Louis: C. V. Mosby Company, 1952), who maintains that the purpose of using any liquid on the hone is about 10 percent for lubrication and 90 percent to remove the cuttings of metal as they accumulate. Using a viscous liquid such as oil on the hone tends to form the metal cuttings into an abrasive paste capable of additional injury to the knife edge. It is preferable to place the hone on the side of the sink, attach rubber tubing to a spigot, and in this way keep a steady stream of water over the stone while honing (Fig. 2-4).

The motion in honing should be from heel (handle end) to toe.

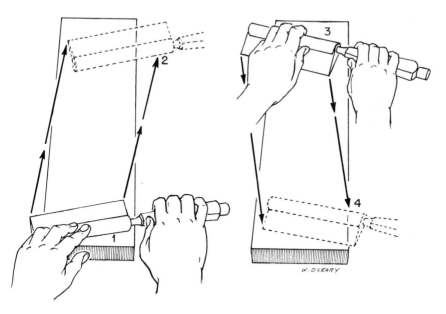

Figure 2-4. Honing technique

The edge of the knife is moved forward, the knife is turned on its back with the edge of the knife upward, and the blade is drawn toward the operator in a diagonal stroke. A right-handed person moves the knife with the right hand while the fingertips of the left hand gently guide it. Always turn the knife on its back without lifting it from the hone. Pressure when honing should be sufficient only to hold the edge evenly against the stone. Inspect the knife edge under the microscope from time to time to check the progress of honing.

STROPPING. *The purpose of stropping is to sharpen the knife.* If the knife has become dull after use but is free of nicks, it is usually necessary only to strop it. A paddle strop, one that is firmly attached to a solid back so that it will not sag, is preferred. When a strop such as a barber's strop is used, there is too much free motion to the strop, and it is very easy to round off the delicate edge of the knife. A good grade of leather strop (horsehide is ideal) with a coarse and a fine side is a worthwhile investment. Because the grade of strops readily available commercially is often inferior, the strop may have to be ordered specially from a leather goods supplier. The initial expense is more than compensated for by the results obtained and the longer life of the strop.

After honing, a wire edge produced by the stone must be removed by stropping. The knife should be clean and dry. The strop must be free of paraffin flecks, dust, or any other abrasive material larger than a few microns in diameter. Very fine abrasives (e.g., levigated alumina or diamond dust) applied to the strop are recommended by some workers as an aid in polishing the knife. The writer finds that such abrasives tend to clog the pores of the strop with metallic particles, causing it to be excessively coarse to the point of damaging a well-honed edge. The "finishing" or fine side of the strop (made of smooth, supple leather) removes the final bits of roughness and polishes the blade edge. This strop can be kept in top condition by an occasional cleaning. With the fingertips work in a rich foam of mild soap, shaving lather, saddle soap, or commercially available strop paste. Massage it well into the leather. Wipe free of moisture with a clean, soft, lintless cloth and allow to stand overnight (on edge, if the paddle-type strop is used). This treatment improves the drag required during stropping to keep the blade edge firmly against the leather.

Stropping Technique. With the back and handle in position, reverse the honing motion and move the knife toward the operator with the edge following. The knife is turned on its back and moved forward in a diagonal stroke. Unless the knife is turned with the edge of the blade upward, it will cut into and damage the strop. Stropping should not resemble a gymnastic maneuver. A very light pressure is used, just the weight of the knife. Speed is not essential or desirable. Instead, establish a rhythmic, flowing motion. Careless use of the strop, *particularly overstropping,* will spoil the best edge. Twenty to 30 double strokes are usually adequate.

Testing for keenness with hairs, skin, and other material merely dulls the edge. The only true test of whether the knife is properly sharpened is whether it cuts the tissue satisfactorily. A well-sharpened knife has a sharp, smooth, and even edge and is without irregularities (Fig. 2-5).

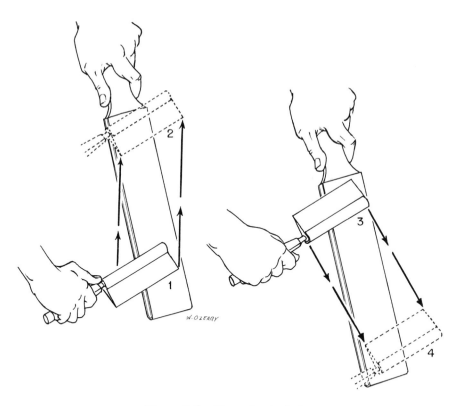

Figure 2-5. Stropping technique

AUTOTECHNICON

Autotechnicon is the commercial name of a machine that automatically fixes, dehydrates, clears, and infiltrates tissue. In some laboratories it is also used for the decalcification of bone and for the staining of tissues. It (or other similar processor) is standard equipment for the hospital with a large volume of tissue to be processed.

Such a machine (Fig. 2-6) consists of a time clock, a circular superstructure that contains the basket carrier, a receptacle basket and receptacles (stainless steel or plastic capsules), and a circular deck which holds the reagent beakers and paraffin baths. Small sections of tissue are enclosed in the perforated capsules. These capsules are placed in the basket, which in turn is attached to one of 12 yokes in the superstructure, while it is in the raised position. The entire superstructure descends, immersing the basket in the first solution and sealing the other reagent beakers to prevent evaporation. To move the basket from one reagent to the next in the processing sequence, the entire superstructure ascends and descends at scheduled intervals controlled by the time clock. During immersion in the fluids, the basket oscillates up and down in a reciprocal motion to keep the tissue and reagents in a state of controlled agitation, which significantly increases the speed of penetration. After the prescribed amount of time in the last paraffin bath, the tissue will remain here until removed manually.

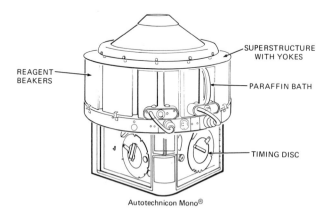

Autotechnicon Mono®

Figure 2-6.   Autotechnicon

Processing takes approximately 16 hours on a routine cycle, so that the machine is usually set for an overnight run with the processed material ready for casting (embedding) when the technician arrives the following morning. Both single (Mono) and double-decker (Duo) models are available which will carry one or several baskets, according to the need.

AUTOTECHNICON ULTRA
(FOR VACUUM EMBEDDING)

Vacuum processing is desirable for any histologic work in which speed is important, for tissues can be received, processed, and diagnosed all in the same day. There are also other advantages. When tissues are infiltrated in paraffin, in vacuo, the impregnation is more thorough. Vacuum embedding in paraffin is particularly valuable for dense tissues, such as fibrous tissue, muscle, and for blood-containing organs, spongy tissue with air spaces, and fibrin. It is also recommended for any tissue that is likely to become overhardened during the usual 2-hour to 3-hour immersion in hot paraffin.

The Ultra is a tissue processor similar to the original Autotechnicon, but in addition it incorporates heat and vacuum in all stages of the tissue processing. The heat and the vacuum increase the speed of fluid exchange within the tissue, permitting the processing time to be greatly reduced. Instead of the traditional overnight processing, the Ultra will fix, dehydrate, clear, and infiltrate tissue in as little as 3 or 4 hours. It has the obvious advantage that in an emergency, e.g., a particular biopsy evaluation, the diagnosis can be delivered much more rapidly (Fig. 2-7).

The reagent beakers are suspended in a bath of mineral oil thermostatically warmed to 38° to 40°C. while the paraffin baths are independently maintained at the usual temperature of 56° to 58°C. The temperature of the mineral oil bath can be changed to suit the laboratory requirements or it can be shut off completely. A vacuum head mounted in the superstructure attaches to the receptacle basket carrying the specimens and provides 15 in. of vacuum throughout the processing cycle. It too can be either adjusted to various pressures or

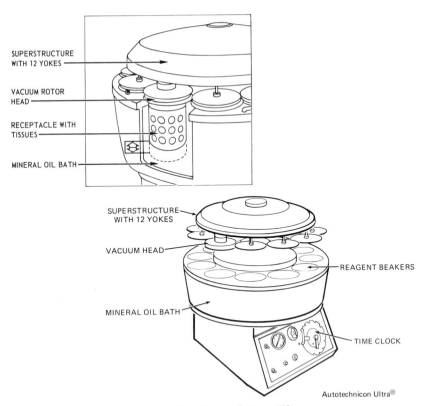

Figure 2-7.   Autotechnicon Ultra

disconnected. There is only one vacuum head so that only one basket of tissues can be processed under vacuum at a given time. The Ultra has the flexibility of running on an overnight schedule without vacuum.

A basic principle has been applied to the rapid scheduling that essentially calls for 1-hour processing for each millimeter of tissue thickness. It must be considered, however, that some unfixed tissues are extremely difficult for the pathologist to cut at less than 3 to 4 mm., so that in our experience nothing less than a 3-hour to 4-hour schedule has been workable for routine diagnostic pathology. See page 66 for schedules.

The processing reagents used with the Ultra may require some modifications of the individual laboratories' preference, for several commonly used dehydrants and clearing agents deteriorate the rubber on the vacuum head and have an adverse effect on the tubing in the vacuum system.

Care of the Autotechnicon

Solutions must be changed two or three times a week, depending on the volume of tissue sent through. Twice a week would represent a reasonable average for changing solutions. If any solution becomes contaminated or cloudy, however, a change is required. When there are three or four beakers containing the same solution, only the last requires a fresh change. Remove the first beaker and discard the solution. Move the others up in place, decanting the reagent from one to the other beaker to replace evaporated liquids, and make the last change a fresh one.

Clean all nylon parts such as beakers and baskets with detergents. Do not use acids. Be sure that no paraffin is sticking to the beaker rims, to the rims of the paraffin baths, or to the beaker cover ring. These must be kept free of paraffin to avoid damage when the superstructure rises. Tissue receptacles and the basket are cleaned of residual paraffin by immersion in xylene.

The Autotechnicon never requires oiling or greasing. All moving parts are designed so as to operate either without oil or grease, or they are permanently packed in suitable lubrication.

SLIDES AND COVERGLASSES

A good grade of slide or coverglass may often be used from the box as it comes from the supplier after only a brief polishing with a soft, lintless cloth. An exception to this rule are slides to be used for fluorescent microscopy. These must be carefully cleaned, rinsed in alcohol, and oven dried. Any dust particles or lint will fluoresce and interfere with the tissue interpretation. Handle slides and coverglasses by the edges to avoid soiling.

Cleaning and Storing Slides and Coverglasses

1. Soak in acid alcohol (page 26).
2. Rinse in water.
3. Place in 95% alcohol.

4. Polish and dry each one with a soft, lintless cloth. Gauze or cheesecloth cut into pieces the size of a handkerchief is convenient.

5. Once cleaned, both slides and coverglasses should be stored in covered clean boxes or in dishes with lids.

Labeling Slides — Choice of Methods

1. The case number of the specimen is etched with a diamond marking pencil along the edge of the right-hand side of all slides.

2. Frosted-end slides are very convenient, for they may be marked with a black glass-marking ink (india ink or Gold Seal black ink) in addition to etching. These inks are designed to resist most of the reagents commonly used. Frosted-end slides are usually marked before the tissue section is picked up. Identifying slides in this manner facilitates staining and handling.

3. If slides do not have frosted ends, the case number is applied to a special paper label available for this purpose. This label is not attached until after the section has been stained and mounted and the slide cleaned. These slides must be diamond-marked initially to provide identification.

4. Just prior to coverslipping, a small slip of paper bearing the identification number may be placed on the slide next to the section. The mounting reagent is applied, and the coverglass placed in position. The number remains permanently sealed with the section.

5. Special self-adhesive labels are available that not only provide identification, but also, when placed on both ends of the slides, keep them far enough apart to prevent their sticking together when stacked (Elman Labels, Inc., 2311 Perkins Place, Silver Spring, Md. 20910).

Containers for Slides

For this purpose, a variety of holders is available:

1. Cardboard trays that accommodate 2, 4, or 20 slides (usually freshly prepared slides).

2. Slotted wooden or plastic or reinforced cardboard boxes ranging in size to accommodate from 12 to 100 slides.

3. Special metal filing cabinets with drawers capable of holding thousands of slides for long-term storage.

PARAFFIN OVEN

Paraffin ovens maintain a more even temperature if equipped with water jackets. The temperature of the oven should be regulated just above the melting point of paraffin (between 50° and 60°C.). The maximum temperature of an oven purchased for this purpose need not exceed 80°C. Ovens with a higher temperature range are not only unnecessary but undesirable. The temperature should be checked regularly, and the oven kept clean of spilled paraffin.

The size of the oven should be large enough to serve several functions: (1) Cakes of paraffin are melted down, filtered, and stored within the oven; (2) Oven may be used for infiltration purposes, rather than the baths on the Autotechnicon; (3) Oven may be used for drying slides; and (4) Oven may be used for heating solutions or stains, or for staining tissue sections at higher than room temperature.

INCUBATORS

Although not an absolute essential, an incubator regulated at 37°C. is a welcome piece of equipment in the pathology laboratory. Sections of the central nervous system require careful drying. Paraffin-embedded brain sections dried slowly overnight (without melting the paraffin) at 37°C. tend to remain more firmly affixed to the slides.

Not only is the incubator an excellent drying oven, but several staining techniques require that the tissue be treated or stained at this temperature. When such an oven is not available, covered Coplin jars may be placed in the water flotation bath (43°C.) to provide a close approximation of the required temperature.

ACCESSORY EQUIPMENT

Balance

A small balance capable of weighing small loads of as much as 100 gm. with a 1 to 2 mg. sensitivity is generally all that is required in preparing solutions for histologic techniques. If an instrument of larger capacity is needed or if it is necessary to use an analytic quantitative balance, one or more of these is usually available in the clinical laboratory of the pathology department. Be sure the weighing pan is protected. After use, wipe the pan free of any corrosive material that is placed or dropped on it.

Tissue Flotation Bath

The water bath is used to float smooth and facilitate separation of embedded tissue ribbons. It is thermostatically controlled to maintain the proper temperature (43°C. is recommended). The bath has a dull black interior to allow high visibility of the floating translucent paraffin ribbons. After utilization, pour the water over the rim *opposite* the electrical element. While the bath is still warm, wipe thoroughly to remove adherent bits of paraffin while they are still soft.

If gelatin has been used in the bath as a slide adhesive, the bath must be washed carefully each day with a good detergent. The use of gelatin encourages the formation of bacteria, and the bath must be kept scrupulously clean; otherwise this bacteria may appear on tissue sections and present a false picture.

Slide Dryers

One type of slide dryer provides a drying chamber within which a steady current of warm air blows over the slides and carries away the moisture. The slide accommodation capacity varies with the model. Although these dryers are thermostatically controlled to prevent overheating, it is a wise precaution to maintain a hand-thermometer check on the temperature. If the paraffin melts rapidly from the tissue, the thermostat is set too high. Overheating adversely affects the tissue sections.

Another type of slide dryer is a warming plate, thermostatically controlled. The surface of the plate is anodized aluminum coated black for greater visibility. The plate will accommodate 58 standard 3″ x 1″ slides. Slides are drained and blotted after mounting and placed directly on the plate. An advantage is that at time of sectioning there is no middle step such as inserting slides individually into the slots of the loading carrier or rack.

Magnetic Stirrers

This piece of equipment offers convenience and efficiency in the preparation of fixatives, reagents, and dye solutions. The most common model employs teflon-coated magnetic spinning bars in a variety of sizes to suit the density or volume of the solution. The stirrers may be purchased with or without a hot plate, thermostatically controlled. Both speed control and heat control are operated by separate switches so that the stirrer can be used with or without heat. A beaker or flask is placed on the platform, the motor supplies the impetus, and the magnetic rods do the mixing.

STORAGE CONTAINERS FOR WET TISSUE AND PARAFFIN BLOCKS

Specimen bottles for storage of tissue in preserving solutions should be wide-mouthed. Bottles with a capacity of 60 to 120 ml. with plastic caps may be used for temporary storage of small specimens. Screw-cap jars such as the ones commercially used for mayonnaise make acceptable temporary storage containers for large tissues and autopsy material.

The bottles require much space, and retrieval problems negate their use. The plastic bag system for collecting, storing, and mailing pathological specimens has superseded the use of bottles. After an appropriate fixation period, nearly all of the fixative may be poured from the specimen and the bag heat-sealed, labeled, and stored. Bags made of plastic of less than 0.004 gauge thickness are not workable. Plastic bags (polyethylene of 0.004 to 0.006 gauge thickness) were selected by the Armed Forces Institute of Pathology for the permanent storage of wet tissue (Broadway, C. B., and Koelle, D. G. *Techn. Bull. Regist. Med. Techn.* 30:17, 1960). Among the advantages reported were (1) smaller volume of fixative required; (2) conservation of space;

(3) greater convenience and economy than traditional methods when shipping tissue; and (4) good preservation of tissue during indefinite periods of time.

Paraffin blocks, clearly identified, are stored in commercially purchased containers, wooden trays, cardboard boxes, or paper or plastic envelopes in a *cool* place free of rodents and insects.

QUIZ

1. Define briefly the use of the following:
   a. light microscopy
   b. dark-field microscopy
   c. electron microscopy
   d. phase contrast microscopy
   e. polarizing microscopy
   f. fluorescent microscopy
2. What is the purpose of the following?
   a. rotary microtome
   b. Autotechnicon
   c. what advantages are there to processing tissue under vacuum?
   d. freezing microtome
   e. paraffin oven
3. Name four kinds of microtomes. What is each used for?
4. What is the purpose of honing a microtome knife?
5. What is the purpose of stropping a microtome knife?
6. What is a magnetic stirrer?
7. If gelatin is used in flotation baths, what precautions must be observed?
8. How is wet tissue stored?
9. How are paraffin blocks stored?

3

Stock Solutions to Have on Hand

The term *stock solutions* actually has two connotations. There are some solutions that are used in bulk every day or nearly every day in the histology laboratory. It is more efficient that these be made up in advance in large quantities, e.g., gallon-size amounts, readily available on need. Daily use of large quantities makes it advantageous to prepare and store these solutions in plastic containers, with or without siphons. Measure the capacity of the container before preparing the solution, since a gallon container is not sufficiently large for 4 liters of solution.

Time is saved in the preparation if each container is marked with a felt marker to indicate the levels to which the various constituents are to be added to make up the desired mixture. Label the container clearly as to contents. Examples of stock solution prepared in large quantities are acid alcohol, sodium thiosulfate, fixatives, and dilutions of alcohol. *If no solvent is specified, water is to be used.*

Stock solutions are also solutions made up in a strength more concentrated than what is actually needed and from which dilutions (or *working solutions*) are prepared at time of use. Stock solutions like these must keep well on storage and not deteriorate on standing. It is more efficient to make dilutions from a prepared stock solution than it is to weigh, measure, mix, and prepare a specified percentage for each individual technique. Some stock solutions serve more than one purpose. Saturated picric acid, e.g., may be used in compounding fixatives or preparing staining solutions. All such stock solutions should be dated and initialed when made. An additional control factor would be to add the discard date (D.D.). The discard date is determined by the approximate life span of the solution.

In the preparation of acid solutions some precautions must be observed. Acids are always poured into the other solutions (*acid to water*), which are usually in bulk. The heat generated by mixing may cause spattering of the acid or breakage of glassware if this rule is not observed. After pouring acid from a bottle, replace the cap securely, rinse off the outside of the bottle with tap water, and dry before returning bottle to shelf.

Acid Alcohol 0.5%

70% ethyl alcohol	1000 ml.
Hydrochloric acid, concentrated	5 ml.

Acid Alcohol 1.0%

70% ethyl alcohol	1000 ml.
Hydrochloric acid, concentrated	10 ml.

Ammonia Water
(For hematoxylin series)

Tap water	1000 ml.
Ammonium hydroxide (58%)	2–3 ml.

Carbol-Xylene 1:3

Phenol (crystals)	25 gm.
Xylene	75 ml.

See additional information on page 50.

Thick Celloidin 11%

Parlodion (celloidin)	1 oz.
Absolute alcohol	125 ml.
Ether	125 ml.

Dissolve the Parlodion in the alcohol and ether in a glass preserving jar complete with rubber ring or some other airtight container. Roll the jar several times a day and reverse the position from time to time until solution is complete. This usually takes from 3 to 7 days. Store in dark away from heat.

D I L U T E C E L L O I D I N S O L U T I O N

Thick celloidin (11%)	5 ml.
Equal parts of absolute alcohol and ether	95 ml.

This solution is used for attaching problem sections more firmly to the slides (page 284). Store in a preserving jar complete with rubber ring. For convenience, keep a screw-cap jar (a size that allows the easy immersion and withdrawal of a 3″ x 1″ slide) containing the dilute celloidin on the staining bench ready for use. Filter once a week.

C L E A N I N G F L U I D
(For chemically cleaning glassware)

Potassium dichromate	20 gm.
Distilled water	200 ml.
Sulfuric acid, C.P.	20 ml.

Pulverize the potassium dichromate. Dissolve this in the distilled water in a Pyrex container with the aid of a little heat. Cool, and then *slowly* add the *sulfuric acid*. Keep the solution tightly covered.

This solution is highly corrosive. Handle with great care.

Before treating beakers, graduates, bottles, and so forth with the acid cleaning fluid, wash them in soap and hot water. Rinse with hot water to remove the soap. Leave in cleaning solution for 2 hours or more. Rinse in running tap water, and dry with opening downward on drying rack. Chemically clean glassware is imperative in all procedures employing silver nitrate techniques.

M A Y E R ' S E G G A L B U M E N

Very satisfactory egg albumen can be procured from laboratory supply houses. For those who prefer to make their own, the formula is:

Egg white	50 ml.
Glycerin	50 ml.

Beat the egg white and glycerin together and filter through coarse filter paper or through several thicknesses of gauze. Add a thymol crystal to preserve the albumen and prevent the growth of molds. Store the stock bottle in the refrigerator. This mixture is commonly used to provide better adhesion of tissue sections to the slides. Albumen is a protein and if present in too large an amount will absorb dye solutions. The mixture should be spread in an even, almost invisible film across the slide.

FORMIC ACID DECALCIFICATION SOLUTIONS
(After Morse)

SOLUTION I

Sodium citrate	200 gm.
Distilled water	1000 ml.

SOLUTION II

Formic acid (88%)	500 ml.
Distilled water	500 ml.

For use: Combine equal parts of Solution I and Solution II. The sodium citrate in this solution acts as a neutralizer to prevent excessive swelling caused by the acid.

1% GOLD CHLORIDE

Gold chloride	1 gm.
Distilled water	100 ml.

Score vial with a clean, fine file, and break glass vial of 15 grains (15 grains = 1 gram) into the distilled water. Store in brown bottle in a dark place or in the refrigerator. It stores well for as long as 6 months.

0.1% GOLD CHLORIDE

1% gold chloride	10 ml.
Distilled water	90 ml.

0.2% GOLD CHLORIDE

1% gold chloride	10 ml.
Distilled water	40 ml.

Solutions are stable for approximately 100 slides.

ALCOHOLIC IODINE SOLUTION 0.5%

Iodine crystals	5 gm.
80% alcohol	1000 ml.

This solution is primarily used to remove mercuric chloride crystals (page 277) following fixation with mercuric chloride-containing fixatives, i.e., Zenker's and Helly's fluids. The dish of iodine solution is added to the series immediately following deparaffinization. The solution may be reused in the staining series until it turns light in color. A portion of a stock solution of greater concentration (10 to 15% solution) than that indicated can be added daily to the dish until it resumes a fairly deep red-brown color which will restore its efficiency. The dish should be washed periodically and replenished with a fresh supply of the 0.5% solution.

Gram's Iodine

Iodine crystals	1 gm.
Potassium iodide	2 gm.
Distilled water	300 ml.

This reagent has multiple uses. It is a stain for glycogen and amyloid. It may serve as an oxidizing agent. It is most commonly used in the Gram techniques for staining bacteria (page 194). It stores well for at least 2 months.

Lugol's Iodine

(For Verhoeff's elastic tissue stain)

Potassium iodide	4 gm.
Iodine crystals	2 gm.
Distilled water	100 ml.

Weigert's Iodine

Iodine crystals	1 gm.
Potassium iodide	2 gm.
Distilled water	100 ml.

Lithium Carbonate (Saturated Solution)

Lithium carbonate	6 gm.
Distilled water	500 ml.

1N (Normal) Hydrochloric Acid

Hydrochloric acid, concentrated, s.g. 1.19	83.5 ml.
Distilled water	916.5 ml.

2N (Normal) Hydrochloric Acid

Hydrochloric acid, concentrated, s.g. 1.19	83.5 ml.
Distilled water	416.5 ml.

Picric Acid (Saturated Solution) 1.22%

Picric acid	1.22 gm.
Distilled water	100.00 ml.

It is a versatile solution with multiple usages, including those as (1) an ingredient of fixing solutions; (2) a postmordant for formalin-fixed tissue; (3) a constituent in many special staining techniques, particularly connective tissue stains; and (4) a counterstain or a differentiator.

Stock Rosin Solution 10%

Colophony or cherry rosin	50 gm.
Absolute alcohol	500 ml.

Store colophony solution away from the light. It is used to differentiate azure-eosin stains like the Giemsa stain and Mallory's phloxine-methylene blue stain.

Sodium Thiosulfate Solution 5% (Hypo)

Sodium thiosulfate	50 gm.
Distilled water	1000 ml.

This is a bleach for the iodine staining produced by removal of mercuric chlorides in that solution. It is also commonly used to remove unreduced silver in nearly all silver nitrate staining methods.

4

Fixation of Tissue

Tissues must be fixed promptly following cessation of circulation to prevent postmortem decomposition and to preserve and set as closely as possible the structure they had in life. Fixation is generally accomplished by immersing the tissues in chemical solutions, although perfusion by the vascular system is occasionally done. Fixatives are categorized in several ways: according to their effect on proteins, precipitating or nonprecipitating, coagulant or noncoagulant; or whether they are organic or inorganic, aqueous or nonaqueous in composition. They may also be classified according to their special ability to alter or make more prominent some particular cell structure. For practical purposes they are perhaps best classified as to whether they are *routine* or *special* fixatives.

Since no single reagent is available that combines all the requirements of a perfect fixative, two or more reagents are usually used in combination to produce the optimum results. For instance, the great shrinkage in tissue caused by ethanol can be offset by combining it with acetic acid, which has a swelling action. The different reagents used for fixing fresh tissue possess in varying degrees the characteristics of penetrating, killing, and hardening. A good fixative is one with the ability to penetrate and kill tissue quickly, and to harden or affect it so that it will not be significantly altered by the various processes of dehydrating, embedding, sectioning, staining, clearing, and mounting.

Fixation begins at the periphery of the tissue and proceeds inward. Slow-penetrating fixatives allow time for postmortem autolysis to occur in the center of the specimen. Sections cut too thick will likewise retard rapid permeation and result in improperly fixed tissues. A well-cut and well-stained section is dependent to a great extent upon proper fixation. Thin blocks of tissue must be placed promptly in an adequate amount of fixative to ensure best results (10 to 20 times the tissue volume). Some shrinkage is inevitable during processing. For this reason very minute specimens should be wrapped in lens or cigarette paper or placed in a special fine mesh capsule before immersing in the fixative. If these measures are not taken, the small segments of tissue may migrate through the perforations in the capsule and be lost in processing.

Effects of Fixation

1. The most marked effect is denaturation of proteins which renders the proteins insoluble and converts them from their natural gel-like state into a semisolid.

2. Concomitantly with the denaturation, the tissues become resistant to the effects of subsequent technical processing, which can cause damage or distortion.

3. Following fixation, tissue blocks are much more permeable to fluids than they were in the natural state.

4. Staining will be strongly influenced, for the fixative can make the tissue more acid or more basic than it was in its natural state.

5. Some fixatives have the disadvantage of inhibiting or interfering with dye reactions, whereas other fixatives act as mordants to enhance or ensure certain staining results.

Selection of Fixing Solution

In a routine diagnostic histopathology laboratory, the selection of a fixative is of necessity determined by practical rather than ideal considerations. The fixative must be rapid in action, must permit a broad range of staining techniques, and must be suitable for a wide variety of tissues which will be processed collectively. The original fixative will determine to a large extent what can and cannot be done with the tissue subsequently. Fats are dissolved out by nonaqueous fixing agents such as alcohol and acetone, while water-soluble carbohydrates are best preserved by them.

The solution in which the tissue is initally fixed will affect its staining reaction to a considerable degree. **Routine** (or general) fixatives are intended for demonstration of general relationships among cells, tissues, and organs. Staining for specific cellular detail (e.g., mitochondria or Golgi apparatus) or for carbohydrates requires *special* fixation. In the diagnostic histopathology laboratory usually one selected general fixative (10% formalin, Helly's fluid, or Bouin's solution) is employed. All tissues received in the laboratory are promptly fixed in this solution. Later, when special stains are required, the technician must work with tissue not always fixed as recommended for a specific staining procedure, and optimal staining results are not always possible. Postmordanting or special treatment, such as deformalinization, of tissue sections will rectify this in some staining procedures.

Postmordanting or *secondary fixation* entails treating the slides or tissue sections in Helly's, Zenker's, or Bouin's fluid after they have been initially fixed in formalin, when one of these other fixatives is essential to a specific staining result. One may likewise use picric acid, mercuric chloride, or chromate solutions for postmordanting (page 276).

A type of sequential fixation may also be employed whereby all surgical tissues are grossed and initially placed in 10% formalin as they accrue. For the final 2 hours of fixation they are transferred to Helly's solution to enhance their cutting and staining properties. The introduction of the Helly's fluid necessitates the extra step of washing out the potassium dichromate before attachment to the tissue processor.

For recommendations on selection of the appropriate fixative, see Fixatives and Their Properties (page 35).

PROCEDURE FOR FIXATION

Small blocks of tissue, ideally not more than 2 cm. square and not more than 4 to 5 mm. thick, are placed in a quantity of selected fixing fluid about 10 to 20 times their volume. Surgical and autopsy specimens should be fixed as soon as possible after removal. Tissues that cannot be processed immediately should be refrigerated to retard decomposition and autolysis. The length of time required for fixation will depend on the size and density of the tissue, the rate of penetration of the fixing fluid, and the temperature at which it is fixed. Refrigerator temperatures require longer fixation time. Small biopsy specimens and loose-textured tissues will fix far more rapidly than masses of fibrous tissue or whole organs (such as a uterus). Chilled fixatives penetrate more slowly than those used at room temperature. In several instances ideal fixation is done slowly over one day or more, but the pace of modern medical technology requires that the fixation time be limited in the interest of prompt diagnosis. It takes roughly 6 to 48 hours to fix tissue adequately. Because this text is designed for use in routine surgical pathology processing, fixative formulas which require days or weeks to complete fixation are not included. (The reader is referred to R. D. Lillie's text *Histopathologic Technique and Practical Histochemistry* for this information.)

Washing Tissue after Fixation

After the tissue is properly fixed, excess fixative must be removed from it to ensure proper staining. The choice of the medium for washing is determined by the fixative.

When tissues have been fixed in *Helly's* or *Zenker's fluid* they must be washed in running water from 1½ to 24 hours to wash out the yellow-staining potassium dichromate. The time required is determined by the size and volume of the tissue or by the Autotechnicon clock setting.

After fixation in *10% formalin,* tissue may be washed briefly in water and then placed in 70% alcohol, or simply placed directly into the 70% alcohol. Formalin is extracted more rapidly in 70% alcohol than in unchanged water.

When tissues have been fixed in *Bouin's* solution, the excess fixative should be washed out in 50% or 70% alcohol until most of the yellow color has been removed. If some coloration remains after the sections have been cut and mounted on the slide, the excess picric acid should be removed by washing slides in water after they have been deparaffinized. Residual picric acid will interfere with the staining reaction.

Tissues fixed in *Carnoy's fluid* and other alcoholic fixatives are transferred directly into absolute alcohol, for the dehydration has been initiated in the fixative.

When tissues are not to be processed immediately after fixation and washing, they may be preserved for future use by storing in 70% alcohol or 10% formalin. The 10% formalin is the most frequently used solution for wet storage.

FIXATIVES AND THEIR PROPERTIES

Buffered neutral 10% formalin and Helly's solution are the most used and perhaps best fixatives for general use. They are rapid-acting and permit the use of a broad spectrum of staining methods. For the same reason glutaraldehyde is achieving recognition as a desirable fixative. In cases in which the differential diagnosis may be dependent on special staining or histochemical determinations, it is not unusual to divide the specimen and fix the tissue in 2 or more fixatives, e.g., 10% neutral formalin, glutaraldehyde, and Helly's fluid. Helly's fluid, often referred to as Zenker-formol, is a slight modification of the original Zenker's fluid which contains acetic acid. Helly substituted full-strength formalin in the same ratio (page 37).

Formalin

10% FORMALIN

Full-strength formalin (37%–40% formaldehyde)	10 ml.
Distilled water	90 ml.

The term "formaldehyde" is often mistakenly applied to formalin. The distinction should be maintained. Formaldehyde is a gas, not a liquid. Formalin (formol) is a trade name for the liquid resulting from the combination of formaldehyde gas and water. The gas formaldehyde is soluble in water to the extent of 40 percent. Formalin is considered a 100% solution when making percentage strength dilutions. The routinely used 10% formalin is made by adding 10 ml. of full-strength (commercial) formalin to 90 ml. of water. This then is actually about 4% formaldehyde or 10% formalin.

The advantages of formalin are that it is comparatively cheap, penetrates rapidly, does not overharden tissue even during long periods of immersion, permits the use of a large variety of staining methods, and penetrates and preserves fatty tissue. For specimens to be mailed, 10% formalin is the preferred fixative.

A disadvantage of formalin is that the vapor is unpleasant and irritating, especially to the eyes and nasal mucosa. Also, rubber gloves should be worn for protection while handling formalin-fixed tissue, since formalin may eventually produce an allergic reaction of the skin of the hands.

Formalin frequently produces an artefact pigment in tissues that may be identified as a fine dark brown or black crystalline precipitate probably derived from laked hemoglobin. (See page 277 for removal of formalin precipitate.)

NEUTRAL FORMALIN (STORAGE BOTTLE)

10% formalin solution   1000 ml.
Calcium carbonate to excess

Formalin is usually slightly acid, and when this is not desirable for certain staining procedures, a neutral formalin may be preferred. Formalin will be neutralized by the addition of calcium carbonate in excess, although this is only an approximate neutrality.

BUFFERED NEUTRAL FORMALIN (pH 7)

Formalin, full strength (37%–40% formaldehyde)	100.0 ml.
Sodium phosphate dibasic (anhydrous)	6.5 gm.
Sodium phosphate monobasic	4.0 gm.
Distilled water	900.0 ml.

Buffered neutral formalin is recommended for hemoglobin and hemosiderin fixation. Use of buffered formalin inhibits the formation of objectionable "formalin pigment." It is widely recommended as the best all-round fixative, for its use allows a number of special staining procedures, including histochemical testing. It is particularly recommended for tissues to be stained for the identification of mucopolysaccharides.

FORMALIN AMMONIUM BROMIDE SOLUTION (FAB)

Formalin, full strength (37%–40% formaldehyde)	15 ml.
Ammonium bromide	2 gm.
Distilled water	85 ml.

This preparation is recommended for central nervous system tissues, particularly when gold and silver impregnations are contemplated.

ALCOHOLIC FORMALIN 10%

Formalin, full strength (37%–40% formaldehyde)	10 ml.
80% alcohol	90 ml.

The alcoholic dilution of formalin gives faster fixation, cutting the fixing time almost in half. Alcoholic formalin preserves glycogen. It will, however, dissolve out fat and lipoids in tissue. It is not recommended for the preservation of iron-bearing pigments. After alcoholic-formalin fixation, store tissue in 70% alcohol rather than in formalin.

ZENKER'S FLUID

Potassium dichromate, granular	25 gm.
Mercuric chloride	60 gm.
Distilled water	1000 ml.
Acetic acid, glacial	50–100 ml.
(added just before use)	

Dissolve the potassium dichromate and mercuric chloride in the water with the aid of heat. Corrosive sublimate, seen frequently in the older literature, is another name for mercuric chloride. In making up small quantities, a mechanical stirrer will dissolve the potassium dichromate and mercuric chloride in 30 minutes at room temperature — more rapidly if the stirrer is equipped with a hot plate. At time of use 5 ml. of glacial acetic acid is added to 100 ml. of the stock Zenker's solution. Current authorities are in disagreement as to the necessity of adding the acetic acid *at time of use.* Davenport and Lillie feel that a C.P. grade of acetic acid will not render the solution unstable on standing, and that it can be made up as the entire formula and kept as a stock solution. For best cytologic preservation, tissues fixed in Zenker's or Helly's solutions should be cut small enough (a 2 cm. square or rectangle, not more than 2–4 mm. thick) to ensure complete fixation in 6 to 8 hours. Prolonged treatment in Zenker's will render the tissue brittle, making sectioning difficult. Excess chromate must be thoroughly removed by washing in running water, for 1 hour or longer. Insufficient washing after Zenker fixation will inhibit or interfere with good staining. After fixation and washing, the tissue may be stored in 70% alcohol or 10% formalin. A deposit of mercuric chloride crystals must be removed before staining the tissue sections. The simplest way to remove the crystals is to immerse cut sections of tissue on the slides in alcoholic iodine after the paraffin has been removed from the sections just prior to staining (page 277).

Zenker-fixed tissues stain brilliantly. Zenker fixation is compatible with most stains; in fact many stains require this fixative as a mordant to ensure a specific staining reaction.

HELLY'S FLUID (ZENKER-FORMOL)

Potassium dichromate, granular	25 gm.
Mercuric chloride	60 gm.
Distilled water	1000 ml.
Formalin, full strength (added just before use)	50–100 ml.

The results obtained with Helly's fluid are essentially the same as those with Zenker's solution. In fact its use is recommended whenever

the original Zenker formula is indicated. There is the additional bene-
fit that the formalin in the Helly's fluid improves penetration and fixation, and granules of certain endocrine glands will be preserved intact
with Helly's fluid, whereas they may be dissolved by the acetic acid in
the original Zenker's fluid. Certain cytoplasmic inclusions, intercellular
bridges, and ground cytoplasm are far better preserved with either
Zenker's or Helly's fluid than with formalin fixation. Helly's produces a
consistency in the tissue conducive to cutting thin sections and its use
enhances staining. It is an excellent fixative for bone marrow and
blood-containing organs. Like Zenker fixation, the excess chromate
must be removed by washing in running water and an alcoholic iodine
bath is required to remove the mercuric chlorides. Fixation will take
4 to 6 hours if sections are not larger than 2 to 4 mm. thick.

BOUIN'S FLUID (PICRO-FORMOL)

Picric acid, saturated aqueous solution, about 1.22%	750 ml.
Formalin, full strength (37%–40% formaldehyde)	250 ml.
Acetic acid, glacial	50 ml.

Bouin's fluid is recommended both for general purposes and for
special study (e.g., glycogen fixation). It provides good penetration
and fixation. Lipids are altered and decreased in this fixative. It is
stable and can be made up as a stock solution. It does not interfere
with the staining qualities of the tissue if the fixative is washed out
thoroughly. Fix tissue for 4 to 18 hours, depending on size and density
of the tissue. Wash in several changes of 50% and 70% alcohol for 4
to 8 hours.

Bouin's fluid precipitates proteins, forming protein picrates which
are said to be water soluble, and so it is traditional to transfer the
tissue directly into several changes of 50% and 70% alcohol. The
alcohol will also remove the excess picric acid. Unless this fixative is
thoroughly removed from them, the tissues in the paraffin blocks will
later undergo undesirable changes. If yellow coloration is exhibited in
the sections after mounting on the slide, it should be washed out with
water after the paraffin has been removed. The wet tissue is stored
in 70% alcohol or 10% formalin.

VAN DE GRIFT'S SOLUTION

Ethyl alcohol, 95% (or isopropyl, 99%)	32.0 ml.
Formalin, full strength (37%–40%)	48.0 ml.
Glacial acetic acid	18.0 ml.
Picric acid	16.0 gm.
Mercuric chloride	0.8 gm.
Urea	2.0 gm.

Combine in order the alcohol, formalin, and glacial acetic acid. Add the picric acid, mercuric chloride, and urea separately, making sure that each ingredient is dissolved before adding the next. A magnetic stirrer is helpful. Because the mercuric chloride is minimal, iodine treatment prior to staining is not necessary. The urea is added to improve the osmotic effect of the fluid. This fixing solution is essentially an alcoholic modification of Bouin's fluid. Fix tissues for 3 to 6 hours. Transfer to 95% alcohol to remove excess picric acid. Dehydration has been initiated in the fixative. Staining reaction is intensified with this fixative owing to the mordanting action of the picric acid and mercuric chloride.

CARNOY'S FLUID

Absolute alcohol	60 ml.
Chloroform	30 ml.
Acetic acid, glacial	10 ml.

Carnoy's is a penetrating and quick-acting fixative. Thin sections of tissue will be fixed in 1 to 3 hours at room temperature or preferably for 12 to 18 hours at refrigerator temperature. Tissue fixed in Carnoy's fluid should be transferred directly into absolute alcohol, since dehydration has already been initiated during fixation. It is suitable only for small pieces of tissue. Carnoy's is a recommended fixative for glycogen, since aqueous solutions are to be avoided. It is a good fixative for chromosomes. *All* alcoholic fixatives are best used at refrigerator temperature.

GENDRE'S FIXATIVE

95% ethyl alcohol saturated with picric acid	80 ml.
Formalin, full strength	15 ml.
Acetic acid, glacial	5 ml.
(Use ice cold)	

Recommended for glycogen fixation. Fix for 1 to 4 hours. Wash in several changes of 95% alcohol to remove excess picric acid. Transfer directly to absolute alcohol.

FLEMMING'S SOLUTION (OSMIC ACID SOLUTION)

Chromic acid, 1% solution	75 ml.
Osmium tetroxide, 2%	20 ml.
Acetic acid, glacial	5 ml.

Combine and allow 2 to 3 days for the fixative to go into solution. This fixative is a strong oxidizer.

Flemming's solution is rarely used in today's *routine* pathology laboratory. As a fixative it has limited use. It interferes with several staining methods. It penetrates very poorly, is very expensive, and is suitable only for very thin sections (not more than 2 mm. thick). Flemming's fluid is a good fixative for cytoplasmic structures, but nuclei stain rather poorly. Fat in tissue will be blackened by it. Since the preparation is unstable, do not keep a stock solution. Fix tissue for 1 to 3 days. The fixative must be thoroughly removed by washing in running water for 6 to 24 hours. If tissue is not processed immediately, store in 80% alcohol.

The use of osmic acid as a fixative has been revived in the *research* laboratory with the development of electron microscopy. It is extensively used for tissues to be studied with the electron microscope. It not only fixes the minute fragments (less than 1 mm. thick) rapidly but also stains tissue structures. The osmium tetroxide is reduced as a gray-black deposit.

Absolute Ethyl Alcohol

Absolute (100%) alcohol is only occasionally used as a fixative. It dehydrates and hardens at the same time. It is used specifically to preserve glycogen, although 10% formalin, Carnoy's fluid or Gendre's fluid is to be preferred. Alcohol causes polarization (streaming to one corner of the cell) and tends to cause glycogen to appear as large, coarse granules. It is recommended for fixation of pigments. Absolute alcohol penetrates rather slowly. Tissues should never be left in it for more than 8 to 10 hours at room temperature, as they become over-hardened and will be very difficult if not impossible to cut. Much of the severe shrinkage produced by absolute alcohol can be eliminated if fixation is carried out at very low temperature (−20°C.). It will take approximately 48 hours to fix tissue at this low temperature, 18 to 24 hours at refrigerator (5°C.) temperature.

Acetone

Acetone is of limited application as a fixative. Some shrinkage and distortion are inevitable with acetone fixation. *Ice-cold* acetone is specifically used as a fixative in fluorescent antibody techniques and for some of the enzymes, particularly the phosphatases and lipases which would be largely or completely destroyed by traditional fixatives. Acetone has been in use for many years as a rapid fixative for brain tissue in the diagnosis of rabies, and is now an acceptable substitute for ether-alcohol in the fixation of Papanicolaou smears.

QUIZ

1. What are the characteristics of a good fixative?
2. How long must tissue be fixed?
3. What volume of fixative is used per block of tissue?
4. Explain difference between a "routine" and a "special" fixative.
5. List four effects of fixation.
6. Give the constituents of the following fixatives:
   a. Zenker's fluid
   b. Carnoy's fluid
   c. Helly's fluid
   d. Bouin's solution
   e. 10% formalin
7. What is the strength of commercial formalin?
8. Since excess fixing fluid must be removed from the tissue, explain how you would remove it from tissue fixed in each of the following:
   a. Zenker's solution or Helly's solution
   b. 10% formalin (aqueous)
   c. Bouin's solution
9. What fixative would you employ for the following?
   a. glycogen
   b. bone marrow
   c. tissue for electron microscopic study
   d. central nervous system tissue
   e. fat or lipoid tissue
   f. enzymes
   g. mucopolysaccharides
10. When tissue is to be sent through the mail, which fixative is recommended?

5

Dehydration, Clearing, and Infiltration of Tissue

Before applying the various steps of tissue processing to a specific embedding procedure, it is best to consider them individually in order to understand their functions better. Since the paraffin technique is the prevailing method of microtechnique, most of the material presented is directly applicable to this embedding procedure.

DEHYDRATION

Dehydration is the removal of water from fixed tissue. It is always carried out in covered containers. It is necessary to dehydrate tissues thoroughly prior to embedding in a nonaqueous medium. Neither paraffin nor celloidin is miscible with water. While many compounds are being tested as substitutes for the traditional older ones, particularly in botanical and animal histologic studies, dehydration is still almost universally accomplished in a routine pathology laboratory by the use of graduated strengths of ethyl alcohol, usually starting at 70% or 80% and going to 95% or 100% (absolute) alcohol. Isopropyl alcohol has been recommended and can be used as a substitute for ethyl alcohol for the dehydration and preservation of fixed tissues in the paraffin-embedding process, but is not recommended for use in celloidin embedding.

When processing delicate objects, dehydration should be gradual. Tissue transferred directly from water or an aqueous solution to highly concentrated alcohol (or vice versa) will undergo some distortion of tissue elements due to the currents produced by the mixing of the alcohol and water. The more delicate the object to be processed, the more numerous are the steps required and the closer in strength the different gradations of alcohol should be.

Length of Processing Time

For special tissues, such as those of cytologic interest, delicate tissues (eyes, embryos, and cystic structures), or very large objects, a longer time than usual in each grade of alcohol is recommended. When working with this type of tissue, it is often better to start the dehydration with a dilution as low as 50% alcohol.

Too long treatment in higher concentrations of alcohol (above 80%) makes tissue brittle and difficult to cut. Too long treatment in lower dilutions of alcohol (under 70%) macerates tissue. Preservation of specimens in alcoholic solutions during a long period of time interferes with the staining properties of the tissue.

Slow dehydration in graduated strength solutions is not necessary in routine surgical pathology, and one may initiate the cycle in 80% or 95% alcohol without detriment to the tissue. Total dehydration time depends on volume and type of tissue and in particular on the thickness of the tissue block. The optimum tissue thickness should not exceed 0.5 cm. Ten times the volume of tissue is an adequate proportion of dehydrant. For more rapid dehydration, tissues should be kept in motion to accelerate diffusion. Without proper dehydration, efficient tissue infiltration by the embedding medium is improbable. In my experience a total 5-hour period of dehydration is reliable, provided that the solutions are changed frequently enough to maintain their strength.

An average length of time on the Autotechnicon cycle for processing paraffin-embedded tissue in a routine pathology laboratory is as follows (for alternate methods of dehydration see page 65):

80% alcohol	1 hour
95% alcohol	1 hour
100% alcohol or acetone	1 hour
100% alcohol or acetone	1 hour
100% alcohol or acetone	1 hour

Dealcoholization

When absolute alcohol is used as the final dehydrant, the tissue must be dealcoholized (usually in xylene) before infiltration with paraffin, as absolute alcohol is not readily miscible with paraffin.

Making Dilutions of Alcohol

When a particular percentage of alcohol is desired, it is generally made by diluting a high percentage of alcohol with distilled water. In order to secure a given percentage, subtract the percentage required from the percentage strength of the alcohol that is to be diluted and the difference will be the amount of water that is to be used.

For example, if 50% alcohol is the percentage required and 95% alcohol the percentage to be diluted, then $95 - 50 = 45$. Therefore, 50 parts of 95% alcohol and 45 parts of water are the amounts to be combined. Simply place 50 ml. of 95% alcohol in a 100 ml. graduated glass cylinder and fill up to the 95 ml. mark with distilled water (Fig. 5-1).

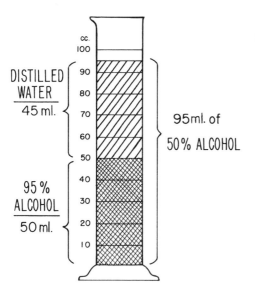

Figure 5-1. Method of alcohol dilution

DEHYDRATING AGENTS—
ADVANTAGES AND DISADVANTAGES

Alcohol

While ethyl, methyl, isopropyl, and butyl alcohols can be used, ethyl and isopropyl alcohols are predominantly used in a routine laboratory for the dehydration of tissues. They are fast-acting, nontoxic, and reliable. There is some distortion of tissue due to shrinkage produced by the alcohol. Long immersion in high concentrates of ethyl alcohol is to be avoided. Absolute alcohol, especially, causes overhardening of the tissue.

Methyl alcohol is toxic. As a dehydrant, it is primarily employed for blood and tissue films and for smear preparations.

Butyl alcohol is recommended for use in plant and animal microtechnique. The dehydrating power of butyl alcohol is low, requiring long periods of immersion to dehydrate. This is an advantage when rapid processing is not required, as there is less shrinkage and hardening than with ethyl alcohol. Both n-butyl and tertiary butyl alcohols may be used in combination with ethyl alcohol in an embedding series. When employed in this manner, the butyl alcohol does not replace the whole dehydrating technique, but serves only as a substitute for the higher concentration of ethyl alcohol. Butyl alcohol also functions as a clearing agent in this series, since it is miscible with paraffin. Tertiary butyl alcohol may also be used to dehydrate slides after staining in dyes that are easily extracted with ethyl alcohol.

Dioxane

Dioxane (diethylene dioxide) is a remarkable reagent. It both dehydrates and clears, and is readily miscible with water, alcohol, xylene, and paraffin. It produces less shrinkage than does alcoholic dehydration. Tissue can be left in this reagent for long periods of time without its affecting the consistency of the tissue or its staining properties. Since dioxane is miscible with both water and paraffin, tissue may be placed directly into dioxane from washing, and it will be both dehydrated and cleared. Or dioxane may be used as the final dehydrant only, in place of absolute alcohol, in order to avoid the hardening effect of the highest concentration of ethyl alcohol.

Dioxane is reported to be slightly toxic to man, and should be used only in a well-ventilated room.

Acetone

Acetone is widely used as a substitute for alcohol in the dehydrating process. It is very rapid in action, and is less expensive than some of the other dehydrants. When haste is necessary, Lillie recommends 20 minutes in four fresh changes of acetone for dehydration of tissue in an embedding series. Or, as an alternate series, not less than four changes of acetone, each of 40 minutes' duration. Of these only the fourth change need be fresh; the others are moved up one in position. From dehydration in acetone, tissue should be transferred to a paraffin solvent to be cleared prior to infiltration, since acetone does not mix readily with paraffin. Although acetone has been reported by some workers to produce extensive shrinkage, we have seen no such effect on direct comparison with ethyl alcohol-dehydrated surgical specimens.

Cellosolve

Cellosolve (ethylene glycol monoethyl ether) dehydrates rapidly and is reported to have no harmful effect on tissue. The tissue is transferred from water or normal saline directly to cellosolve. The series for dehydrating consists of four baths: 30 minutes, 30 to 60 minutes, 60 minutes, and 90 minutes. The tissue must be cleared in xylene, and then may be infiltrated with three changes of paraffin of 1 hour each. Tissue may be stored in cellosolve for months without distortion.

Triethyl Phosphate

Triethyl phosphate may be used in the paraffin-embedding technique. Tissues are fixed, washed, and transferred directly into triethyl phosphate for dehydration (three changes in 24 hours). It displaces water readily and produces very little distortion in tissue. It does not harden tissue. It is soluble in alcohols, benzene, ether, chloroform, and xylene. It may also be used to dehydrate sections and smears following certain stains.

Tetrahydrofuran

Tetrahydrofuran is a reagent that both dehydrates and clears tissue, since it is miscible with water and paraffin. It is miscible with lower alcohols, water, ether, chloroform, acetone, benzene, and xylene. In its properties and use, it is much the same as dioxane, with the exception that it is reported to be nontoxic. Tetrahydrofuran has a rather offensive odor, has been known to engender conjunctivitis in personnel, and should be used only in a well-ventilated room.

CLEARING

Although the term *clearing* refers especially to the rendering transparent of tissue elements, whereas *dealcoholization* refers to the removal of alcohol prior to embedding in paraffin, very often the same reagent may be used for either purpose, and in consequence the term clearing has come to be used in either sense. The liquids employed for these purposes are not always interchangeable, however, for not all dealcoholizing agents can be used as clearers and not all clearing agents are solvents of the resins used in mounting media.

We speak of clearing in two procedures. In each of these instances clearing serves a slightly different purpose. In the embedding process, we clear tissue after dehydration with alcohol, and in the mounting procedure, we clear after sections have been stained and dehydrated.

Clearing in Embedding

After the tissue has been dehydrated with alcohol, we employ a clearing agent the function of which is to dealcoholize; consequently, it must mix readily with alcohol. It must also be a solvent of paraffin in order to facilitate the penetration of this embedding medium. In other words, we replace the dehydrant with a liquid that will mix with the paraffin. Of course, when paraffin is readily soluble in the dehydrator (e.g., dioxane) this step is not necessary.

When essential oils, such as oil of cedarwood, are used to clear tissue, the specimen becomes translucent, hence the name of the process. Although the use of saturated solutions of paraffin in the solvent (clearing agent) is sometimes recommended as an intermediate step between clearing and paraffin infiltration, this is not generally required for the processing of routine pathology specimens, and need only be resorted to for special projects of a research nature.

The most frequently used clearing agents for dealcoholization in the embedding process are xylene, toluene, dioxane, and chloroform. Other clearants are oil of cedarwood, terpineol, and aviation gasoline.

Clearing in Mounting

Clearing agents make microscopic preparations transparent and are always liquids with a high index of refraction. After tissue sections have been stained, they are dehydrated and then dealcoholized (cleared) prior to mounting. The clearing agent employed here must not only be capable of removing the alcohol, it must also be a solvent of Permount and other resins used in mounting media. The most frequently used clearing agent in mounting is xylene. Others are toluene, terpineol, and carbol-xylene.

Glycerin, gum syrup, or Brun's solution is used when the tissue is to be cleared directly from water (e.g., frozen sections). In this instance, no dealcoholization is involved. These clearing agents merely improve the refractive index of the tissues and hold the coverglass in place.

CLEARING AGENTS— ## ADVANTAGES AND DISADVANTAGES

Xylene

Xylene is a colorless reagent. It is the clearing agent in most common use today. It is used for clearing both in the embedding process and in the mounting procedure. However, prolonged treatment in xylene in the embedding process is to be avoided, since it will overharden tissue. Tissues are cleared best from absolute alcohol. Xylene is relatively rapid in its displacement of alcohol and is readily miscible with paraffin. Used in the mounting procedure, xylene does not dissolve celloidin, nor does it affect aniline dyes. Brain or central nervous system tissues become overhardened if xylene is used in the embedding process. Toluene is preferable for processing brain sections.

Toluene

The properties of toluene are similar to those of xylene. Toluene clears less rapidly than xylene or chloroform, but does not harden tissue; consequently it is a good clearing fluid in which to leave tissue overnight. It is a colorless reagent. It is readily miscible with paraffin. It clears best from absolute alcohol. It is used for clearing in both embedding and mounting procedures.

Dioxane

Dioxane is a colorless, somewhat toxic reagent used primarily in the embedding process. It is capable of both dehydrating and clearing directly from water. It is miscible with paraffin. Very long periods of immersion in dioxane will not alter tissue (see Dehydration).

Oil of Cedarwood

Oil of cedarwood is used to clear both paraffin and celloidin sections in the embedding process; it is very penetrating. It produces no shrinkage, and tissues may be left in it indefinitely without harm. Immersion in oil of cedarwood often improves cutting. Clearing in oil of cedarwood must be followed by immersion in xylene and three changes of paraffin to ensure removal of the oil. It is a rather expensive clearing agent, and its use is rapidly being replaced with terpineol, which is similar in properties.

Chloroform

Chloroform is used in clearing tissue in the embedding process. Since chloroform penetrates a little more slowly than xylene, it will take a little longer to clear tissue. It does not make tissue quite as brittle as xylene, but does produce some hardening. It is dangerous to inhale chloroform, since it may affect the liver. Its use should be avoided when possible.

Benzene

Benzene is preferred by some workers as a clearer in the embedding process of tissue because it penetrates and clears tissue very rapidly. It also evaporates from the paraffin bath very rapidly. Benzene produces a minimum of shrinkage. Avoid use when possible, as excessive exposure to benzene damages bone marrow and may be carcinogenic.

Amyl Acetate

Amyl acetate produces no hardening effect on tissue even after long periods of immersion. Tissues are usually cleared from 90% or 95% ethyl alcohol. Amyl acetate is recommended for large pieces of tissue which would become overhardened in the time required for penetration of absolute alcohol and the usual clearing agents. It is also recommended as a clearing agent for embryologic material (Drury, H. F. *Stain Techn.* 16:21–22, 1941). It is well to use all amyl derivatives in a well-ventilated room. Specimens may even be stored in amyl acetate without damage to the tissue.

Terpineol

Terpineol (artificial oil of lilac) is particularly recommended for clearing celloidin sections in the mounting procedure. Terpineol is pleasant to use. It clears tissue from 80% and 90% alcohol. In the paraffin-embedding process it has been recommended as a worthy substitute for oil of cedarwood. Terpineol may be used for clearing both in embedding and in mounting procedures. It is not to be confused with terpinol (artificial oil of hyacinth), which is unsuitable.

Carbol-Xylene

Carbol-xylene (a 1:3 part ratio of phenol and xylene) is used prior to mounting stained tissue sections. It clears very rapidly. The use of carbol-xylene is usually reserved for material that is difficult to clear, e.g., a thick mucinous Papanicolaou smear. Avoid leaving slides in this clearing agent for more than 5 to 10 minutes. After they are cleared, the slides should be *thoroughly* rinsed in xylene before mounting in order to remove all traces of the carbolic acid, which later would leach out the stain.

INFILTRATION

After tissues have been thoroughly cleared with a clearing agent (xylene, dioxane, chloroform, oil of cedarwood), it is necessary to infiltrate the tissue with a supporting medium. To understand this better, consider this analogy. If a piece of sponge were cut into slices, the sections would be compressed and distorted. However, if the same sponge were put in a container filled with liquid paraffin and allowed to soak up or become infiltrated with the paraffin, then to cool in the container until the paraffin hardened, and then were sliced, the supporting paraffin would keep the various components of the sponge in proper relation to each other.

Fixed tissues are not firm or adhesive enough to allow thin sectioning without some supporting medium to hold the cells and intercellular structures in proper relation to each other. For this purpose two major embedding media are used, paraffin and celloidin. Two more recently introduced embedding mediums, not used routinely, are Carbowax (water-soluble wax) and plastics.

EMBEDDING MEDIA

The term *embedding media* designates all materials used by the histologic technician to infiltrate, support, and enclose specimens which are to be subsequently cut into thin sections. Of necessity embedding media must be substances capable of being converted readily from liquid to solid form. In the fluid state the embedding medium penetrates into the interstices of the tissue and then is converted into a solid. The conversion may be brought about by *crystallization* (paraffin and Carbowax), *evaporation* of the solvent (celloidin), or by *polymerization* (plastics).

Paraffin

In the paraffin technique, blocks of refined, white, filtered paraffin to which has been added beeswax, rubber, plastics, or some other medium to facilitate ribboning are supplied by laboratory supply houses. The addition of rubber reduces the brittleness of paraffin, increases the stickiness of the wax, and makes it easier to secure continuous ribbons. Bayberry increases the firmness of paraffin at high room temperatures, which facilitates securing of very thin sections. All additives increase the plasticity of the paraffin necessary for histologic work. I have had best results with paraffins sold under the trade names of Paraplast, Bioloid, and Histowax.

Paraffin is solid at normal room temperature. Heat renders paraffin fluid so that it can permeate the tissue. Ideally the hardness of the paraffin used for infiltration is matched to the hardness of the tissue. However, the hardness of the paraffin selected is most usually determined by the temperature in which the tissue blocks are to be sectioned. Soft paraffins (low melting point of about 45° to 50°C.) have the advantages generally of being finer grained and less brittle, but they can be used only in cool temperatures (59°F.). Hard paraffins (melting point of about 56° to 62°C.) allow thinner sections to be obtained, provide better support of hard objects, and *are suitable for laboratory temperatures of 72°F.* While both have their own virtues, it is not surprising that paraffin with a high melting point, 56° to 58°C., is adopted for routine work.

Cakes of paraffin are placed in clean metal or enamel pitchers and melted down in a paraffin oven regulated at a temperature just above the melting point of the paraffin. Coarse filter paper is folded into a cone and placed in a funnel set into another pitcher. The molten paraffin is filtered within the oven and is then ready for use. Even the commercially prefiltered paraffin especially prepared for histologic work will yield grit and dirt on filtering. *Careful filtering of the paraffin reduces injuries to the knife edge,* when sectioning the tissue. Paraffin trimmed from the blocks around the specimens may be saved, melted down, filtered, and reused. The new electric modular embedding units store, filter, and dispense paraffin. They are efficient and time saving.

After tissue specimens have been completely dehydrated and cleared, they are immersed in melted paraffin for 2 to 4 hours. Usually two or more changes of paraffin are required to eliminate traces of the solvent (clearing agent) which would prevent the paraffin from hardening properly. The liquid paraffin infiltrates the tissue, and when cold and solidified it provides the support necessary for cutting thin sections. Rapid chilling of the melted paraffin is recommended on the principle that slow cooling of a liquid which normally crystallizes on cooling results in the formation of large crystals. Rapid cooling will provide a fine crystalline structure capable of fitting closely to the individual cells, thus providing adequate support. Of equal importance to the busy laboratory, rapid cooling saves time.

For complete paraffin-embedding procedure, see Chapter 6.

Celloidin

The celloidin used in embedding is a purified form of pyroxylin nitrocellulose. This is available in two forms: hard platelets (Parlodion) and alcohol-moistened lint (low-viscosity nitrocellulose, or LVN).

Parlodion is usually supplied in 1-ounce quantities (approximately 28 gm.) in brown bottles. As it comes from the supplier it looks like short, stiff, curled strips of transparent celluloid, light amber in color. These strips are dissolved in equal parts of absolute alcohol and ether. Stock solutions (page 81) are prepared in advance and stored in tightly stoppered containers, such as Mason jars, away from light and heat until they are to be used.

Low-viscosity nitrocellulose (nitrated lint variety) when received from the supplier is wet with alcohol. Because of this LVN requires extra calculations for proportioning the solvents (ether and alcohol). Allowance must be made for the alcohol (35%) which has been added by the manufacturer at the time it is packaged. The lint is best stored by removing it from its metal container (which is subject to rust contamination) and transferring it to airtight jars to prevent the evaporation of the alcohol.

LVN, as the name indicates, is a nitrocellulose preparation of low viscosity making it possible to use higher concentrations of this medium and still have a fluid that will penetrate rapidly. Embedding in LVN will take approximately one-half to three-fourths of the time it would require to embed the same material in Parlodion, which is very viscous in high concentrations. For this reason, it is preferred by some histologic technologists. For both forms of nitrocellulose, the solvent is the same, i.e., equal parts of absolute ethyl alcohol and ether.

Whether solid or in solution, both types of nitrocellulose embedding media must be stored in the dark; they will deteriorate if exposed to the light.

After thorough dehydration through the alcohols and a mixture of equal parts of absolute alcohol and ether, tissues are slowly infiltrated with first a thin and then a thick solution of celloidin. The final hardening of the celloidin is accomplished by gradual evaporation of the solvent (ether and alcohol) until the embedding medium is the correct consistency for cutting on the microtome.

For complete celloidin-embedding procedures, see Chapter 7.

Carbowax

A more recent embedding medium (not used routinely) is a water-soluble wax preparation (solid polyethylene glycol) sold under such trade names as H.E.M. (Harleco Embedding Medium) and Carbowax. Carbowax is a soft, white wax compound usually supplied in round jars bearing the identifications Carbowax 4000 and Carbowax 1500. The numbers are assigned to different groups to indicate the approximate molecular weights. The higher the molecular weight, the harder the wax. Carbowax may also be procured in solid particles resembling Tissuemat flakes. The recommended formula for preparing the embedding mixture is a combination of 9 parts of Carbowax 4000 and 1 part of Carbowax 1500, melted down in the paraffin oven at 56° to 58°C. This is not a rigid formula, and the quantity or type of Carbowax may be varied by the individual laboratory to suit its needs. The mixture should be prepared in advance and stored in the paraffin oven or incubator.

Tissues are transferred directly to the water-soluble wax after fixation and washing. No alcoholic dehydration is necessary. The tissues are placed in the melted wax within the incubator and usually require three changes of Carbowax, each of 1 hour's duration, to complete infiltration.

For complete Carbowax-embedding procedure, see page 105.

Plastic Embedding Media

Butyl methacrylate was introduced into microtechnique as an embedding medium in 1949. Its main application was in the preparation of the ultrathin sections required for electron microscopy, for which it is particularly well suited. Epoxy resins like Epon 812, Maraglas, Cardolite, and other polyester plastics such as Vestopal W have superseded the use of butyl and methyl methacrylates. For additional information see page 116.

The plastic embedding medium is a pale liquid monomer. Following complete infiltration in the liquid state the plastic is solidified by polymerization. While the plastic would gradually polymerize if left at room temperature, the process is too slow for practical use and generally it is caused to solidify by the addition of a catalyst (initiator and activator), by heat, or by a combination of both.

Advantages of Plastic Embedding Media

1. It permits ultrathin sectioning (down to 10mμ).
2. It causes very little distortion.
3. Blocks can be stored indefinitely.

Disadvantages

1. The embedding process is rather complicated.
2. The process is very slow.
3. It requires the use of special expensive equipment.

The tissues are fixed in osmium tetroxide or are initially fixed in glutaraldehyde or paraformaldehyde, with postfixation in osmium tetroxide. They are washed, dehydrated in graded alcohols, cleared, and transferred to the liquid plastic. After thorough infiltration, the plastic is allowed (or activated) to polymerize and in doing so becomes a solid. (See Electron Microscopy, page 111.)

QUIZ

Dehydration

1. Define dehydration.
2. How is dehydration routinely accomplished?
3. What effect will prolonged treatment in high concentrations of ethyl alcohol have?
4. What determines the length of time for dehydration?
5. How would you make 190 ml. of a 35% solution of alcohol using 95% alcohol?
6. Name three reagents besides ethyl alcohol that are used for the dehydration of tissue.
7. List several advantages and one disadvantage of dioxane as a dehydrant.

Clearing

1. What is the purpose of clearing?
2. In what two procedures do we "clear" tissue?
3. List three or more clearing agents used in each of the procedures in question 2.

Infiltration

1. What is the purpose of infiltration?
2. a. What kind of paraffin is used in histologic work?
   b. How is it prepared for use?
3. a. What is celloidin?
   b. How is it prepared for use in the celloidin-embedding procedure?
4. a. What is Carbowax?
   b. How is it prepared for use?

6

Paraffin Tissue–Processing Method

Identification of the specimen is controlled by an accession number which is applied to paper chits (typewritten in advance or marked with a graphite pencil) or by the use of a prenumbered stamped label. The accession number is enclosed with the tissue in the embedding capsule at the time it is grossed (macroscopically examined) by the pathologist. With the newer dual purpose process/embedding cassette, this accession number is marked directly on the plastic rim. The identifying numbering system will accompany the tissue through all the steps of processing. Remember that if the accession number is not clear or is lost during processing, the tissue cannot be properly identified. Also, if the number is applied to the wrong tissue, a grave error in diagnosis may result.

Best results are obtained with paraffin sections if the pieces of tissue to be processed are soft, small, and of uniform consistency.

ADVANTAGES AND DISADVANTAGES OF PARAFFIN

Advantages

1. Very thin sections may be obtained.
2. The process is very rapid (sections can be prepared in 24 hours).
3. It is easy to get serial sections (page 71).
4. The tissue blocks can be easily stored, and for an indefinite period of time.

Disadvantages

1. *Overheated* paraffin renders the specimen brittle, making sectioning difficult.

2. Prolonged treatment in paraffin causes shrinkage and hardening of the tissue.

3. Tissues that are difficult to infiltrate (bone, teeth, eyes, brain) need long immersion for proper support; otherwise they crumble on sectioning. But long immersion in paraffin is not possible without the deleterious effects produced by heat.

4. Paraffin processing removes fats — the dehydrants and clearing agents used in the process are fat solvents.

STEPS IN PARAFFIN-EMBEDDING TECHNIQUE

Below is an outline of the steps in the paraffin-embedding technique.

1. Fixation
2. Dehydration
3. Clearing
4. Infiltration
5. Embedding (casting)
6. Sectioning

FIXATION

Tissues for paraffin embedding, ideally not more than 2 cm. square and not more than 4 mm. thick, are placed in a perforated capsule with the identifying paper chit. They are covered with any preferred routine fixative (10% formalin, Zenker's, Helly's, or Bouin's solution) for 4 to 24 hours. Most properly cut surgical specimens are well fixed in 4 to 6 hours. After fixation in Zenker's or Helly's fluid, tissues are washed for 1½ to several hours (depending on the volume of tissue being processed or on the Autotechnicon clock setting) to remove the excess fixative. If tissue has been formalin-fixed, it can be placed directly into 70% alcohol, which will extract the formalin readily, or it can be washed briefly in water and then placed in the alcohol. Bouin-fixed material is transferred directly into 70% alcohol.

DEHYDRATION

The purpose of the dehydrating agent is to remove water from the tissues in order that a solvent of paraffin, not miscible with water, may be substituted. Both acetone and dioxane are suitable dehydrants and may be used in place of alcohol, the traditional dehydrant. Routinely, with the Autotechnicon or some similar processing machine, the tissue is dehydrated in a series of graduated changes of different strengths of alcohol for approximately 1 hour each. (See also alternate methods of processing on page 65.) A typical processing schedule to prepare for paraffin embedding (fixation, washing, dehydration, clearing, and infiltration) is shown in Figure 6-1. The fluids are kept in

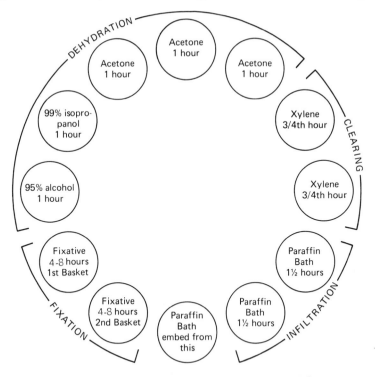

Figure 6-1. Autotechnicon processing schedule

motion to speed up diffusion, thereby shortening the time required for complete processing. The least time necessary to do the job satisfactorily is the ideal time. Tissues should be immersed in the reagents no longer than the minimum time to accomplish their purpose.

CLEARING

When absolute alcohol is used as the dehydrant, it is followed by xylene, chloroform, or oil of cedarwood to clear out the alcohol, which is not readily miscible with paraffin. When oil of cedarwood is used to clear, it is followed by immersion in xylene (30 minutes to 2 hours) to remove the excess oil. From xylene the tissue can go directly into melted paraffin, xylene being readily miscible with and a solvent of paraffin. If dioxane is used as the dehydrant, the tissue is transferred directly from dioxane into paraffin since dioxane both dehydrates and clears and is miscible with paraffin.

INFILTRATION

After immersion in a clearing agent, the tissue is submerged in melted paraffin, either in the paraffin bath on the tissue-processing machine or in the paraffin oven. Paraffin replaces the clearing agent in the tissues. Two or three changes of paraffin are employed to eliminate traces of the clearing agent, which soften the paraffin and make sectioning of tissues difficult. Since prolonged treatment in molten paraffin causes shrinkage and hardening of the tissues, they should be left in this medium no longer than necessary. Infiltration in overheated paraffin also produces shrinkage and hardening and is to be avoided. The temperature of the molten paraffin should be checked routinely with a thermometer.

At least two and sometimes three or more changes of paraffin are required in certain embedding series. Duration of the bath depends on the size, thickness, density, and nature of the specimen. Skin and nervous tissue infiltrate slowly with paraffin. Muscle, fibrous tissue, blood, and fibrin will become overhardened in paraffin if left in this medium for more than 3 hours. Tissue from the brain and spinal cord, due to its compact nature, needs relatively longer treatment in paraffin and requires 4 to 6 hours impregnation for medium-sized sections. Allowing for the exceptions noted, two changes of paraffin, each 1½ hours long, are adequate for proper infiltration.

CASTING (BLOCKING; EMBEDDING)

Following complete infiltration the specimens are cast in a mold. *Casting* is the enclosing of the tissue or specimen in a solid mass of the embedding medium. Generally speaking, the surface of the section to be cut should be placed parallel to the bottom of the "boat" — the container in which it is cast. To orient tissue for proper embedding, the pathologist may notch with a scalpel or mark with india ink the side of the tissue opposite that to be cut.

The technician's ability to recognize tissue provides assurance that the sections will be embedded in the proper plane. For instance, cross sections of tubular structures are properly stood on end. Sections of skin and cervix must be positioned so that the cut surfaces bordered by the epithelial edge are flat against the bottom of the container. Using skin as an example, it must be positioned so that the epithelial edge, the subcutaneous tissue, and the deeper layers are all flat to the bottom so that all strata will be seen in the finished slide. For training purposes, we keep a daily, simple log identifying the type of tissue with the accession number, e.g., S-71-5210 = skin. This log is always close at hand at time of casting (page 63).

Tissues may be embedded in L-shaped strips of metal, paper boats, or a variety of plastic embedding molds designed specifically for this purpose. The relatively inexpensive plastic molds have almost entirely replaced other types of embedding containers. In addition to convenience, these plastic molds support the block while it is being sec-

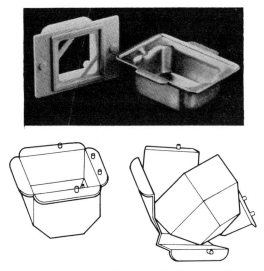

Figure 6-2.   Plastic embedding molds

tioned, and are designed to fit the microtome vise, eliminating the step of mounting the specimen on a block holder (Fig. 6-2).

The most current design of the newer molds is a dual carrier which serves as both the perforated capsule for the fresh tissue and as a casting mold for the processed tissue. The tissue remains in this carrier/mold throughout the entire cycle from fixation to storage, and is never removed from its original container (Fig. 6-3).

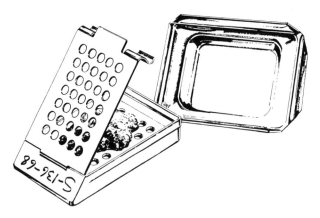

Figure 6-3.   Tissue-Tek II Process/Embedding Cassette

CASTING TECHNIQUE

1. After the tissue has been thoroughly infiltrated, a single capsule is removed from the paraffin bath and opened.

2. Warm paraffin is poured, about midway, into the plastic container or base mold of appropriate size.

3. With warm forceps, the tissue is oriented in the bottom of the container in the correct plane of sectioning.

4. The mold is transferred to a chilled enamel tray in order to anchor the tissue firmly in place and held flat with a forceps until it holds its position. Quickly pour in the remainder of the paraffin to the top of the mold. Set aside on the tray. (Have 2 or 3 of these flat trays in the refrigerator at all times when not in use.)

5. When the tray is filled with molds, transfer to the refrigerator or to an ice tray to complete hardening of the paraffin. This will take approximately 15 to 30 minutes.

Sophisticated thermoelectric modular embedding units have been designed to increase the efficiency of this phase of tissue processing. These units embody paraffin reservoirs with dispenser faucets, hot and cold plates (hot for orientation and cold for securing the tissue into position), and larger refrigerated plates or drawers to complete solidification of the paraffin or for storage until ready to cut.

ORIENTATION OF SPECIMEN (EMBEDDING OR CASTING)

1. Select proper size mold to allow segments of specimens to be embedded all flat to the bottom of the container and still have a margin of *a few millimeters* around all edges. The mold must also be deep enough to allow paraffin to be added to about twice the thickness of the specimen.

2. Do not layer specimens. All pieces of tissue should be embedded firmly to the bottom of the container so that the cut section will present a valid representation of the tissue submitted. All segments of cervical cone, skin, and so on should be embedded individually, only a few

millimeters apart, at the same level and preferably with the epithelial edges all in the same parallel placement. For instance the epithelial edges would all be positioned to the left within the mold. Have an order to the embedding.

3. Light, loose textured materials such as cell blocks and scanty endometrial curettings are best stirred up (whirled toward the center of the mold with warmed forceps) until they aggregate in the approximate center of the mold, while the paraffin is still warm. Then the mold is set on the chiller plate where the aggregate can be gently tamped to the bottom.

4. Stratified tissues like cyst walls, gallbladder wall, ovarian wedges, and skin sections must be carefully oriented *on edge* so that the side of the tissue from which it is desired to take sections is positioned vertically to the bottom of the mold.

5. It is best not to embed a very small soft specimen in the same mold with a large dense block. In order to obtain a full section of the larger specimen you may shave completely through and lose the small specimen.

Following casting, the hardened blocks are inverted so that the tissue is near the uppermost surface with the greater thickness of paraffin beneath it. The appropriate size mold should be used whenever possible. A margin of paraffin in excess of a few millimeters around the tissue is unnecessary and may cause compression as the sections are cut. If paraffin surrounds the tissue in excess of 2 mm. around the object, it may be trimmed after it is mounted on the microtome with a single edged razor blade.

Once tissues have been "blocked," they may be stored in a cool place indefinitely. In fact this is the best way to preserve specimens. If blocks are dipped in or coated with melted paraffin after they have been sectioned on the microtome, the paraffin will seal the tissue, and they will remain in a better state of preservation during long intervals of storage.

METHODS OF PROCESSING IN PARAFFIN
(Dehydration, Clearing, Infiltration)

METHOD I

95% isopropyl alcohol		1 hour
99% isopropyl alcohol		1 hour
Acetone	3–4 changes	1 hour each
Xylene	2 changes	¾ hour each
Melted paraffin	2 changes	1½ hours each

METHOD II

80% alcohol		1 hour
95% alcohol		1 hour
100% alcohol	3–4 changes	1 hour each
Xylene		1 hour
Melted paraffin	2 changes	1½ hours each

METHOD III: DIOXANE

95% alcohol		1 hour
Dioxane	4 changes	1 hour each
Melted paraffin	3 changes	1 hour each

METHOD IV: BUTYL ALCOHOL

80% alcohol		3 hours
90% alcohol		6–12 hours
Butyl alcohol	1 change	3 hours
Butyl alcohol	2 changes	3 hours
Butyl alcohol	3 changes	12–15 hours
Melted paraffin	3 changes	1 hour each

METHOD V: VERY SLOW PROCESSING

80% alcohol		6–24 hours
95% alcohol	2 changes	6–24 hours
100% alcohol	2 changes	6–24 hours
100% alcohol and xylene, equal parts		6–24 hours
Oil of cedarwood or terpineol		6–24 hours
Xylene to remove oil of cedarwood or terpineol	2 changes	1 hour each
Melted paraffin	4 changes	3–6 hours in all

METHOD VI: RAPID PROCESSING

(With the Ultratechnicon)

	2 mm. Tissue Thickness	4 mm. Tissue Thickness
Solution	2-Hour Cycle	4-Hour Cycle
10% alcoholic formalin	25 min.	55 min.
95% alcohol	5 min.	10 min.
Absolute alcohol	5 min.	10 min.
Absolute alcohol	5 min.	10 min.
Absolute alcohol	5 min.	15 min.
Absolute alcohol	10 min.	20 min.
Absolute alcohol	10 min.	20 min.
Absolute alcohol	5 min.	10 min.
Xylene	10 min.	15 min.
Xylene	10 min.	15 min.
Paraffin 56° to 58°C.	10 min.	20 min.
Paraffin 56° to 58°C.	20 min.	40 min.

CUTTING AND MOUNTING PARAFFIN SECTIONS

Since this is largely an acquired manual skill, experience is far more essential than directions in learning how to cut sections skillfully. Paraffin-embedded sections are cut on a rotary microtome. The beginner should be provided with a type of tissue that will be fairly easy to cut, such as kidney. The tissue blocks are best kept chilled on a block of ice or in a special refrigerated tray designed for this purpose. The chilled paraffin block is mounted in the vise of the microtome with the identification number clearly visible. Carefully adjust the block to the microtome, making certain that it is completely behind the knife edge. The broad side of the block should be parallel to the knife. Be certain that the block holder is rigid. Screw back the feed mechanism. Fix the knife in its proper position and adjust the indicator that regulates the thickness of the sections.

The sizes of different cells vary from a few to 100μ in thickness. Routinely, sections are cut at 6μ, although the recommended thickness may vary with the technique from 2 to 15μ, depending on the specific cell or component to be studied. A micron (μ) is $\frac{1}{1000}$ of a millimeter or $\frac{1}{25,000}$ of an inch. It is best for the beginner to practice cutting at a greater thickness (10 to 12μ) until the technique of handling the delicate tissue ribbons has been mastered.

Next, make sure that both the upper and lower edges of the paraffin block are parallel to the knife edge. The *parallel edges are essential for ribboning.* If there is an excess of paraffin surrounding the block, trim it off with a single edged razor blade so that a margin of paraffin not exceeding a few millimeters thick is left surrounding the tissue. The excess of paraffin will cause wrinkling and hinder flattening of the sections. If small triangular wedges are cut from the four corners of the paraffin block, the resultant ribbon that is formed will have notches between each individual section that will aid separation of the sections.

If the block does not ribbon, the knife may be improperly sharpened or the angle of the knife may be wrong. The recommended clearance angle is between 5° and 10°; the recommended bevel angle is between 27° and 33°. If such instruction is not meaningful to you and you wish to set the knife angle to give the best possible sectioning, use this trial and error adjustment method: Take a paraffin block of old autopsy or student material. Cut and observe a ribbon. Tilt or straighten knife position by very small increments until the ribbons fall easily from the block and are free of all compression, pleating, or other distortion. Once the ideal angle is achieved, leave the set screws in this position or mark the knife holder with a felt marker at the correct angle setting.

The angle will remain constant for a long time, indeed until repeated sharpenings alter the bevel. At this time, repeat the procedure given above to find the new optimum angle. Nearly all cutting problems are directly attributable to a dull knife and/or incorrect knife angle.

While securing the block holder, icing the block, or making other adjustments, keep the microtome locked to prevent knife injury to the tissue or hands. Before ribboning, wipe the knife edge clean and free of tissue or paraffin with cloth toweling or xylene-moistened Q-Tips. Blot ice water from the block and knife after chilling.

With the hand wheel bring the block up to and immediately behind the knife edge. Shave into the block gingerly, taking thin cuts (approximately 10 to 25μ) until the outer layer of paraffin is removed and the tissue is fully in contact with the knife edge. The smaller the specimen, the more care is required, since the risk is increased. A biopsy the size of a "period" could be completely lost with careless shaving into the block.

Icing the block briefly to harden the paraffin will aid cutting. Keep an ice cube in a shallow container next to the microtome. Ice any hard or fibrous tissue a little longer or chill block with Cryokwik freon aerosol spray. Soft tissue, on the other hand, often cuts more easily and without wrinkling if the block is not too cold. Heat produced by rubbing the thumb over the block will often help in cutting soft tissue and will prevent compression of sections.

To cut sections, revolve the flywheel with an even and somewhat rapid motion. Generally a hard tissue, e.g., cervix, is best cut with a firm, relatively rapid stroke, while soft tissue, e.g., brain, is best cut with a slow, gentle motion. As each new section is cut, it displaces the previous one. These individual sections adhere to one another by one edge to form a ribbon. As the section begins to fold onto the knife edge, lift the free end of the ribbon gently with a pair of fine forceps and draw it toward you, taking care to avoid pulling the ribbon too taut, as this breaks the chain. When the ribbon reaches a length of 6 to 8 inches, detach it from the microtome by supporting the far end of the ribbon with the blunt end of a histologist's pick or a camel's-hair brush. When cutting *serial sections,* use a fine camel's-hair brush to support the leading edge of the tissue instead of forceps, for forceps may damage the first section. Take care to separate the sections from the machine at a safe distance from the knife edge. Never allow forceps, pick, or any other hard object to come in contact with the knife edge.

Lay the sections on the surface of a dish of warm water or on the surface of a constant-temperature hot water bath (approximately 43°C.). An overheated water bath or excessive stretching will produce artefactual separation of tissue components, mimicking edema. Lower one end first and then the other. Stretch the ribbon out evenly by gently pulling the ends of the paraffin ribbon with the forceps and pick. Wrinkles and small folds can be flattened out by quick but cautious stretching and gentle tapping with the blunt end of the instruments. Remove any air bubbles that may have formed under the paraffin ribbon. With a pick that has been bent at an angle, reach under the ribbon and cautiously break up the bubbles by drawing the air bubble to one side, taking great care not to puncture the ribbon. If air bubbles are not removed, the tissue may later float off the slides.

Some workers mount the tissue section on a clean glass slide, relying on capillary attraction to hold it in place. Most technicians, unwilling to take the chance of losing one or more sections, apply a thin coat of egg albumen or one of the commercially available slide adhesives to affix the section to the slide. These are spread thinly so that the protein will not pick up the stain and detract from the appearance of the slides. (See Gelatin Method, page 287.)

To Mount Sections on Slides

Have ready clean slides which have been thinly and evenly coated with a drop of egg albumen-type fixative. Frosted-end slides will have been prelabeled; others are etched at this time on the far right corner. Visually, select the best sections in the ribbon on the water bath and carefully tease these away from the other sections with the blunt end of the instruments. Sections may also be separated by cutting with a clean, heated scalpel, taking care not to bring the heated knife too close to the tissue. I do not like this technique because the melted paraffin coats the water bath with a film of oily residue.

While holding the strip of ribbon to be mounted steady with the pick in the right hand, with the left hand slip a clean slide directly under the ribbon. Lift the slide from the bath, center the section on the slide, and stand it upright for a few seconds to allow the water to drain off. Blot the end of the slide and transfer to dryer or slide warmer. Carefully wipe the surface of the water bath with strips of paper toweling after each section is cut. If this is not done, residual cells or segments from one case may be picked up and incorporated with tissue from another patient. Wipe knife edge clean of tissue or moisture.

When multiple sections are cut, a warming table is desirable and convenient. The warming table will hold the slides until all of the sections are cut and ready to be transferred to the oven for complete drying. Place the mounted sections on a warming table regulated slightly below the melting point of the paraffin (about 43°C.) Heat causes sections to expand and thereby flattens out some folds and creases. Ideally, to prevent artefacts produced by too rapid drying and

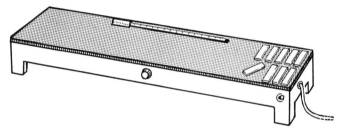

Figure 6-4.   Ranson warming plate

to encourage better adhesion, sections should be dried slowly without melting the paraffin (Fig. 6-4).

When the operation of cutting and mounting all of the sections is finished, drying may be completed in a 60°C. paraffin oven, in a commercially available hot-air slide dryer, or on the Ranson warming table. Allow to dry for a minimum of 30 to 40 minutes for better adhesion. When the sections are properly dried, they can be deparaffinized and stained by any of the standard staining methods (see Chapter 14).

Sections of the central nervous system require careful drying. Leave them overnight in a 37°C. oven.

Brittle or Hard-to-Cut Tissue

Brittle or hard-to-cut tissue may be caused by any of the following:

1. Prolonged treatment in certain fixatives.
2. Prolonged immersion in high concentrates of ethyl alcohol.
3. Prolonged treatment in certain clearing agents.
4. Prolonged treatment in molten paraffin or infiltration in overheated paraffin.
5. Drying out of tissue before it is placed in the fixative (e.g., biopsy specimens left in the operating room and allowed to dry out before immersing in fixative).
6. Failure to give special handling to some tissues (e.g., animal or brain tissue) which when treated with routine methods become hard and brittle.

The technician usually discovers that the tissue is hard and difficult or impossible to work with at the time she is sectioning it on the microtome. At this stage the tissue has already been infiltrated and embedded. Very often the following method will help the technician to secure a section:

1. Shave into the block on the microtome until the tissue is exposed.
2. Place the shaved block in a shallow dish containing water to which has been added a small amount of detergent (½ teaspoon of any dry detergent to 100 ml. tap water).
3. Leave the shaved block in this solution only until it can be cut successfully. This usually takes from 45 minutes to 1½ hours. If tissue cannot be sectioned after 3 hours, transfer to plain tap water and leave overnight. (See also Chapter 15.)

Static-Electricity Interference in Cutting

Cutting paraffin-embedded tissue sections in very dry weather is often made difficult by the formation of static electricity, which causes the tissue to curl over the instruments or become affixed to the metal parts of the machine or to the knife. When this condition occurs, try one of these remedies:

1. Breathe out or blow gently on the section as it is being ribboned to break up the static electricity formed.
2. Boil water in the room to increase the humidity.

Cutting Serial Sections

When serial sections are required, it is important that every section be saved so that there will be a true series. In cutting, use a fine camel's-hair brush instead of forceps to support sections in order to prevent any injury or loss of sections. Place convenient lengths of the paraffin ribbon on a flat cardboard surface — a shallow box lid makes a good receptacle. Many rows of sections may be arranged in order, with proper identification numbers marked directly on the cardboard. Store undisturbed and free of drafts in a cool place or in a refrigerator. When ready to mount and stain, cut ribbons into the desired number of sections with a sharp knife. To keep them in correct order, float only a few sections at a time on the hot water bath. Pick up the sections on a clean glass slide which has been previously coated with a thin, even layer of egg albumen. Mark the slide with identifying number and series number, drain off excess water, and dry as usual. One average size block of tissue can produce as many as 300 or more slides when processed serially.

Difficulties Most Commonly Encountered in Cutting Ribbons

1. Failure of block to ribbon:
    block not parallel to knife edge
    knife dull
    paraffin too hard
    knife tilted too much
    sections too thick
2. Uneven and crooked ribbons:
    wedge-shaped or irregularly trimmed blocks
    edge of block not parallel to knife edge
    irregularity in knife edge
    paraffin not homogeneous
3. Compressed, wrinkled, or jammed sections:
    knife dull
    paraffin block too warm
    paraffin on knife edge
    sections too thin
    microtome set screws loose
4. Tearing and crumbling of sections:
    incomplete fixation of tissue
    incomplete dehydration or clearing of tissue
    incomplete infiltration of tissue with paraffin
    paraffin too hot for bath and/or embedding
5. Split ribbon or lengthwise scratches in ribbon:
    nicks in knife edge
    knife edge dirty
    too much knife tilt
    grit, dirt, mercuric chloride crystals, calcium, sutures, or foreign
        bodies in the paraffin or tissue
6. Lifting of sections from knife on upstroke:
    too vertical a knife tilt
    knife dull
    paraffin too soft or room too warm

7. Sections clinging to knife:
    static electricity
    knife edge dirty
    knife dull
    knife tilt too vertical
8. Varying thickness of sections:
    clamp set screws on block or knife holder not tight
    knife not tilted enough to clear bevel
    blocks too large
    blocks too hard
    microtome not adjusted correctly

QUIZ

1. How long do we normally infiltrate tissue in molten paraffin?
2. What is the effect of prolonged treatment in paraffin?
3. How many changes of paraffin are made routinely?
4. How is tissue "cast" or "blocked"?
5. What are paraffin sections cut on? At what thickness?
6. Why are parallel edges of the block necessary to cutting?
7. What is the purpose of coating slides with egg albumen fixative?
8. At what temperature is the hot water bath maintained if the melting point of the paraffin is 56° to 58°C.?
9. a. How are paraffin sections dried?
    b. For how long?
    c. Why do we dry slides?
10. What is meant by "serial sections"?
11. List two or more complete methods of processing tissues in the paraffin technique.
12. Give three advantages and three disadvantages of the paraffin-embedding technique.

7

Celloidin Tissue–Processing Method

Although originally a trade name for a nitrocellulose compound (supplied by the Schering Company in Europe), the name *celloidin* has become a general term designating any kind of nitrocellulose employed in embedding procedures. For histologic purposes, nitrocellulose is available in two forms, one an alcohol-moistened lint, generally designated as LVN (low-viscosity nitrocellulose), and the other hard-curled amber chips (Parlodion).

The celloidin method is not as popular as the paraffin technique, due in great measure to the long period of time required to process celloidin-embedded material. Paraffin sections can be prepared in 24 hours. Celloidin sections take several days to several months to prepare. The celloidin method is still employed for large objects, for very delicate and extremely hard material, for tissues that contain spaces that tend to collapse, and for special research studies. Celloidin is not ordinarily removed from the sections; therefore in delicate specimens (as in embryology) the celloidin will support and hold together the fragile structures until the time that they are mounted on the slide. For hard tissue such as bone, long infiltration will afford greater support and will not affect the consistency of the tissue.

ADVANTAGES AND DISADVANTAGES OF CELLOIDIN

Advantages

1. Shrinkage is negligible, since no heat is required for infiltration. There is minimal distortion of tissue.

74

2. The consistency of large tissues, which must be immersed for long periods of time, is not affected by celloidin. The same objects treated with paraffin would become very hard due to the heat. Celloidin permeation is carried out at room temperature.

3. Celloidin provides better support for material which is hard to infiltrate (eyes, bone, large sections of brain, etc.), and for material which tends to collapse easily due to air spaces, so that it does not crumble in sectioning.

Disadvantages

1. The celloidin process is very slow (several days to several months).

2. Very thin sections are difficult to obtain, and in some thicker sections, cell details may be obscured.

3. Serial sections are difficult to prepare.

4. Photomicrographs are difficult to obtain.

5. The sections age poorly.

FIXATION

For celloidin embedding, tissue may be fixed in any of the preferred fixatives. After fixation, it must be washed thoroughly to remove the excess fixative.

DEHYDRATION

Specimens are dehydrated very slowly in ascending-strength solutions of ethyl alcohol, ending with equal parts of absolute alcohol and ether. Infiltration with the celloidin is impossible unless tissue is completely dehydrated. At no time should the solution be contaminated with water or moisture. No clearing step is necessary in the celloidin series, since the infiltrating medium is held in solution by an ether and alcohol combination. Thus, the transition between the last dehydrant (absolute alcohol and ether) and the embedding medium is completely compatible.

INFILTRATION

Infiltration is carried on without heat. This is one of the major advantages of the celloidin method. The tissue is infiltrated with a celloidin-ether-alcohol solution, using at least two strengths. Exact strengths are not of prime importance so long as the tissue is first infiltrated with a thin and then a thick celloidin. The celloidin must remain fluid and not be allowed to gel until the tissue specimen is completely infiltrated. Gelation occurs when the solvent is allowed to evaporate. A convenient method is to prepare in advance three jars containing thin celloidin 6%, thick celloidin 12%, and thick celloidin 14% (the last is for embedding).

The completely dehydrated material is immersed in a thin, syrupy celloidin (6%) in a closed airtight container. Wide-mouth bottles, screw-cap jars, preserving jars complete with rubber rings, or glass dishes with sealed or airtight covers may be used. The time required for complete infiltration will depend on the size and density of the tissue, and will take several days for small pieces of loose-textured material, several weeks for large sections of brain, and as long as 6 months to process sections of one-half hemisphere of brain. Dilute solutions of celloidin remain fluid longer than the more concentrated ones.

After the tissue has been impregnated with thin celloidin (6%) this is drained off and thick celloidin (12%) is poured over the tissue to continue infiltration. It is important that the tissue be completely immersed in the celloidin throughout the process. It will take several more days to one or more weeks for infiltration to be completed. Up to and including this stage, the infiltration is carried on in a tightly stoppered container to prevent evaporation, and the celloidin is allowed to remain in its fluid state.

EMBEDDING

Tissues may be embedded in relatively shallow tin or enamel pans which are covered by sheets of weighted glass, or in any glass dish that has a fitted cover. Adhesive tape may be applied to glass dishes with loosely fitting covers to produce a seal at the cover line. When tissue is to be exposed to the air to aid evaporation, the strips of adhesive tape are easily removed and reapplied. If tissues are to be embedded in a vessel that is not covered, they must be placed under a bell jar to control the rate of evaporation of the solvent.

Hardening the Tissue Block

To attain the consistency necessary for cutting the celloidin, the solvent (ether and alcohol) must be evaporated. This evaporation must be very gradual to achieve a consistent, uniform degree of hardness throughout the block and to prevent the formation of air bubbles. The specimen is removed from the infiltrating celloidin (12%) and transferred to an appropriate embedding vessel containing freshly poured, thick embedding celloidin (14%). Evaporation of the solvent is carried on until the syrupy fluid is hardened or "jelled." The evaporation in this stage is still continued under a cover. However, the cover may be lifted from the specimen for a few minutes once or twice a day to aid in hardening the celloidin. The celloidin is hard enough if the ball of the finger no longer leaves an impression on it (Bolles Lee), and approximates the consistency of an art gum eraser, firm but rubbery.

MOUNTING THE TISSUE ON THE MICROTOME BLOCK

The mass of hardened celloidin is loosened and removed from the embedding vessel. It is trimmed of excess embedding medium. It is then attached to a grooved vulcanized fiber or rubber block. Before mounting, the fiber block is labeled with a soft lead pencil to show the proper identification. To mount, place the block with the side to be cut uppermost in a Petri dish containing a small amount of ether and alcohol (equal parts). This will soften the celloidin a little on the underside of the block. With an applicator stick, coat the fiber block with a layer of thick celloidin, pushing the mixture well into the grooves. Quickly attach the softened surface of the tissue block to the fiber mounting block, pressing it firmly into place. Air-dry for a few minutes, and then place the block in a wide-mouth jar of chloroform for 2 hours to harden the celloidin completely. Transfer the block to a jar containing 80% alcohol for several hours or until it is ready to be sectioned. The 80% alcohol will produce the consistency necessary for cutting.

CUTTING AND STAINING CELLOIDIN SECTIONS

Celloidin sections are cut on a special sliding microtome. On most models the knife is mounted horizontally and is moved down across the stationary block. On some celloidin microtomes, the knife is stationary and the block is moved against it. In the "wet" celloidin technique, both the knife and block must be kept wet with 70% alcohol while cutting. Some technicians have a drip arrangement for both knife and block, while others prefer to use a camel's-hair brush moistened with the alcohol. Sections are usually cut 10 to 25μ thick as compared to 4 to 10μ with the paraffin method. In experienced hands, however, sections may be cut as thin as 6 to 8μ. Sections may be picked up from the knife with a moistened camel's-hair brush and transferred to a dish of 80% alcohol. Cut sections are stored in 80% alcohol until they are ready to be stained.

Cutting Serial Sections

If sections are to be mounted serially, as they are cut they are arranged in order on the surface of the knife. Serial sections may be removed from the knife with the aid of pieces of tissue paper cut to the size of the dish or jar in which the sections are to be stored. The papers are moistened with 70% or 80% alcohol and placed on the knife over the section or sections, pressing down until they adhere. Each paper is carefully lifted with its attached section and stacked in numerical order in 80% alcohol, or the sections may be transfered directly to the slide. When a dish is used for stacking the series it should be large enough to permit the papers to lie flat and small enough to prevent their moving about. The bottom of the dish is initially covered with 70% or 80% alcohol only a few millimeters in depth (to prevent the sections from floating out of order), and more alcohol is added as the series accumulates. The tissue papers can be numbered serially on one corner in advance.

Labeling

For indefinite storage of celloidin-embedded blocks, write identification in india ink on a small piece of paper and attach this to one side of the block, using thick celloidin as the adhesive. Harden this label into place with chloroform or 80% alcohol. When tissues from several patients are to be stored in a common receptacle, bag the blocks in gauze, with one ticket bearing the identification within the bag and another attached to the string on the outside for rapid recognition and retrieval.

Staining

Unlike paraffin sections, celloidin sections can be stained by nearly all methods without removing the celloidin. When it is desirable to remove the celloidin, the sections may be placed in equal parts of absolute alcohol and ether for 5 to 10 minutes. This will dissolve the celloidin. Hydrate the sections by immersing in absolute alcohol followed by 95% alcohol.

Celloidin sections are usually stained in Stender dishes, finger bowls, or watch glasses. They are usually not attached to the slides until after staining. The free sections are carried through the staining series on a bent glass rod or a section lifter. It is more difficult to differentiate celloidin sections than paraffin sections; they tend to overstain. Counteract this by diluting the stain or shortening the staining time.

If it is preferable to stain the sections on slides (e.g., serial sections), they may be attached in this manner. Transfer the sections to a slide and dry by blotting with fine filter paper. Cover the section with absolute alcohol for ½ minute to soften the celloidin and blot again. Dip the slide in thin celloidin (see page 80) in a Coplin jar and drain it.

Breathe over the tissue briskly, and then immerse the slide in 80% alcohol for 5 minutes to harden the celloidin coating.

To make the thin celloidin used for attaching sections to the slide, combine:

Thick celloidin (12%)	5 ml.
Equal parts of absolute alcohol and ether	95 ml.

Clearing Sections After Staining

Formerly, oil of origanum was used to clear celloidin sections after they were stained. The oil of origanum discolored the celloidin and was rather messy to work with. Most celloidin technicians prefer to work with clear, pleasant-smelling terpineol. After sections have been stained, they are dehydrated through 95% alcohol and transferred directly into a dish containing terpineol. Dehydration in absolute alcohol is avoided, since it will dissolve the celloidin. As they clear, the celloidin sections will float to the bottom of the dish containing terpineol. They are then placed in xylene, where they are left until they are to be mounted on slides. Any preferred mounting reagent may be used: Permount, neutral Canada balsam, or Harleco synthetic resin. A weight is placed on the coverslip and left for 24 to 72 hours to prevent contraction of the celloidin and resultant distortion, if the cut sections are over 10μ thick.

TO PREPARE CELLOIDIN SOLUTIONS FOR EMBEDDING

Celloidin * is supplied in 1-ounce (approximately 28 gm.) and 1-pound brown bottles (page 53). Originally celloidin strips were preserved in water. Before using these strips, it was necessary to wash carefully and to dry thoroughly the celloidin before making up solutions. The new purified Parlodion may be used just as it is received from the supplier.

When only small quantities of the celloidin solution are needed in the laboratory, both thin and thick celloidin can be conveniently made from the 1-ounce bottles by dissolving the dry celloidin in the amounts of ether and alcohol given below. The slight difference from the recom-

* Trade name Parlodion; supplier Mallinckrodt Chemical Works.

mended 6% and 12% will not affect results. If preferred, a large quantity of concentrated stock solution may be prepared and diluted for use.

T H I N   C E L L O I D I N   5 . 6 %

1 ounce Parlodion
250 ml. absolute alcohol
250 ml. ether

T H I C K   C E L L O I D I N   1 1 %

1 ounce Parlodion
125 ml. absolute alcohol
125 ml. ether

A glass preserving jar (Mason jar) complete with rubber ring makes a good airtight receptacle for this preparation. Place Parlodion chips in a dry Mason jar. Add alcohol (from a previously unopened new bottle). Cover; leave at room temperature to allow celloidin to swell. When swelling is complete (24 to 48 hours approximately), add anhydrous ether to jar. Rolling the jar several times a day and reversing the position from time to time is necessary until solution is complete. It usually takes from 3 to 7 days for the celloidin to go into solution.

When large quantities of celloidin are to be used, the preparations given below will better serve the purpose.

T H I N   C E L L O I D I N   6 %

90 gm. Parlodion
750 ml. absolute alcohol
750 ml. ether

T H I C K   C E L L O I D I N   1 2 %

180 gm. Parlodion
750 ml. absolute alcohol
750 ml. ether

E M B E D D I N G   C E L L O I D I N   1 4 %

210 gm. Parlodion
750 ml. absolute alcohol
750 ml. ether

The celloidin may be dissolved in the same manner as previously mentioned, or the celloidin may be bagged in gauze, tied with a string, and suspended in very large preserving jars containing equal parts of absolute alcohol and ether. When the celloidin is completely dissolved the gauze bag is removed and the jars are rolled on the bench to mix the solution evenly.

Stock celloidin solutions should be stored away from light, sun, or heat.

P R O C E D U R E   F O R   T H E   W E T   C E L L O I D I N   M E T H O D

The wet celloidin method is used primarily on bone, teeth, large sections of brain, and whole organs. Tissues embedded with the "wet" celloidin method are stored "wet" in 80% alcohol and must be cut wet, that is, both the knife and the tissue block are kept moist with 70% alcohol while cutting. For illustration purposes the method below is designed for *tissue not more than 3 to 5 mm.* thick. Longer time in each solution would be required for thicker blocks.

1. After fixation and washing, harden and dehydrate tissue blocks in 80% alcohol for 24 hours.

2. Repeat in 95% ethyl alcohol for 24 hours.

3. Place in absolute alcohol for 24 hours.

4. Place in equal parts of absolute alcohol and ether for 24 to 48 hours.

5. Infiltrate in thin celloidin (6%) in tightly stoppered container for 4 to 6 days or longer depending upon type of tissue.

6. Continue infiltration in thick celloidin (12%) in tightly stoppered container for 3 to 6 days or longer.

7. Embed tissue in proper embedding vessel in a fresh change of thick (embedding) celloidin (14%). The embedding vessel must have a cover or be placed under a bell jar. The cover may be removed once or twice a day for a few minutes to aid in hardening the celloidin. Gradual evaporation of the solvent to the correct consistency will take approximately 4 to 7 days.

8. Loosen the celloidin block from the mold, trim, and mount on rubber or vulcanized fiber blocks.

9. Place block in a wide-mouth jar of chloroform for 2 hours to harden the celloidin completely. Or harden the block by exposing it to chloroform vapor — place a wad of chloroform-soaked cotton under the bell jar with the tissue blocks. The chloroform vapor will harden the celloidin in from 2 hours for small blocks to several days for larger ones. From the chloroform, transfer blocks to 80% alcohol for storage until they are to be sectioned.

DRY CELLOIDIN PROCESS

The dry celloidin process is preferred for embedding whole eyes (see procedure on page 85). Material embedded by the dry method can be cut without alcohol because of the presence of oil of cedarwood in the block, but the knife is lubricated with oil of cedarwood. Follow the wet celloidin process and mount the tissue on rubber or fiber blocks as usual. The wet celloidin method is followed up to and including step 8. Then, instead of hardening in chloroform and storing in 80% alcohol, place the blocks in Gilson's mixture (equal parts of oil of cedarwood and chloroform) for 12 to 24 hours depending on the size of the blocks. Transfer the blocks to a mixture of 3 parts of oil of cedarwood to 1 part of chloroform for 12 to 24 hours. Transfer the blocks to 100% oil of cedarwood and leave for 24 hours or until ready to cut. Or, if preferred, from this stage the blocks may be removed and allowed to dry in the atmosphere prior to sectioning. These are stored dry in an airtight container.

CELLOIDIN-PARAFFIN (DOUBLE-EMBEDDING) METHOD

This is the so-called double-embedding process, in which the tissue is first infiltrated with celloidin and subsequently embedded in a paraffin mass. It is far easier to cut serial sections from celloidin-embedded material treated in this way.

The tissue is infiltrated with celloidin by the *dry celloidin method.* The celloidin blocks are trimmed directly from the oil of cedarwood and carried through two changes of chloroform. The excess chloroform is blotted from the blocks, and they are then placed in melted paraffin in the oven at 56° to 58°C. for about 2½ hours (two changes of paraffin of 1¼ hours each). The blocks are cast in a fresh change of paraffin and allowed to cool and harden. They are then cut on a rotary microtome, following the paraffin-sectioning technique. The rotary microtome produces ribbons rather than the single cuts that are delivered on a sliding microtome with the traditional celloidin technique. Because the celloidin inhibits the stretching obtained with paraffin ribbons, it may be necessary to float the sections on 95% alcohol to soften the celloidin and allow flattening.

NITROCELLULOSE (LVN) METHOD FOR EMBEDDING EYES

Low-viscosity nitrocellulose (nitrated lint variety of celloidin) when received from the supplier is wet with alcohol. Because of this LVN requires extra calculations for proportioning the solvents (ether and alcohol). Allowance must be made for the alcohol (35%) which has already been added by the manufacturer at the time it is packaged. The lint is best stored by removing it from its metal container (which is subject to rust contamination) and transferring it to airtight jars to prevent evaporation of the alcohol. The jars must be stored in a cool, dark place. Exposure to light deteriorates nitrocellulose, whether in the solid state or in solution.

CAUTION. LVN is more explosive than the Parlodion type of celloidin and should be handled with care. When dry it will explode if hit. The nitrocellulose as it is received is wet with alcohol. The container must be kept tightly covered and stored away from sunlight to avoid evaporation of the alcohol. Any nitrocellulose not required for future use should be carefully destroyed, as the material becomes increasingly hazardous as the alcohol evaporates.

Since LVN solutions, as the name indicates, are of low viscosity, it is possible to use higher concentrates of this medium and still have a fluid that will penetrate rapidly, thereby shortening the time required for infiltration by as much as 50 percent in some cases. For this reason, many technicians prefer to use it rather than the usual celloidin (Parlodion) preparation.

The nitrocellulose is dissolved in equal parts of absolute alcohol and ether, allowing for the alcohol already present in the lint. Recommended concentrations of the solutions are thin (10%) and thick (20%).

20% STOCK SOLUTION OF LOW VISCOSITY NITROCELLULOSE (LVN)

Nitrocellulose	140 gm.
Anhydrous ethyl ether	250 ml.
Absolute alcohol	210 ml.

It will take 4 to 5 days with occasional agitation to dissolve the nitrocellulose. The stock 20% concentration is diluted to the preferred strengths with equal parts of absolute alcohol and ether.

One of the disadvantages of the use of LVN is that it contains a grit that must be removed, in order to prevent injury to the knife edge when cutting the sections. Filtering is impractical. It is best to allow the solution to settle for a week or more and then pour off the clear supernatant portion of the LVN solution for use.

The celloidin type of embedding is preferred to paraffin for whole eyes. Celloidin embedding furnishes greater support for the delicate layers of the eye; when eyes are sectioned using the paraffin method, the retina may become detached from the harder tissues (sclera and choroid) that encircle it. The oil of cedarwood used in the dry technique aids in softening the brittle layers.

The following method for eye embedding is used at the Massachusetts Eye and Ear Infirmary, Boston, Massachusetts:

1. Fix whole eye, without opening it, in 10% formalin for 24 hours.
2. Transfer directly to 40% alcohol and leave for 24 hours.
3. Slowly dehydrate in 50% alcohol for 24 hours.
4. Continue dehydration in 60% alcohol for 24 hours.
5. Dehydrate in 70% alcohol for 24 hours.
6. Dehydrate in 80% alcohol for 24 hours.
7. Dehydrate in 95% alcohol for 24 hours.
8. Open the eye: The eye is placed with the cornea downward and the nerve uppermost. Parallel vertical cuts are made so as to provide a center slice which includes the nerve head (optic disc), lens, iris, and cornea (Fig. 7-1).
9. Dehydrate in absolute alcohol for 24 hours.
10. Dehydrate in absolute alcohol and ether, equal parts, for 24 hours.
11. Infiltrate with 8% nitrocellulose for 5 days.
12. Infiltrate with 12% nitrocellulose for 5 days.

Figure 7-1.   Eye in cross-section

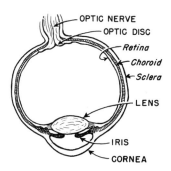

13. Infiltrate with 20% nitrocellulose for 5 days.

14. Embed in 20% nitrocellulose and evaporate solvent slowly for 2 to 4 weeks. Embedding is carried out in sealed glass dishes or in covered glass dishes beneath a bell jar. The embedding container should be coated with a thin, almost invisible film of mineral oil, to prevent the LVN from sticking to the sides of the dish.

Orient the specimen so that the side to be cut is on bottom. Cover with solution to depth of twice the height of the specimen.

15. When nitrocellulose has acquired the correct consistency (firm but not brittle), loosen edge and cut out celloidin blocks. Mount on fiber blocks, using 20% nitrocellulose as the adhesive, and place in a covered wide-mouth jar of chloroform for 1 hour to harden.

16. Transfer to large covered jars of equal parts of chloroform and oil of cedarwood. Leave for 24 hours.

17. Transfer to covered jar containing 3 parts of oil of cedarwood to 1 part chloroform. Leave for 24 hours.

18. Transfer to covered jar of oil of cedarwood (100%). Leave for 48 hours or until ready to cut.

Sectioning

1. Sections may be cut on a standard rotary microtome (Spencer) with a special clamp attachment for holding the celloidin block. While cutting, keep the block or knife lubricated with oil of cedarwood applied with a camel's-hair brush. Cut sections 14μ thick.

2. As the sections are cut, transfer them to large, flat dishes containing 95% ethyl alcohol, where they will flatten out.

3. Individual sections of the eye may be picked up on any hard-faced paper or floated onto small ($1\frac{1}{2}$ inch) squares of fine filter paper. Stack the sections, tie with thread, and mark with proper accession number. Store the bundles in 80% alcohol until ready to be stained.

Staining

1. Before placing the sections in the staining solutions, remove excess oil of cedarwood by washing in two or more changes of 95% alcohol.

2. Float the sections on water for a few minutes.

3. Stain in hematoxylin and eosin by transferring individual sections from dish to dish with a bent glass rod or a perforated section lifter.

4. Dehydrate the sections through two or three changes of 95% alcohol. Avoid absolute alcohol.

5. Carry sections directly from the 95% alcohol into terpineol to clear.

6. Mount sections of the eye directly from the terpineol onto a clean glass slide. Blot the section and rinse it gently with xylene from a flow bottle while it is on the slide. Coverslip in Permount.

Storage

When series of sections are cut, but are not to be stained immediately, they may be stacked in order on small papers, tied with thread, bagged in gauze and stored in large jars of 80% alcohol. It is wise to include in the gauze bag the celloidin block from which the sections were cut and the sections removed from the gross specimen when the eye was opened.

QUIZ

1. a. What is celloidin?
   b. Describe the two forms in which it is available for histologic work.
2. Give in outline form the procedure for the wet celloidin process.
3. How does the dry celloidin technique differ from the wet?
4. What is meant by the double-embedding process?
5. a. What are celloidin blocks mounted on?
   b. What are celloidin blocks cut on?
   c. How are celloidin blocks stored?
6. What is the average thickness of celloidin sections?
7. What is the solvent for LVN?
8. What is the main advantage of LVN over Parlodion?
9. What percent solution is considered a thin solution for LVN? What percent solution is considered a thin solution for Parlodion?
10. List three advantages and three disadvantages of the celloidin-embedding technique.
11. How are sections stained?

Processing of Frozen Sections

I.   Freezing Microtome
II. Cryostat

Before any tissue specimen can be cut into thin sections suitable for microscopic interpretation, it must be supported by some medium. Freezing the water in the tissue hardens it and is one way of providing the necessary rigidity.

Frozen sections are of great value both to the pathologist and to the patient. With frozen sections the pathologist can often make a diagnosis in a few minutes (generally when the patient is anesthetized in the operating room) rather than have to wait the many hours or days necessary to prepare tissue by other methods. Frozen sections are also used in a routine histology laboratory for the study of fatty or lipoid material that would be dissolved out in the paraffin or celloidin process, both of which methods employ alcohol and other fat solvents. Certain impregnation methods of the central nervous system require the use of frozen sections. Enzymes also are best demonstrated in frozen sections, since most are destroyed at temperatures above 53°C.

In 1932 Schultz-Brauns introduced the cold-knife technique, which at that time represented a great advance in frozen section microtomy, and since then modifications of equipment and techniques have improved the thinness and quality of the sections produced, ultimately resulting in the evolution of the cryostat. In practice the standard freezing or clinical microtome has many disadvantages. The freezing microtome has almost entirely been replaced, even in the smallest hospital, by the open-top cryostat developed by Chang, Russell, and Moore in 1961. The freezing microtome provides a cumbersome method of handling tissue. The cryostat provides ease of preparation and, more importantly, superior quality and thinness of the sections. The freezing microtome technique will be described briefly with more detailed information provided on cryostat methods.

I. *Freezing Microtome*

Fresh, completely unfixed tissues can be cut directly, without embedding, on a carbon dioxide or other freezing microtome. Frozen sections of fixed tissue do not adhere well to the slide and stain poorly. Fresh tissues are preferable. Freezing microtomes generally utilize a cylinder of liquid carbon dioxide, with a feed pipe leading from it to the freezing chamber of the table-mounted microtome. A simple lever-operated valve releases jets of carbon dioxide which cool the chamber and rapidly freeze the specimen mounted on its surface.

METHOD OF PREPARING FROZEN SECTIONS

1. The piece of fresh tissue from which the frozen sections are to be cut should not be thicker than 4 or 5 mm.

2. Place a drop of water on the block holder under the tissue on the freezing box to aid in attaching it securely.

3. Carbon dioxide (freon, or some other refrigerant) is used to freeze (solidify) the tissue. The tissue is held flat on the stage with a glass slide and the carbon dioxide released in short bursts. The consistency of the frozen tissue is important. It should be frozen just to the point at which it will be hard enough to section, and will appear white and firm. Adjust height of object carrier to bring the face of the block a hair below the knife edge. Adjust the feed mechanism to produce the desired section thickness. Sections are not ordinarily cut much thinner than 10 to 15μ on a freezing microtome. Move the knife into the tissue slowly. Completely frozen tissue will usually be too hard to cut without producing sections that will fracture over the edge of the knife. Reject fractured sections; continue to cut sections at short intervals until the tissue softens and produces satisfactory samples.

Ideally the cut is made through unfrozen tissue just above the "frost line." Keep the knife edge wiped clean and dry while cutting.

4. With the dampened tip of the little finger, lift the sections from the knife and float them on a wide dish of normal saline, distilled water, or 10 to 20% alcohol. Place the water dish on a dark or a black background in order to see the sections; they are usually colorless or very light in color.

METHOD OF HANDLING AND STAINING FROZEN SECTIONS

Thinner sections that curl and unroll in the water are selected for use. They may be handled as *free floating sections* or may be **mounted** on the slides.

FREE FLOATING SECTIONS. These may be stained by transferring each section through the different solutions with a bent glass rod or a perforated section lifter; or if they are to be stained in quantity, the free floating sections may be transferred to small paper cups perforated with pin pricks, and the cups may be used to carry the sections through the various solutions.

MOUNTED SECTIONS. They may be floated onto albumenized slides and dried quickly over a gentle flame before staining, or they may simply be mounted and stained directly on the wet slide with an eyedropper.

Mounting Technique for Free Floating Sections

From the water bath, float a single section onto an albumenized slide, guiding it with a bent, finely tapered glass rod. Holding the slide at a slant, draw it from the water. If any portion of the section does not lie flat, dip that side under the water again, float it smooth, and withdraw again.

To Flatten Curled Sections

If a section is folded over on itself, it can be flattened by transferring it first to a weak alcoholic solution (30% to 50%) and then to a bath of fresh water. The change in surface tension of the water will spin the section flat. Pick up on slide immediately.

STAINING

All fat stains require frozen sections and special oil-soluble dyes (pages 259 and 375). Frozen sections for rapid diagnosis are usually stained with metachromatic, polychrome stains or with a rapid hematoxylin and eosin method (page 100). The first two are temporary stains, with aqueous mounts. The hematoxylin and eosin stain is permanent because it is postfixed, dehydrated, cleared, and mounted in a permanent resin.

If sections are to be treated with alkaline solutions, i.e., metallic stains, float the section onto a slide. Blot with hard filter paper. Immerse briefly in a thin celloidin solution, drain, breathe over section to promote drying of the celloidin mixture, and harden in 80% alcohol before proceeding with stain. The step by step procedure for collodionization is on page 284.

Rapid Eyedropper Staining Method

1. Float the frozen section onto a clean glass slide.

2. With an eyedropper, place a drop or two of a *metachromatic stain* such as toluidine blue or thionine directly on the tissue. Leave stain on for about 10 seconds or slightly longer.

3. Rinse gently with water from eyedropper to remove excess stain. Keep slide in a fixed horizontal position during steps 2 and 3.

4. Drain the slide, and coverslip with an aqueous mountant. If desired, the coverslip may be sealed with clear nail polish after it has been wiped free of all water.

TOLUIDINE BLUE 0.5% ALCOHOLIC

Toluidine blue	0.5 gm.
20% ethyl alcohol	100.0 ml.

Combine and filter. Solution improves on standing.

THIONINE 0.5% ALCOHOLIC

Thionine	0.5 gm.
20% ethyl alcohol	100.0 ml.

Combine and filter. Solution improves on standing.

Rapid Giemsa Staining Method (Polychrome) Stain for Free Floating Sections

1. Float the frozen sections on normal saline solution.

2. Pick up the section on a bent glass rod. Drop directly onto the tissue 1 to 2 drops of Giemsa stain (commercially prepared, ready to use). Allow the tissue to stain for 10 to 15 seconds.

3. Rinse the tissue in a dish of water which has been slightly acidified with acid alcohol (a few drops of 1% acid alcohol to approximately 200 ml. of distilled water).

4. As soon as a pink color starts to appear, stop differentiation immediately by transferring the tissue to plain distilled water.

5. Rinse in another change of water, pick up on slide, and mount in an aqueous mountant.

Coverslipping

After staining, the sections are mounted directly in glycerol, gum arabic, Brun's fluid, or some other *aqueous* mounting medium. Commercially available water mountants are Clearcol, Viscol, Abopon, and the Paragon water mountant.*

BRUN'S CLEARING FLUID

(For mounting frozen sections from water)

Glucose	24 gm.
Glycerine	6 ml.
Spirits of camphor	6 ml.
Distilled water	84 ml.

Combine in a bottle, shake well, and filter. Keep the solution stoppered. This mountant will keep indefinitely.

* Clearcol, available from H. W. Clark, 33 South High St., Melrose, Mass. 02176. Abopon, available from Valnor Corporation, Brooklyn, N.Y. Paragon Aqueous Mountant, available from Paragon C. & C. Co., Bronx, N.Y.

II. Cryostat (*Cold Microtome*)

The main advantage of the cryostat is that it provides a technical refinement of frozen section methods and produces fresh-frozen sections of quality. The sections obtained with this method are of a precise micron thickness, a technical advantage not possible with the traditional freezing microtome. The added improvement in design is that the **knife**, the **microtome**, and the **tissue** are all maintained at the same temperature. An enclosing chamber eliminates the undesirable sensitivity to atmospheric pressure and humidity that is encountered with the traditional freezing microtome and cold-knife technique. The cryostat furnishes a completely controlled environment while cutting.

The cryostat is essentially a refrigerated chest that contains a rustproof rotary microtome. Although a variety of European- and American-made models are available, two main types of cryostat are in general use. One is operated with gloved arms and hands inserted through side portholes, and visual observation is possible by means of a front panel of Lucite or glass. The quick frozen section is mounted, attached to the microtome, sectioned, and transferred to a cold glass slide, **all within the chamber.** The slide is then removed from the chamber to room temperature, and the tissue section is affixed to the slide by thawing, gentle heat drying, or immersion in a fixative. This model cryostat is rather bulky, very expensive, and more difficult to operate.

The second type of cryostat consists of a microtome mounted in a portable open-top cold chamber with a double-hinged lid that provides access to the microtome. Fairly constant temperatures are maintained with the lid half open. The machine is operated by means of an external hand-controlled wheel. No gloves are required to be worn with this open-top model, except while making the initial adjustments, placing the cold knife, or moving the knife to another position. A fast-freeze platform is incorporated into the chamber to bring the tissue to cutting temperature.

Advantages of the cold-microtome technique are multiple. Alterations of tissue caused by fixation, dehydration, and heat are avoided, since fresh tissue is processed. The sections permit a wide variety of histochemical procedures, particularly work with enzymes that require fresh sections and with fluorescent antibody techniques. Of equal importance, cryostat-cut sections are of better quality and enhance the accuracy of the frozen section diagnosis. In summary, rapid pathologic diagnosis, fluorescent microscopy, autoradiography, and histochemistry all are possible with cryostat microtomy. In fact the cryostat is used for any tissue study in which the traditional fixation and paraffin-embedding would cause histochemical change.

Learning to operate a cryostat requires only minimal training and is easier if the operator has had previous experience with the standard microtome. As is not the case with the paraffin technique, fibrous tissue cuts easily, whereas soft tissue requires more technical skill. The ideal temperature for cutting cryostat sections will differ somewhat with the type of tissue. When tissues are cut at colder than the optimal cutting temperature, they fragment. Tissue sections cut at warmer than ideal cutting temperature may collapse at the edge of the knife. Tissues cut at the ideal temperature produce consistently acceptable sections that lie flat on the knife edge. Although optimal cutting temperatures vary with different tissues, in practical application and for convenience the majority of workers find a cryostat setting of $-20°C$. satisfactory. Tissues requiring supercooling to $-35°C$. or lower can be brought to this temperature with the ancillary carbon dioxide quick-freeze apparatus, or they can be initially snap frozen to this temperature with dry ice or chilled isopentane (page 134).

HANDLING SMALL FRAGMENTS OF TISSUE FOR CRYOSTAT FROZEN SECTIONS

Obtaining a frozen section of very minute fragments of tissue, like needle aspiration biopsies, presents the hazard of hitting the knife against the metal object holder. To avoid this, the fragments are grouped and cushioned on a cube of moistened paper toweling; or a commercial embedding matrix may be applied under, around, and over the tissue. When rapid diagnosis is not required, some workers embed the tissue segments in 10% gelatin for 24 hours prior to cutting the frozen sections.

Block Mounting Methods for Frozen Sections

Method I

Moisten a small folded cube of filter paper, freeze this to the object holder by immersing in a beaker of cracked *dry ice,* and mount and freeze the tissue block on this elevated base with the aid of water, O.C.T.* compound or some other embedding matrix commercially available for this purpose. The object holder is held with a forceps during immersion.

Method II

This method is most often used for the preparation of frozen sections for rapid diagnosis.

1. Lightly wet the bottom of the heat extractor with the cryostat lubricant. This will prevent it from sticking to the tissue.
2. Apply a few drops of O.C.T. (which will serve as a foundation for the tissue) to a cold object disc and set disc on quick-freeze platform.
3. Bring heat extractor over the disc for quick freezing to press the matrix well into the grooves. This will prevent the tissue from popping from the disc on impact with the knife edge.
4. Remove object holder, add another drop or two of embedding matrix, position tissue on object disc, support it by framing the periphery with the O.C.T., and return disc to freezing platform. Bring heat extractor over the surface for a 30-second fast freeze.

* O.C.T. This is a compound which provides convenient specimen matrix for cryostat sectioning at temperatures of $-10°$C. and below. It is a commercial water-soluble glycol and resin-embedding media supplied by Lab-Tek, Westmont, Ill.

CRYOSTAT TECHNIQUE

The complete technique given below is for use with the open-top cryostat (Fig. 8–1). Much of the material contained herein has been gleaned from the *Handbook on the Microtome-Cryostat* (by J. R. Baker, published by International Equipment Company, Boston, Mass., 1961) with the kind permission of the publisher.

Preparation of Equipment

1. A *cold* knife is essential for the preparation of cryostat sections. The knife may be either stored in the cryostat chamber or prechilled within it for 1 hour before cutting.

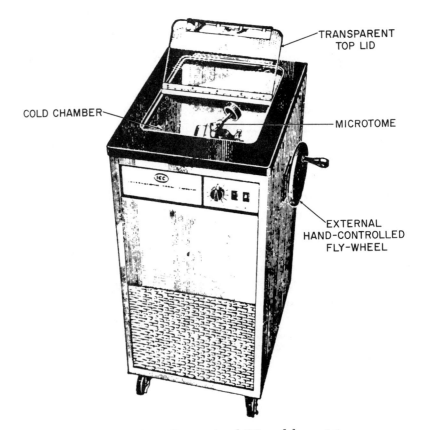

TRANSPARENT TOP LID

COLD CHAMBER

MICROTOME

EXTERNAL HAND-CONTROLLED FLY-WHEEL

Figure 8-1.   International CT model cryostat

2. With hands protected by cotton gloves, the cold knife is set at the approximate angle of 30°, and the lid closed.

3. A bottle of cryostat lubricant, a camel's-hair brush, and a supply of Q-Tips should also be stored within the refrigerated chamber. The Q-Tip swabs are used for cleaning frost residue and debris from the knife edge.

Preparation of Tissue (Freezing)

1. Select fresh (or previously refrigerated) **unfixed** tissue blocks several millimeters thick, so that the knife edge while cutting will be kept clear of the metal object holder. Elevate small fragments with cubes of moistened paper or support with O.C.T. compound.

2. With an eyedropper place a few drops of water or squeeze a few drops of O.C.T. on the metal object holder. Center tissue, surround base of tissue with a few more drops of water (or O.C.T.), and freeze rapidly with dry ice, freon, or carbon dioxide, or with the fast-freeze device mounted in the cryostat chamber (see page 95). When the tissue is completely frozen, the block will appear opaque and white. Blocks that have been quick frozen or mounted or both may be stored in the freezer if they are protected by an airtight covering such as Saran wrap.

Alternate Method

When tissues are not to be cut promptly, they may be quick frozen and stored in the freezer. Flatten thin slices of fresh tissue against the wall of a test tube; then immerse test tube into a slush made by placing cracked dry ice into a wide-mouth vacuum bottle or beaker and adding 95% isopropanol until semisolid. When the tissue is immersed, it will freeze almost instantaneously. Cap tube and store in freezer until ready to mount and section.

Sectioning

1. Transfer object holder with frozen tissue to the microtome, which should be in the locked position. Tighten clamp on object holder securely. Set feed mechanism to desired thickness (2 to 16μ).

2. Bring stage holding knife forward to allow a $\frac{1}{4}''$ clearance be-

tween the subsequent down-travel of the block and the knife edge.

3. Release drive wheel lock and line up tissue block to knife, bringing knife to within 1 to 2 mm. of the tissue. The relationship of the block to the knife edge should be *exactly parallel.*

4. When the face of the block is almost in contact with the knife, release ratchet from micrometer wheel. Turn wheel with hand, a fraction of a turn at a time to advance the tissue until it begins to section.

5. Continue trimming off the face of the tissue block until a full section representative of the tissue is present on the edge of the knife.

6. Return ratchet to the teeth of micrometer wheel.

7. Brush knife clean of debris, moisture, or ice film with prechilled Q-Tips.

8. Turn wheel slowly until leading edge of tissue begins to cut. Frozen sections do not really ribbon, consequently operation of the fly wheel instead of being a continuous motion consists of taking a single cut. With a fine camel's-hair brush, gently stroke the section onto the microtome blade as it travels downward, while turning the drive wheel slowly. Smooth and flatten the section as necessary with brush. Alternatively, an antiroll device may be used. This accessory consists of a glass or plastic plate attached to the knife and designed to prevent the specimen from rolling or curling as it is sliced. This device, originally troublesome, has been redesigned and refined to a considerable degree.

9. Transfer section to a "warm" slide (room temperature) or a "cold" slide (cryostat temperature), depending on mounting technique to be used (see below).

10. Brush knife clean and dry between each section cut.

MOUNTING OF SECTIONS

WARM SLIDE. Take a clean slide at room temperature and hold it a fraction of an inch over the frozen section on the knife. The section will be attracted directly to the warm slide and will transfer itself from the cold knife to the slide. Direct pressure is undesirable and results in distortion or artefacts. Once mounted, the section is ready for immediate processing (i.e., rapid diagnosis) or cold storage.

COLD SLIDE. Place clean slides in a small, open, slotted box within the cryostat chamber until they reach cryostat temperature (a few minutes). The frozen section is placed on the cold slide, oriented, smoothed and flattened with a camel's-hair brush, and then removed to room temperature. A finger is rubbed against the underside of the slide beneath the section, and the slight warmth causes the section to flatten out and become affixed to the slide. Once the section has been thawed and has adhered to the slide it is ready for immediate processing or cold storage. There are fewer artefacts produced with the cold-slide method and it is a preferred technique for enzyme studies.

COVERSLIP OR SLIDE SUCTION PICK-UP. A suction pick-up accessory that holds a coverslip or slide in position to remove the tissue slices as they are cut is available commercially.

SALVAGING THE FROZEN SECTION BLOCK AFTER SECTIONING

The block from which the frozen section has been cut may be removed from the object holder, defrosted at refrigerator temperature for 1 hour, fixed, and processed automatically on the Autotechnicon. This method prevents artefacts produced by rapid or simultaneous thawing and fixing of tissue. A permanent section may be cut from the material from which the frozen section diagnosis was made, or the paraffin block can simply be stored with the other material submitted on the case.

STAINING CRYOSTAT SECTIONS

Fat stains are always done on frozen sections and mounted in an aqueous mountant. See pages 259 and 375 for oil-soluble staining methods. Following brief fixation, most special staining procedures can be employed on frozen sections with little or no modification. For rapid diagnosis, sections may be stained for a few seconds in an 0.5%

toluidine blue or thionine (page 91), or they may be stained with commercial products like the Paragon frozen section stain. These are temporary mounts. Alternatively, a rapid hematoxylin and eosin technique may be used. This is a permanent mount and may be stored. *Note:* Sections mounted directly from water or from aqueous stains must be coverslipped using a water-soluble mountant (page 92). Sections which have been dehydrated and cleared may be mounted in a permanent synthetic mountant such as Permount or Histoclad.

Rapid Biopsy Technique with Hematoxylin and Eosin

This method takes only 5 to 10 minutes and produces well-differentiated sections which are permanent. Set up the usual solutions in the series in screw-cap Coplin jars in a position convenient to the cryostat.

1. Immerse frozen section on the slide in the fixative at room temperature for 30 to 60 seconds (10% neutral formalin recommended).

2. Rinse briefly in 70% alcohol.

3. Rinse in water.

4. Stain for 10 to 15 seconds in Harris' hematoxylin, rinse in water, and immerse in 1% lithium carbonate to blue. Rinse in two changes of water. If desired, hematoxylin may be differentiated in 0.5% acid alcohol and washed prior to blueing.

5. Counterstain 2 to 10 seconds in 1% alcoholic eosin.

6. Dehydrate through two fresh changes of 95% ethanol (approximately 5 to 10 dips each or until alcohol sheets off the section).

7. Dehydrate in two changes of absolute ethanol or in acetone (approximately 5 to 10 dips each, agitating slide constantly).

8. Transfer and clear in two changes of xylene and mount in a permanent mountant like Permount or Histoclad.

SPECIAL HANDLING METHODS FOR CUT FROZEN SECTIONS

Sections for rapid diagnosis are generally picked up with the warm-slide technique and stained immediately. Frozen sections of fresh tissue to be processed for histochemical purposes require special handling. No one method of processing is suitable for all purposes. However, it is generally agreed that immediate fixation at moment of thawing in a cold fixative (5° to —20°C.) is applicable to most methods.

Pearse cites several methods of handling cryostat sections:

1. Pick up section on warm or cold slide or coverslip. Fix by immersion at moment of thawing.
2. Pick up section on warm or cold slide or coverslip, thaw, and dry in air.
3. Pick up on warm or cold slide, thaw, dry, and postfix.
4. Transfer free-floating section while thawing into warm or cold incubating medium (for enzyme histochemistry).
5. Transfer free-floating section while thawing into warm or cold test reagent solution (especially protein or inorganic histochemistry).
6. Transfer free-floating sections into warm or cold fixative.

For most purposes the first three are the methods of choice. For histochemical studies on labile enzymes, methods 2 or 4 are absolutely necessary. If the enzyme under consideration can withstand fixation, methods 1, 3, or 6 may be applied. Pearse points out that "choice of method must be dictated by practical, rather than theoretical, considerations."

In most instances, fixed mounted cryostat sections can be stored in closed plastic boxes within a standard laboratory refrigerator at approximately 5°C.

FIXATION

Rapid Method for Histochemical Procedures

Immerse thin cryostat sections in chilled (refrigerator temperature) fixatives for 30 seconds to 10 minutes. Recommended fixatives are acetone, acetic-alcohol, ether-alcohol, formol-alcohol, Carnoy's solution, and 10% neutral formalin. When allowed for enzyme histochemistry, a 30-second to 2-minute fixation period is often recommended to prevent diffusion of the enzymes into the surrounding tissues or into the incubating medium. When the precise localization of chemical substances is to be preserved, the choice of fixative will be dictated by the subsequent technique. For fat studies 10% neutral formalin is the recommended fixative.

Fixative Formulas

Acetic-Alcohol

Absolute ethyl alcohol	95 ml.
Glacial acetic acid	5 ml.

Carnoy's Fluid

Absolute ethyl alcohol	60 ml.
Chloroform	30 ml.
Glacial acetic acid	10 ml.

Ether-Alcohol

Ethyl ether	50 ml.
Absolute ethyl alcohol	50 ml.

Formol-Alcohol

Absolute ethyl alcohol	80 ml.
37–40% formalin (full strength)	10 ml.
Distilled water	10 ml.

10% Neutral Formalin

37–40% formalin (full strength)	10 ml.
Distilled water	90 ml.
Sodium phosphate, monobasic	0.4 gm.
Sodium phosphate, dibasic anhydrous	0.65 gm.

CARE OF THE CRYOSTAT

The cryostat will need to be defrosted, cleaned, dried, and oiled on a regular maintenance schedule. Depending on the amount of use it receives, it can generally be operated for 2 to 6 weeks between defrosting. After defrosting and drying, the microtome should be thoroughly lubricated with low temperature silicone oil (stored in the chamber). A hair dryer will speed up the drying process. Following cleaning and drying, it will take approximately 2 to 3 hours to cool the cryostat to cutting temperature. This can be accelerated by placement of dry ice on the microtome and knife. Occasionally the moving parts of the microtome will freeze on recooling. When this occurs apply a few drops of alcohol to these areas, work the hand wheels until they are freely movable, and add additional lubricant. Also, in addition to the above, the cryostat chamber and microtome should be sterilized periodically or when necessary by washing down with Amphyl or some other disinfectant.

A cryostat in constant demand may necessitate training the night engineer to perform this function so that the equipment is always available for early morning frozen sections of diagnostic pathology.

QUIZ

Frozen Sections

1. What are the advantages of frozen sections?
2. With what is the tissue infiltrated?
3. What are sections cut on?
4. Give in outline form two methods of handling and staining frozen sections.
5. List two or more dye solutions used for frozen sections.
6. What preparation is used for coverslipping sections?
7. Why are frozen sections used for the demonstration of fat in tissue?

Cryostat Sections

1. What is the cryostat?
2. Why does it represent a preferred technique for frozen sections?
3. How may tissue blocks be quick frozen?
4. Give two methods of mounting cut sections on slides.
5. Give in outline form a method of staining for rapid biopsy diagnosis.
6. For special histochemical methods, how are tissue sections fixed and for how long?

REFERENCES

Adamstone, F. B., and Taylor, A. B.   The rapid preparation of frozen tissue sections. *Stain Techn.* 23:109, 1948.

Baker, J. R.   *Handbook on the Microtome-Cryostat.* Boston: International Equipment Co., 1961.

Chang, J. P., Russell, W. O., Moore, E. B., and Sinclair, W. K.   A new cryostat for frozen section technic. *Amer. J. Clin. Path.* 35:14, 1961.

Chang, J. P., Russell, W. O. and Moore, E. B.   An improved open-top cryostat. *J. Histochem. Cytochem.* 9:208, 1961.

Klionsky, B., and Smith, O. D.   Application of the refrigerated microtome in surgical pathology. *Amer. J. Clin. Path.* 2:144, 1960.

Murray, M., Jaeschke, W. H., and Stovall, W. D.   Rapid technique for frozen sections. *Amer. J. Clin. Path.* 31:419, 1959.

Pearse, A. G. E.   *Histochemistry: Theoretical and Applied.* (2d ed.). Boston: Little, Brown, 1960, pp. 13–23.

Schultz-Brauns, O.   Verbesserungen und Erfahrungen bei Anwendung der Methode des Gefrieschneidens Unterfixierter Gewebe. *Zbl. Allg. Path.* 54:225, 1932.

Thornburg, W., and Mengers, P.   An analysis of frozen section techniques: I. Sectioning of fresh-frozen tissue. *J. Histochem. Cytochem.* 5:47, 1957.

9

Special Tissue–Processing Methods

I. Carbowax Technique
II. Electron Microscopy
III. Fluorescent Microscopy

I. Water-Soluble Wax (Carbowax) Technique

Unlike paraffin and celloidin, this newer preparation, Carbowax (page 54), is water-soluble, and consequently no dehydration of the tissue is required prior to infiltration. The tissues are fixed, washed, and transferred directly into the melted wax. Carbowax provides a rapid method for embedding tissue for histologic study, with the special advantage that deleterious dehydrating chemicals can be avoided. Also, some enzyme histochemical studies are possible with this technique.

Unlike paraffin and celloidin techniques, the water-soluble wax method has been used successfully for the demonstration of fat in tissue. However, the standard formula for Carbowax impregnation will not adequately infiltrate tissues containing large amounts of gross fat or large sebaceous glands. Rinehart and Abul-Haj (see below) report good results obtained by infiltrating tissues of high lipid content with Carbowax 1000 rather than with the usual formula. If fat is not the component to be studied, the tissue can be treated with a fat solvent such as acetone prior to infiltration with water-soluble wax.

Since the workers who have published their experience with water-soluble wax differ somewhat in their methodology, references for further reading are listed at the end of this section (page 110).

ADVANTAGES AND DISADVANTAGES OF CARBOWAX

Advantages

1. The embedding process is rapid (dehydration time is eliminated).

2. Fat components may be demonstrated, since dehydration in alcohols and other fat solvents is unnecessary.

3. There is less shrinkage and distortion of the tissue than in methods which require dehydration.

4. Excellent cytologic detail is possible.

5. In experienced hands, with proper embedding, sections may be cut as thin as 1 to 3μ.

6. The method does not require any mechanical device (i.e., tissue processor).

Disadvantages

1. Water will dissolve the embedding medium; great care must be taken to keep the blocks free from water.

2. To obtain good sections, more care is required than with paraffin.

3. Sectioning on the microtome is more difficult than with paraffin. Cutting requires greater technical ability.

4. Tissue containing large amounts of gross fat is not adequately penetrated.

5. In warm and humid areas an air-conditioned laboratory is a requisite because of the hygroscopic nature of Carbowax.

6. The determination of the ideal proportions of the different compositions of wax for a particular climate is a major problem.

TO PREPARE THE MEDIUM

The formula usually given for the embedding mixture is 9 parts of Carbowax 4000 and 1 part of Carbowax 1500. This is not a rigid formula and the quantities or the use of different compositions of Carbowax (e.g., Carbowax 1000 or 1540) may be varied by the individual laboratory to suit its needs. The temperature often determines the amounts to be combined, and the prescribed formula may be too soft for sectioning in very hot climates. The higher room temperatures require a harder wax. The mixture should be prepared in advance and stored in a humidity-controlled paraffin oven or incubator. If the Carbowax is overheated, the blocks tend to be crumbly when being sectioned (additional information on page 54).

FIXATION

The tissue is fixed in any good fixative. Wash out fixative thoroughly in running water.

INFILTRATION

The tissue blocks, not more than 3 to 4 mm. thick, go directly from the wash into melted water-soluble wax in the paraffin oven at 56° to 58°C. Leave approximately 3 hours. Agitate the tissue from time to time, for the wax does not take up and diffuse the water from the tissues readily. If tissues rise to the surface of the embedding vessel, lay filter paper over the top of the melted Carbowax to hold the tissue well into the embedding medium.

The tissue is impregnated with three changes of Carbowax, each for 1 hour. The last change should be in a shallow embedding container or mold (glass container or paper boat).

HARDENING

From the last change remove the mold from the oven, cast the block, and harden Carbowax rapidly by transferring the embedding container to the refrigerator for 15 to 30 minutes.

MOUNTING ON BLOCK HOLDER

If paper cups or glass are used, remove the tissue block from the embedding container. Trim away excess wax and mount on block holder for rotary microtome. To attach the tissue, dip the block in melted Carbowax, press firmly to the block holder, and cool and harden in the refrigerator. If a plastic embedding mold has been used, simply insert chilled mold in vise of microtome.

CUTTING SECTIONS

There are divided opinions as to whether sections should be cut at room temperature or whether the blocks should be thoroughly chilled for 15 to 30 minutes in the refrigerator before cutting.

Sections are cut on a rotary microtome. Material does not always ribbon. Handle sections with a camel's-hair brush instead of metal instruments.

CAUTION. Neither the block nor the knife may be iced during cutting. *All contact with ice or water must be avoided* due to the solubility of the wax.

MOUNTING CARBOWAX SECTIONS ON SLIDES

There are various methods of mounting the sections on slides.

1. Place section directly on a dry slide and press down with a rolling motion of the index finger.

2. Spread 3 or 4 drops of flotation medium on a horizontal slide. Deposit strip of ribbon on slide. Drain carefully.

3. Float the sections on Pearse's formula (diethylene glycol flotation medium) or on the Blank and McCarthy formula (gelatin-potassium dichromate flotation medium). The media help to prevent shredding of the sections. Pick up on gelatinized slides. Because of the solu-

bility of Carbowax in water, the preferred mounting method is flotation on special media.

Flotation Media for Carbowax

PEARSE FORMULA

Diethylene glycol	40 parts
Distilled water	50 parts
Full-strength formalin (38–40%)	10 parts

BLANK AND MCCARTHY FORMULA

Mix equal parts of 0.02% gelatin and 0.02% potassium dichromate. Boil for 5 minutes in daylight. Cool and filter.

Gelatin Slide Adhesive

Gelatin (granular)	10 gm.
Distilled water	60 ml.
Glycerol	50 ml.
Phenol	1 gm.

Slides are thinly coated with this preparation.

DRYING AND STAINING

Dry sections in a 37°C. oven for 10 to 30 minutes. Stain as desired. Most routine stains can be applied with very little modification. Sections usually require slightly longer staining time. It is unnecessary to deparaffinize sections in the usual manner with xylene and the alcohols. If the flotation medium has not already dissolved the wax, the slide may be dipped in water to remove the wax, and then drained and dried again before staining. After staining, use the routine dehydrating agents (unless fat stains are employed), and clear and mount in any neutral mounting medium. If fat stains are used, avoid all contact with the higher grades of alcohol and xylene.

STORAGE

After sectioning, the cut surface of the block should be coated with the Carbowax to protect the embedded tissue. Wrap the blocks in Saran wrap or seal in plastic bags with the use of heat or by tying with strings. Store in a closed container in a cool place.

QUIZ

1. How is Carbowax prepared for use?
2. How is infiltration accomplished?
3. In what manner are blocks hardened?
4. What are Carbowax sections cut on?
5. Give two alternate methods of mounting Carbowax sections on slides. Which is preferred?
6. How are sections dried?
7. In what manner are sections stained?
8. Give three advantages and three disadvantages of the Carbowax method.

REFERENCES

Blank, H., and McCarthy, P. A general method for preparing histologic sections with a water-soluble wax. *J. Lab. Clin. Med.* 36:776, 1950.

Firminger, H. I. Carbowax embedding for obtaining thin tissue sections and study of intracellular lipids. *Stain Techn.* 25:121, 1950.

Jones, R. M., Thomas, W. A., and O'Neal, R. M. Embedding of tissues in Carbowax. *Techn. Bull. Regist. Med. Techn.* 29:49, 1959.

McCormick, J. B. Improved tissue embedding method for paraffin and Carbowax. *Techn. Bull. Regist. Med. Techn.* 29:15, 1959.

Rinehart, J. F., and Abul-Haj, S. Histologic demonstration of lipids in tissue after dehydration and embedding in a polyethylene glycol. *Arch. Path.* 51:666, 1951.

Wade, H. W. Notes on the Carbowax method of making tissue sections. *Stain Techn.* 27:71, 1952.

II. *Electron Microscopy*

Electron microscopy makes it possible to examine cells and tissues at magnifications far beyond the range of the light microscope (page 6). In the 1930's the electron microscope was developed, and although direct magnifications of 500,000 times are possible, it too has its limitations. Because it transmits electrons through the object under study, it projects a silhouette image. A camera installed within the microscope photographs this image. The electron micrographs produced are used for interpretation of the fine structural components of the cells, rather than the conventional slides. The electron microscope has revealed much of the ultrastructure of cells and modified our knowledge and concepts about cell structure. It is actually a step beyond cellular morphology to the macromolecular level.

Many laboratories and hospitals are exploring the field of fine structural changes in cells. Most such laboratories require the full-time services of trained electron-microscopy technicians. The development of electron microscopy has been so rapid that a number of techniques have been learned either by experience or by personal instruction. What is practiced or taught in one laboratory may be quite unpopular in another. On this account the brief description that follows is intended to give some basic information mostly of an introductory nature.

Due to the low penetrating power of electrons, electron microscopy demands ultrathin tissue sections in the range of 100 to 600 A thick (thin as one-millionth of an inch). Their preparation involves careful fixation and embedding of the tissues in plastics. Specimens are most generally fixed in osmic acid (or doubly fixed in glutaraldehyde-osmic acid), dehydrated, embedded in liquid plastics, polymerized to the solid state, and cut on a special ultramicrotome.

FIXATION

Tissue fixation must be as immediate as possible, because early autolytic changes not visible by light microscopy may render cells that were fixed improperly or too late, useless for electron microscopy. The conventional use of single fixation with buffered osmium tetroxide (Palade's fluid) has been largely replaced by the double fixation method, i.e., initial fixation with buffered glutaraldehyde or paraformaldehyde, followed by postfixation with buffered osmium tetroxide. Glutaraldehyde followed by osmium tetroxide maintains fine structures and adds contrast. Both fixatives are buffered to a pH of 7.2 to 7.4 for optimal preservation.

Initial fixation in glutaraldehyde will permit both light microscopy and, if desired later, electron microscopy on the same tissue specimen. For instance a surgical specimen may be fixed in glutaraldehyde from which suitable paraffin sections may be prepared. Later, if the specimen warrants additional study with the electron microscope, a portion of the fixed specimen (wet stock) may be diced into 1 mm. cubes, postfixed in osmium tetroxide, dehydrated, and embedded in the plastic resins. For electron microscopy, fixation at refrigerator temperature is recommended. Tissues fixed in buffered glutaraldehyde, paraformaldehyde, or a combination of the two can be stored for several weeks or months, permitting one to postpone processing until convenient.

With the double fixation method, the glutaraldehyde should be rinsed out of the tissue with a suitable cold buffer before completing fixation in osmium tetroxide. Blocks of 0.5 to 2 mm. size for electron microscopy study or enzyme localization need be fixed only for 30 minutes to 4 hours.

OSMIC ACID FIXATION

Preparation of Osmic Acid Solutions

Observe cautions noted on page 126 in the preparation of all solutions containing osmic acid.

Rinse the clean glass stoppered bottle (which is to be used for storing the solution) thoroughly with glass distilled water. If the bottle is not scrupulously clean the solution will rapidly become discolored. Scrub the vial of osmium tetroxide with an abrasive cleanser and rinse thoroughly in water followed by distilled water rinses. Dry vial well. Under a hood, with fan running, score the vial of osmic acid with a clean fine file. Snap vial in two and drop into the bottle of distilled water or buffer solution. Stopper and shake vigorously.

Allow the bottle to remain at room temperature for 24 hours, shaking occasionally. Prepare the osmic acid solution at least 1 day before required, for it is slow to dissolve. This is a stable solution and will keep for some weeks at refrigerator temperature if stored in an airtight container. Label and date bottle. Three traditional formulas for osmium fixatives are given below.

PALADE'S FIXATIVE

VERONAL ACETATE BUFFER (STOCK SOLUTION A)

Sodium veronal (barbital)	14.7 gm.
Sodium acetate	9.7 gm.
Add distilled water to make	500.0 ml.

Combine and store in refrigerator. The buffer is stable and will keep for some months.

2% OSMIUM SOLUTION (STOCK SOLUTION B)

Osmium tetroxide	1.0 gm.
Distilled water	50.0 ml.

Prepare according to instructions for osmic acid solutions p. 112.

0.1N ONE-TENTH NORMAL HYDROCHLORIC ACID (STOCK SOLUTION C)

Concentrated hydrochloric acid	8.0 ml.
Distilled water to make	1000.0 ml.

Store in refrigerator. Stable for several months.

PALADE'S WORKING SOLUTION

Solution A	5.0 ml.
Solution B	12.5 ml.
Solution C	5.0 ml.
Distilled water	2.5 ml.

Combine. Adjust the pH to 7.4 with a few drops of buffer. This solution is relatively unstable. It will keep under refrigeration for a week or more. Just before use, 0.045 gm. per milliliter of sucrose solution may be added (optional).

For use: Place specimen in a vial with enough fixative to cover the specimen (2 to 3 ml.) After sections are immersed in the fixative in stoppered vials, place the vials in a bowl of ice or refrigerate to prevent autolysis. Fix for 1 to 3 hours.

ZETTERQVIST OSMIUM FIXATIVE

VERONAL ACETATE BUFFER (SOLUTION A, PAGE 113)

2% OSMIC ACID (STOCK SOLUTION B, PAGE 113)

0.1N HYDROCHLORIC ACID (STOCK SOLUTION C, PAGE 113)

RINGER'S SOLUTION

Sodium chloride	8.05 gm.
Potassium chloride	0.42 gm.
Calcium chloride	0.18 gm.
Add distilled water to make	100.0 ml.

ZETTERQVIST WORKING SOLUTION (pH 7.2–7.4)

Veronal acetate buffer	(Solution A)	10.0 ml.
Stock 2% osmium	(Solution B)	25.0 ml.
Ringer's solution		3.4 ml.
0.1N hydrochloric acid	(Solution C)	approx. 11.0 ml.

The pH is adjusted to 7.2 to 7.4 with solution C.

Add distilled water to make	50.0 ml.

The molarity of this fixative is 0.34M and it is used at 0° to 4°C. The solutions are kept in glass stoppered bottles in the refrigerator.

MILLONIG'S OSMIUM TETROXIDE FIXATION SOLUTION pH 7.2–7.4

Solution A: prepare 2.26% sodium phosphate monobasic in distilled water. Stable for several weeks at refrigerator temperature.

Solution B: prepare 2.52% sodium hydroxide in distilled water. Stable for several weeks at refrigerator temperature.

Solution C: prepare 5.4% glucose (dextrose) in distilled water. Stable for several weeks at refrigerator temperature.

Solution D: *isotonic disodium phosphate buffer.* Prepare by mixing 41.5 ml. of Solution A and 8.5 ml. of Solution B. The pH is adjusted to the required value (7.2–7.4) with Solution B.

WORKING SOLUTION

Osmium tetroxide	0.5 gm.
Solution D	45.0 ml.
Solution C	5.0 ml.

Following the instructions for preparation of osmic acid solutions given on page 112, score the vial of osmic acid, snap it in two, and drop into the bottle containing the buffer solution. Store in refrigerator where it will be stable for some weeks. Fix tissues for 2 to 4 hours at 0° to 4°C.

DOUBLE FIXATION METHODS

Glutaraldehyde Fixation

CACODYLATE BUFFER 0.2 M (pH 7.4)

Sodium cacodylate	4.28 gm.
Distilled water	30.00 ml.
0.1N hydrochloric acid	8.00 ml.

Fill up to 100 ml. with distilled water. Store in refrigerator.

Prepare glutaraldehyde fixative by mixing 25 percent aqueous glutaraldehyde with sodium phosphate buffer (above) or sodium cacodylate buffer to give a final concentration of 1.5 to 6.0 percent glutaraldehyde in 0.5 to 0.1 M buffer at pH 7.2 to 7.4. Fix tissues for 1 to 4 hours at 0° to 4°C. followed with 1 hour's postfixation in Millonig's fixative, page 115.

Paraformaldehyde-Glutaraldehyde Fixation

Heat 25 ml. of distilled water to 60° to 70°C. Remove from heat and add 2 gm. of paraformaldehyde slowly, stirring constantly until dissolved. Allow solution to cool and add 5 ml. of 50% aqueous glutaraldehyde. Solution is made up to 50 ml. with sodium phosphate buffer pH 7.2 to 7.4 (page 115). Fix tissues for 1 to 2 hours at refrigerator temperature, rinse with buffer solution, and postfix in osmium tetroxide.

PLASTIC EMBEDDING MEDIA

Methacrylate, originally in widespread use as an embedding media for electron microscopy, has been largely replaced with epoxy resins. With epoxy resins there is less damage from polymerization, and sections appear to be more resistant to degradation when irradiated by the electron beam. Plastic media in common use are Vestopal W, Maraglas, Araldite, and Epon-812. Epon-812, an epoxy resin, is the method given preference here. It has a viscosity lower than some of the other resins and consequently penetrates more rapidly. The hardness of the embedding matrix is controlled so that its consistency can be adjusted to the kind of tissue embedded.

Degrees of hardness can be varied by changing the proportions of the curing agents used in making up the formulas. The embedding resin must be strong enough (hard, brittle consistency) so that the ultrathin sections required for electron microscopy can be cut without distortion of the subcellular structures. Epon-812 is a mixture of diepoxides and triepoxides. The liquid resin is hardened by acid anhydride curing agents such as nadic methyl anhydride (NMA) and dodecenyl succinic anhydride (DDSA) in the presence of an amine accelerator 2,4,6, − tridimethylaminomethyl phenol (DMP-30) and polymerized (fused to a solid) by heating.

EPON EMBEDDING MEDIA

EPON-812 STOCK SOLUTIONS
(After Luft, 1961)

Mixture A:	Epon-812	62 ml.
	DDSA (dodecenyl succinic anhydride)	100 ml.
Mixture B:	Epon-812	100 ml.
	NMA (nadic methyl anhydride)	89 ml.

It is important that the viscous liquids in these solutions be thoroughly mixed either manually or with a mechanical mixer. Store the stock solutions of Epon in the refrigerator or freezer.

EPON-812 WORKING SOLUTIONS
FORMULA 1

Mixture A	80.0 ml.
Mixture B	10.0 ml.
DMP-30 (2, 4, 6, tridimethylaminomethyl phenol)	1.5 ml.

Mix thoroughly before use.

FORMULA 2

Mixture A	80.0 ml.
Mixture B	20.0 ml.
DMP-30	1.5 ml.

Mix thoroughly before use. This mixture contains a higher concentration of nadic methyl anhydride. The NMA together with the DMP-30 increases the hardness of the plastic. Too soft a mixture may cause folding or chattering when sectioning the block. The higher the proportion of NMA, the harder the block.

EPON-812 — MINICK'S MODIFICATION OF LUFT

In his article (*Stain Techn.*, Vol. 38, No. 2, March 1963), Minick presented a method of one-step mixing followed by low temperature storage of Epon-812 embedding solution. His method is as follows:

1. Start magnetic stirrer (glass mixing rods) at low speed and maintain at this speed throughout.

2. Pour *220 ml.* of Epon-812 into a 1 liter beaker on the stirrer.

3. Add *185 ml.* of dodecenyl succinic anhydride (DDSA).

4. Add *94 ml.* of nadic methyl anhydride (NMA).

5. Allow the three ingredients to mix for 15 minutes.

6. With the stirrer still running, add *7.5 ml.* of 2,4,6, tridimethyl-aminomethyl phenol (DMP-30) and allow mixing to continue for 30 minutes.

7. Turn off stirrer and pour finished resin into 2-ounce bottles, allowing a small margin at the top for expansion.

8. Line caps with aluminum foil and tighten securely. Store in freezer at −20° to −30°C. Label and date bottles. Remove from freezer as needed and allow to stand at room temperature for a minimum of 1 hour, then *use in the same manner as freshly mixed resin.*

An advantage to this method is that the complete embedding media can be prepared in sizable quantities, packaged in small aliquots suitable for 1 day's use, and frozen until needed. The frozen media stores well for as long as 2 months. The proportions of DDSA, NMA, and DMP-30 are equivalent to a 6:4 mixture of Epon-anhydride as recommended by Luft (*J. Biophys. Biochem. Cytol.* 9, No. 2, pp. 409–414).

EPOXY RESIN EMBEDDING SCHEDULE WITH EPON-812

1. Following fixation, dehydrate in 70% ethyl alcohol. 15–30 min.

2. Dehydrate in 85% ethyl alcohol. 15–30 min.

3. Dehydrate in 95% ethyl alcohol. 15–30 min.

4. Dehydrate in absolute ethyl alcohol. 60 min.

5. Clear in propylene oxide. 60 min.

6. Replace with a 50:50 mixture of propylene oxide and the working (catalyzed) solution of Epon-812 60 min.

7. Decant and complete infiltration in a change of fresh, 100% Epon-812 mixture. Several hours

8. Remove block of tissue with a pipette and embed (cast) in a fresh change of Epon in heat-dried gelatin capsules.

9. Polymerize the plastic matrix for 24 hours at 45°C. followed by 24 hours at 60°C.

Glutaraldehyde, DDSA, NMA, propylene oxide, DMP-30, and Epon-812 are all available from Fisher Scientific Company.

PROCESSING SEQUENCE (STEP BY STEP)

Fixation

The tissue for electron microscopy is carefully diced (less than 1 mm.) with a very sharp razor blade with a minimum of pressure. The tissue is then suspended in a drop of fixative on a paraffinized surface or in a plastic mincing dish. Great care is taken not to squeeze the tissue. The specimen is placed in a vial with enough fixative to cover. Vials are stoppered and packed in ice or refrigerated promptly. Fixation will take one-half to 4 hours.

Dehydration

Although acetone dehydration is used with certain resins, alcohols are primarily used to remove the water from the tissue blocks. The vials are decanted and the tissues are treated with increasing strengths of alcohol to absolute, at room temperature.

Clearing

Tissues for Epon-812 embedding are cleared in propylene oxide, which is miscible with the alcohols and epoxy resins. It is a transitional stage between dehydration and infiltration and accelerates infiltration. Propylene oxide replaces most of the alcohol and diffuses out of the tissue to be replaced with the liquid resin. Propylene oxide is stored in the refrigerator but allowed to come to room temperature before use.

Infiltration

To make the tissue firm enough to cut, it is necessary to infiltrate it with the resin. The tissues are impregnated with the liquid resin which has been combined with liquid anhydrides, carefully proportioned so as to produce the required consistency. The initial infiltration is transitional and consists of a 1:1 mixture of propylene oxide/ Epon-812. It is followed by infiltration in a change of fresh, 100% Epon mixture. If the resin mixture has been frozen or refrigerated it is allowed to come to room temperature before the bottle is opened. Up to and including the final stage of infiltration the tissues are processed in stoppered containers.

Casting

Once the final stage of infiltration is reached, the heat-dried gelatin capsules (or commercially available BEEM plastic capsules) are arranged vertically in a special holder. The tissue is transferred to the bottom of the capsule and the embedding resin added. *Alternate method:* The capsules are filled nearly to the brim with fresh resin mixture with a 5 cc. syringe. The bit of tissue is removed from the processing vial with a pipette and drained on filter paper, and one piece of the tissue is placed on the surface of each capsule and allowed to sink to the bottom.

Polymerization

Complete hardening of the plastic is encouraged by oven heat and takes a minimum of 24 hours. *Typical incubation schedules include* (1) incubation at 35°C. for 12 hours, followed by 45°C. for 12 hours, followed by 60°C. for 12 hours; (2) 24 hours at 45°C. followed by an additional 24 hours at 60°C., or (3) complete incubation carried out at 60°C. for 24 hours.

At the final stage of polymerization, the resin will be solid but may still be dented slightly through the capsule on pressure from the fingernail. The capsules are removed from the oven, and as they cool they become more rigid. It is best to allow these blocks to remain at room temperature overnight or longer before trimming. The gelatin capsule is removed by immersion in warm water for 5 to 10 minutes. After cooling, the base of the solid resin is marked with a diamond marker for identification of the specimen.

Trimming

The blocks are trimmed to a blunt pyramidal form and mounted in holders. The tissue is trimmed very close on all sides with a razor blade using visual control at magnifications of $6\times$ to $20\times$, available with the microscope attachment of the ultramicrotone.

Sectioning

Microtomy for electron microscopy involves the use of special precision instruments and techniques. The ultrathin sections are cut under microscopic visual control. Glass or diamond knives are used for sectioning tissue.

GLASS KNIVES. The size, shape, and width of the knife will depend on the kind of microtome to be used. To make equilateral triangular glass knives, plate glass ¼″ to ³⁄₁₆″ thick in 5″ × 8″ sheets is carefully washed, scored with a glass cutter, and broken by stress to produce strips. The strip is then placed on a flat surface and scored at 45° and 90°. The mark is made up to about 1 mm. from the edge which will form the knife edge. Either with a white-hot Pyrex glass rod touch the score mark about ¼″ from the edge or break the glass with glazier's pliers held in each hand. The strip should break cleanly into equilateral triangles. The glass is broken emphasizing pulling with the pliers, not bending. With a little practice enough glass knives for two days' work can be broken in less than an hour. The cutting edge of the glass knife should be straight across and not particularly concave or convex in any direction. To avoid dust contamination, store the knives in clean, covered dishes. Most modern electron microscopy laboratories have knife-making machines which save much technician time. Occasionally, specially made diamond knives are used for those materials which are difficult or impossible to cut with the glass knives.

Once a suitable glass knife is chosen, an arrangement for flotation of the ribbon is prepared by attaching masking tape or tinfoil across the front and to the two lateral sides of the knife (Fig. 9-1). This forms a cup on the near slope of the knife. Dental wax or paraffin is used to make a watertight seal along the bottom edges where the

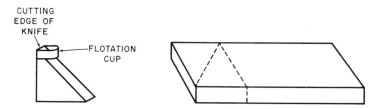

Figure 9-1.   Left: Equilateral triangular glass knife. Right: Sheet of scored plate glass

tape meets glass. Absolutely clean glass-distilled water (with or without a small amount of acetone or alcohol) is dispensed from a syringe needle to fill the cup to the top of the knife edge. *All instruments used for sectioning (forceps, syringes, and so forth) should be carefully cleaned before use.*

CUTTING FOR ONE MICRON EPOXY SECTION

Under magnifications with the microtome microscope attachment, the block is brought to the knife edge by coarse and fine micrometer screw adjustments, and sample tissue sections, perhaps 0.5 to 1.0μ thick are taken. These are picked off the water and placed on ordinary glass slides, stained for 1 minute with toluidine blue (0.5% in 20% alcohol) or with the Paragon stain, and the samples examined directly with the light microscope to identify and verify the type of tissue structure to be studied. When these thick samples have proved suitable, one proceeds to cut ultrathin sections for electron microscopy.

"Thick" or "Adjacent" Sections

In addition to their use for orientation and screening for electron microscopy, these so-called thick or adjacent sections offer much more. They may be used by the diagnostic pathologist to bridge the gap between the conventional paraffin-embedded sections studied with the light microscope and the electron micrographs. The 1-μ sections either may be handled as *wet mounts,* i.e., transferred to a drop of water on a slide, dried thoroughly at room temperature, and then stained; or they may be stained *free floating* by transferring the sections with a platinum wire loop to the surface of the staining solutions. These 1-μ epoxy resin sections can be stained successfully with the periodic acid-Schiff stain, azure II-methylene blue, aldehyde fuchsin, hematoxylin and phloxine, PAS-methenamine, and other techniques with only minor modifications of the conventional staining methods. Owing to the nature of this text, only a sample method will be given in detail. For other methods consult references at the end of this chapter.

Rapid Polychrome Stain for Epoxy-Embedded Tissue

A simple polychrome staining technique for 1-μ sections that closely approximates conventional hematoxylin and eosin paraffin sections was proposed by J. H. Martin, J. A. Lynn, and W. M. Nicky (*Amer. J. Clin. Path.* 46:250, 1966).

1. The section is cut on the ultramicrotome at 0.5 to 2.0μ, and picked up and floated on a drop of distilled water on a clean glass slide.

2. The slide is placed on a low temperature hot plate and the section is allowed to flatten and affix itself to the slide as the water evaporates.

3. When dry, a drop or two of Paragon multiple stain for frozen sections (with a few granules of sodium borate added to increase intensity of staining reaction) is placed on the still warm slide and the slide left on the hot plate for 10 to 20 seconds.

4. Slide is removed, gently washed off with a stream of distilled water, blotted with bibulous paper, and then air dried.

5. The slide is coverslipped with the appropriate catalyzed but unpolymerized resin mixture.

6. Sections are examined either with the conventional light microscope or by phase optics.

SECTIONING FOR ULTRATHIN SECTIONS

All ultramicrotomes have an automatic feed mechanism and hand micrometer. Ribbons of increasing thinness (in the range of 100 to 600 angstrom units) are cut and floated onto the water surface of the metal boat or improvised plastic tape cup. The tissue sections are now picked up from the water onto grids (thin copper screens about 3 mm. across). The grids have previously been coated on one side with a thin film of Formvar plastic or collodion and allowed to dry, and then the film is strengthened by evaporating carbon onto the film surface. Once mounted on the grid, the tissue section is blotted dry and is then ready for staining.

Formvar Film for Grids

Make up a 0.25% solution of Formvar in ethylene dichloride. A clean glass slide is dipped into the filtered solution for one-half to 1 minute and allowed to dry over the vapors from the solution. The film will be thinner if it is dried in this fashion. It is then stripped from the slide and floated on a clean water surface. The copper grids are placed on the film. A piece of Parafilm is then positioned to cover the whole membrane, and the grids become sandwiched between the Parafilm and the Formvar membrane and will not come loose when the Parafilm is picked up from the water bath surface. The grids may be stored in this state and removed from the Parafilm as they are needed.

STAINING ULTRATHIN SECTIONS

The sections which have been mounted on the grids are stained with a solution of uranyl acetate or other heavy metals. A double staining method employing both uranyl acetate and lead citrate is often desirable.

2% URANYL ACETATE STAINING SOLUTION

Uranyl acetate	2 gm.
Distilled water	100 ml.

Dissolve the crystals in the water. Let stand for several days before using. Filter through very fine filter paper into a small dropper bottle.

Staining Procedure

1. Place several drops of freshly filtered uranyl acetate into a small flat dish.
2. Carefully lower grids into staining solution, and stain for *one-half to 2 hours.*
3. Remove grids and rinse in sterile distilled water by dipping grids several times sideways into a beaker.

4. Drain grids on lens paper. Allow to dry, sections facing upwards, in a labeled container. Sections are now ready for examination with the electron microscope.

Double Staining Procedure

1. Stain grids with a saturated solution (approximately 7%) of uranyl acetate in distilled water for *1 to 2 minutes* (see detailed instructions, page 124). Rinse in distilled water.

2. When dried, stain for *1 to 3 minutes* in lead citrate. Rinse carefully in distilled water.

LEAD CITRATE SOLUTION
(After Reynolds, 1963)

1. Lead citrate is prepared by mixing 1.33 gm. of lead nitrate and 1.76 gm. of sodium citrate. Add 30 ml. of distilled water in a 50 ml. volumetric flask. The resultant suspension is shaken vigorously for 1 minute and then allowed to stand for 30 minutes with intermittent shaking to ensure complete conversion of lead nitrate to lead citrate.

2. A total of 8.0 ml. of 1N sodium hydroxide is added. The suspension is diluted to 50 ml. with distilled water and mixed by inversion. The lead citrate dissolves and the staining solution is ready for use. If faint turbidity remains, centrifuge the solution. The pH is 12.0 ± 0.1. Store in a glass or polyethylene bottle. The solution is stable for several months. After fixation in glutaraldehyde and osmium tetroxide this stain is very intense. To prevent overstaining, the solution may be diluted from 1:5 to 1:1000 times with 0.01N sodium hydroxide. The diluted lead citrate solution cannot be kept for more than 2 weeks.

The grid is floated onto a droplet of the staining solution with the sections face downward. After staining for the necessary time, the grid is picked up with a forceps and *immediately* washed by dipping the grid in several changes of distilled water.

Following staining and drying, the grid is inserted in a special holder in the electron microscope, the column of which is under a high vacuum. The specimen is introduced into and moved about in the electron beam under visual observation on a fluorescent screen in a darkened room. Of course only the parts of the specimen not resting on the wires of the copper screen grids can be visualized. Some areas may be too thick or folded, torn, or affected by "knife chatter." Elsewhere flat thin areas are to be found suitable for study. These are photographed and the enlarged prints are used for final study and interpretation, at magnifications of 13,000 to 250,000 times, which are far beyond the range possible with the light microscope. The resolving power of the electron microscope is about 200 times that possible with the light microscope.

CAUTIONS

1. In the preparation of osmic acid fixatives avoid inhaling the osmium because of danger of exposure of the eyes and respiratory tract to osmium vapor. Wear gas-tight goggles and work under a hood with the fan running.

2. Because uranyl acetate is radioactive, it should be handled with the precautions for radioactive materials.

3. Lead-containing staining solutions are poisonous and should be handled carefully.

4. Epon epoxy resin combined with the accelerator DMP-30 is a skin irritant and can cause dermatitis. Avoid contamination of skin, surface of containers, or the laboratory bench. Wash hands thoroughly and promptly with soap and water if contact is accidentally made.

5. Because the epoxy resins cannot be completely removed, all glassware should be labeled and used only for the Epon solutions. Acetone is a solvent for Epon.

6. Flush propylene oxide surplus down the sink drain with copious amounts of cold running water. Avoid inhaling the vapors.

7. Waste epoxy resins are allowed to set for months and are then disposed of as solid waste.

QUIZ

1. What advantage does the electron microscope have over the light microscope?

2. How are tissues fixed? Explain double-fixation method.
3. What size tissue sections are embedded when processing for electron microscopy?
4. What embedding medium is used for infiltration of tissue?
5. What type of knife is used for cutting sections?
6. What are "thick" or "adjacent" sections? What is their purpose?
7. How are 1-μ sections stained?
8. What is the thickness of ultrathin sections?
9. How are the ultrathin sections mounted prior to staining? What staining methods are used?
10. What part does photography play in electron microscopy?

REFERENCES

Handbook. *Thin Sectioning and Associated Techniques for Electron Microscopy.* Norwalk, Conn.: Ivan Sorvall, Inc., 1959.

Kay, D. H. *Techniques for Electron Microscopy.* Philadelphia: F. A. Davis, 1967.

Pease, D. C. *Histological Techniques for Electron Microscopy.* New York: Academic Press, 1960, p. 274.

Porter, K. R. The fine structure of cells. *Fed. Proc.* 14:673–682, 1955.

Sjostrand, F. S. Ultrastructure of cells as revealed by electron microscopy. *Int. Rev. Cytol.* 5:455–533, 1956.

Fixation

Bennett, H. S., and Luft, J. H. s-Collidine as a basis for buffering fixatives. *J. Biophys. Biochem. Cytol.* 6:113–114, 1959.

Millonig, G. Advantages of phosphate buffer for osmium tetroxide solutions in fixation. *J. Appl. Physics* 32:1637, 1961.

Palade, G. E. A study of fixation for electron microscopy. *J. Exp. Med.* 95:285–298, 1952.

Sabatini, D. D., Bensch, K. G., and Barnett, R. J. Cytochemistry and electron microscopy, preservation of cellular ultrastructure and enzymatic activity by aldehyde fixation. *J. Cell. Biol.* 17:19–58, 1963.

Embedding Resins

Finck, H. Epoxy resins in electron microscopy. *J. Biophys. Biochem. Cytol.* 7:27–30, 1960.

Lee, R., and Neville, K.   *Epoxy Resins: Their Application and Technology.* New York: McGraw-Hill, 1957.

Luft, J. H.   Improvements in epoxy resin embedding methods. *J. Biophys. Biochem. Cytol.* 9:409–414, 1961.

Minick, O. T.   Low temperature storage of epoxy embedding resins. *Stain Techn.* 38:131–133, 1963.

Staining

Kingsley, W. B., and Lynn, J. A.   Thin epoxy sections of needle biopsies of kidneys. *Bull. Path.* Chicago: American Society of Clinical Pathologists, 1968.

Lynn, J. A., Martin, J. H., and Race, G. J.   Recent improvements of histologic techniques for the combined light and electron microscopic examination of surgical specimens. *Amer. J. Clin. Path.* 45:704–713, 1966.

Martin, J. H., Lynn, J. A., and Nickey, W. M.   A rapid polychrome stain for epoxy embedded tissue. *Amer. J. Clin. Path.* 46:250–251, 1966.

Munger, B. L.   Staining methods applicable to sections of osmium-fixed tissue for light microscopy. *J. Biophys. Biochem. Cytol.* 11:502–506, 1961.

Reynolds, E. S.   The use of lead citrate at high pH as an electron-opaque stain in electron microscopy. *J. Cell. Biol.* 17:208–212, 1963.

Richardson, K. C., Jarett, L., and Finke, E. H.   Embedding in epoxy resins for ultrathin sectioning in electron microscopy. *Stain Techn.* 35:313–323, 1960.

Trump, B. F., Smuckler, E. A., and Benditt, E. P.   A method for staining epoxy sections for light microscopy. *J. Ultrastruct. Res.* 5:343–348, 1961.

III.   Fluorescent Microscopy

Fluorescence is common in nature. It is found naturally (autofluorescence) in many tissues. Bacteria, fungi, ceroid, riboflavin, lipofuscin, and certain pigments all fluoresce. These substances are unique in that they emit light of a longer wavelength when excited by light of a shorter wavelength. Molecules exist in particular stable or ground states. When energy is introduced, the level of excitation is raised. As the molecule returns to its ground state, the energy is lost. This change is reflected by light, and it is this light that is referred to as fluorescence. Tissues and bacteria, stained or tagged with special fluorescent dyes, can be made to fluoresce or make themselves visible and identifiable.

Fluorescent antibody techniques, once a research tool, are now becoming established as a diagnostic method of increasing value in both the microbiology and histology areas of medical technology. Fluorescent antibody (FA) techniques attempt detection and identification of substances causing disease by means of antigen-antibody reactions. FA testing has been highly successful in some areas but still presents problems in others.

ADVANTAGES OF FA TECHNIQUES FOR TISSUES

Nonviable acid-fast organisms will stain with fluorochromes when they cannot be stained with the traditional carbol fuchsin methods. In kidney disease, fluorescent antibody studies are used to identify gamma globulin localized particularly in glomeruli. Different types of renal lesions have different patterns of uptake of the antisera. In diseases of the pancreas, morphological examination alone cannot identify the hormones that the cells are producing, whereas immunofluorescence can. Tumor identification is enhanced because this technique can distinguish the type of cell which is predominant and active in a functioning tumor. With the use of transplanted organs, fluorescent microscopy provides information that contributes directly to patient therapy. Morphological findings (or features) are not paramount in immunofluorescent work; the uptake of the fluorescent tagged antisera is distributed in linear or granular patterns peculiar to the specific disease entity, and the ability to distinguish and interpret these patterns is sometimes diagnostic.

DISADVANTAGES AND PROBLEMS OF FA TECHNIQUES

Fluorescent antibody techniques require special skill and training both in the preparation of the material and in the interpretation. The necessary equipment is expensive. Suitable equipment is imperative for good fluorescence. One must have a high quality optical system, proper filters, and specific antisera. Personnel need careful training. The success of the FA techniques depends on the purity of the antigen and antibody. There are still problems to be resolved with this technique. Antisera are very expensive. If obtained commercially (which is usual), they are not always as advertised. Making the antisera instead of buying them already prepared is very time consuming. The antisera require careful purification and meticulous conjugation with the fluorescent dyes (fluorochromes).

Autofluorescence and other nonspecific fluorescence caused by dust, tissue debris, pigments, and background material create problems by interfering with clear antigen-antibody fluorescence. Slides stained with FA techniques are *impermanent.* The intensity of the reaction decreases with exposure under the microscope and with time. Long storage of sections will produce autofluorescence, and diffuse fluorescence is inherent in certain organs. One must work around these problems.

EQUIPMENT

In addition to a high-quality optical system, the energy (light) source is of paramount importance — the intensity of the fluorescence is proportionate to the intensity of the light source. The most commonly used source of such high intensity light is a 200-watt mercury vapor lamp, rich in ultraviolet light, carefully housed (for the vapor is under pressure), and always ventilated to dissipate the heat generated. Mercury vapor lamps are expensive and have a short life span.

Because intensity above the absorption band is undesirable, series of filters are used. Usually a *heat absorbing filter* is located just in front of the lamp to remove light near and beyond 600mμ and to prevent breakage of the primary filter. The *primary* or *excitation filter* usually passes light from 300 to 425mμ wavelengths, depending on the particular filter used. This filter, located between the light source and the specimen, selectively passes exciting wavelengths through the microscope condenser and into the specimen to stimulate the latter's specific fluorescent characteristics. To phrase it another way, the exciter filter transmits the wavelength of light which the fluorochrome is capable of absorbing and bars unwanted wavelengths. A yellow *barrier filter* is interposed between the microscope objective and the viewer (usually mounted in the eyepieces) to absorb unwanted ultraviolet rays which can cause ocular damage. This filter is for the protection of the observer.

The choice of the excitation or primary filter depends on the fluorochrome used, since the different fluorescent dyes are sensitive to different light spectra. The absorption and emission spectra are evaluated and a variety of filters are inserted and removed to change the wavelength of the light and to eliminate unwanted background. Selection of the proper filter combination will also reduce autofluorescence. These filters are available in a variety of colors with variable light transmission capacity.

The microscope should have high resolving power and a lens system of good quality. Most observers use microscopes with a dark-field condenser for orienting, in order to avoid bombardment of the specimen and loss of fluorescence. With dark-field observation only the fluorescent material is visible. It is necessary to place a drop of fluorescent-free immersion oil on the condenser to help the illumination. For observation of the morphological features most fluorescent microscopes are equipped so that the dark-field condenser can be removed and the microscope used with bright-field illumination. One must be careful not to expose the specimen more than is necessary. A 10-second to 15-second look is generally permissible. The fluorescent pattern can be documented with Anscochrome 500 or Kodachrome fast film at 30-second to 60-second exposures. Fluorescence is dissipated by continual exposure to bombardment by the light source.

FIXATION FOR FA TECHNIQUES

Fixation denatures and thereby alters proteins. Consequently the choice of fixative is important if the material to be studied is to be preserved as nearly as possible to what it was in life. Different fixatives are designated, depending on the antigen-antibody system (or protein) to be used. Choice of method depends on the stability of the antigen and its resistance to denaturation. It is best to follow directions given with each conjugate. Some viruses are amenable to formalin fixation with the built-in disadvantage that formalin has its own autofluorescence. Zenker fixation or any fixative containing heavy metals or compounds is to be avoided, for they quench or destroy fluorescent material. Since *frozen or cryostat sections are used in immunofluorescent techniques,* it may be wondered why fixation is necessary at all. The fixative tends to localize the antigen and prevent its diffusion into the surrounding tissue. Where allowed, the two most commonly used fixatives are acetone and 95% ethanol. The tissues are fixed after the sections have been cut on the cryostat and transferred to the slide. Because the sections are very thin, fixation time can be kept to a minimum. The slides may be fixed in acetone for 5 to 10 minutes or in ethanol for 15 to 30 minutes. Fixative solutions should be used at refrigerator temperature. Antigens are more stable at lower temperatures. Following fixation, the sections are stained. If fixation is not necessary or desirable, the cryostat sections are air dried for 20 minutes and placed in cold storage until time of staining.

FLUORESCENT DYES

With increased interest in FA techniques, newer, more stable fluorescent dyes are being manufactured. Both acid and basic dyes are used, mostly orange and yellow. The color that comes through is on a longer wavelength so that there is a change of color generally to apple green or red.

The most stable and most commonly used labeling agent is fluorescein isothiocyanate. At a special wavelength of maximal absorption, the compound fluorescein will absorb light when the level of excitation is raised with the high intensity mercury vapor lamp. After the exciting force is removed, the material will continue to fluoresce (yellow green.) *Fluorescence* is the emission of light by a substance that has been excited by a beam of light. The fluorescent dyes or fluorochromes are conjugated (joined or tagged) to the antibodies and serve as tracers. For a listing of the fluorochromes in popular usage, see page 213.

TERMINOLOGY

The nomenclature is quite different from what we are used to in the histology laboratory, and definitions may promote a clearer understanding of the processes involved.

Antigen: a substance foreign to the host which stimulates the formation of a specific antibody. All classic antibodies are modified serum globulins.

Antibody: a substance that joins with or neutralizes the antigen. Antibodies can be produced for laboratory use by giving the antigen to an animal, waiting until it has stimulated production of antibodies, bleeding the animal, and obtaining sera. Antibody preparations are also available commercially.

Antiserum: a serum containing antibodies. Because it is troublesome to produce and absorb the antiserums, if the needed antiserum is available commercially, it is purchased. Antiserum must always be tested for pertinent properties, especially specificity. Even commercially available antisera are not always as advertised, and they too may require appropriate absorption techniques to remove cross-reacting antibodies.

Conjugates: The absorbed antiserum containing the specific antibody is conjugated (joined) with fluorescein to produce a reagent that will localize antigen, by which for example one may identify an organism. The terms "labeled globulins" and "conjugated antisera" are used interchangeably when referring to fluorescent conjugates.

CUTTING SECTIONS FOR FA TECHNIQUES

Paraffin sections are of little value. Blocks of fresh tissue are quick-frozen to avoid alteration and preserve the histologic detail. These blocks are cut on the cryostat and stained fresh or following brief postfixation in acetone or ethanol. Care must be taken to avoid the introduction of O.C.T.* (or some similar matrix), or dust on the slides,

---

* With frozen section techniques O.C.T. is frequently used instead of water to keep the block of tissue on the chuck.

both of which elements would interfere with the fluorescence. Slides should be alcohol cleaned and scrupulously free of dust and lint. The tissue is mounted on a cold slide with the aid of a camel's-hair brush, and affixed to the slide by rubbing the finger on the underside of the slide beneath the tissue. The slides are labeled with a diamond marker and air-dried for 20 minutes before storage or processing.

Quick Freezing

Tissue blocks may be frozen on dry ice (−70°C.), in liquid nitrogen, or in isopentane-propane mixture chilled with liquid nitrogen, depending on the intended use of the sections. The tissue may be quick-frozen directly onto the object holder (chuck) ready for sectioning, or it may be quick-frozen, stored in the deep freeze, and mounted on the object holder at a later time.

Method I: Dry Ice

With gloved hands, crack ice and place in a wide-mouth vacuum bottle or beaker. Add 95% isopropanol until a slush is formed. The tissue is mounted on the object holder, the object holder is held with forceps, and its underside is immersed momentarily in the slush. When the tissue is completely frozen, the block will appear opaque and white. The procedure of freezing is very rapid, which is desirable. Blocks of tissue that have been quick-frozen and/or mounted may be stored in the freezer if they are protected by an airtight covering, such as Saran wrap.

Method II: Dry Ice

Flatten thin slices of fresh tissue against the wall of a test tube; then immerse the test tube in the dry-ice slush. Tissue will freeze almost instantaneously. Cap tube and store tissue in freezer until ready to mount and section.

Method III: Isopentane

Small blocks 4–5 mm. square are plunged into an isopentane-liquid nitrogen mixture (slush) for 1–2 minutes. (Take 50 ml. of isopentane and add liquid nitrogen until it is somewhat semisolid.) Transfer the snap-frozen blocks to small airtight containers which have been pre-cooled. Store in deep freeze until ready to section.

If Method II or Method III has been used, the tissue blocks will have to be mounted prior to sectioning. When ready to cut on the cryostat, remove the frozen block from the freezer and mount on the microtome object holder with the aid of water, without thawing. Moisten a small square of folded paper towel, place on the object holder, and orient specimen on this. Surround toweling and base of tissue with a few drops of water. Freeze tissue to chuck by immersing in a beaker of cracked dry ice or by subjecting it to a jet of carbon dioxide. Cut sections on the cryostat at 3 to 6μ at $-20°$ to $-30°C$. Air dry for 20 minutes.

STORAGE OF CUT SECTIONS PRIOR TO STAINING

Long storage causes unwanted autofluorescence. Make slides as they are needed or store cut sections for as long as 7 to 10 weeks in the crisper section of the refrigerator. Ideally slides should be made shortly prior to staining. The antigen remains in situ and reactive for variable times; reactivity depends on the material being used.

ANTIBODY-DYE CONJUGATION

The conjugation is a long, involved chemical procedure requiring special technical training. The serum containing the antibodies is fractionated, usually by precipitation with half-saturated ammonium sulfate. The precipitated globulin is separated by centrifugation and carefully washed (dialyzed) until it is free of the sulfate. Fluorescein isothiocyanate or some other fluorochrome is added and allowed to react. Dialysis or treatment with cellulose columns or tissue powders is performed to purify the antibodies and to remove unconjugated dye and nonspecific antibodies.

Outline of Globulin Labeling Procedure

1. The protein content of the immune globulin must be accurately determined.

2. The protein content must be adjusted to a concentration of 1 to 3 percent before conjugation.

3. The globulin solution is adjusted to a pH of 9 with buffered carbonate. The efficiency of the conjugate decreases with decreased pH.

4. With a ratio of 0.05 mg./mg. of protein, the dye fluorescein isothiocyanate is added during a 15-minute period, at refrigerator temperature, with constant stirring. The antibody and fluorochrome join. This conjugation will take approximately 12 to 18 hours. Conjugation with rhodamine is similar but takes less time. Step 4 is carried out at refrigerator temperature.

5. The conjugate must be freed of unbound dye, a carefully controlled pH should be maintained, and the dye should not be overdiluted. The conjugate is dialyzed or column cleaned with Sephadex G-25 in a phosphate buffer of pH 7.1, or the cellulose DEAE (diethylaminoethyl) may be used to purify and remove unbound dye and reduce nonspecific staining.

6. Once the conjugate is free of unreactive dye, it is concentrated by centrifugation, put up in small aliquots, fast frozen and stored in the freezer until use. Prior to use the aliquot is defrosted at refrigerator temperature.

Even with commercial conjugated antisera, acetone-ground tissue powders are frequently required to absorb nonspecific antibodies and thus purify the specific antibodies. Antisera vary and absorption may or may not be necessary.

Procedure for Absorption with Tissue Powders

The dried tissue powder (animal or human liver) is placed in a conical test tube. The fluorescent-labeled antibody solution (antiserum) is added, mixed, and allowed to stand for 5 to 15 minutes. Absorption time varies with the amount of nonspecificity. The material is then centrifuged for 10 to 15 minutes at 2000 RPM and the supernatant (purified conjugate) is recovered by careful aspiration. This is filtered through a Millipore filter into a clean container and stored in the freezer. It is best to absorb small amounts as they are needed. The ratio of tissue powder added to the aliquot of antiserum is 100 mg. per milliliter.

Storage of Conjugated Serum

Conjugated serum will last for years if properly stored. Freeze in small aliquots what would be used daily. Freezing and thawing will lessen fluorescence or destroy the dye if the stock solution is repeatedly frozen, thawed, and refrozen. The small aliquots are fast frozen to —70°C. and stored in the deep freeze. When an aliquot is removed for use, defrost and store it in the refrigerator. It will keep for about 4 days.

BASIC ATTACHMENT PROCEDURES

Direct Staining Method

With direct attachment of a particular antibody to its specific antigen, the antibody coats the antigen. With this technique one needs a known labeled antibody for each individual antigen. *Procedure:* (1) The test slide is treated with *fluorescent labeled* antiserum, used as a staining agent, and the homologous antigen adsorbs it. (2) Following this, the slide is washed to remove all nonantibody globulin. What is left is antibody attached to antigen. The preparation is coverslipped and examined with the fluorescent microscope. (See Fig. 9-2.)

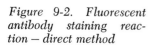

Figure 9-2. Fluorescent antibody staining reaction — direct method

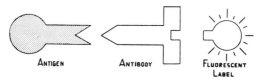

Indirect Staining Method

There are several advantages to this "sandwich method." Non-conjugated antibody can be used, staining is more specific, the number of labeled antisera needed is reduced, and sensitivity is increased. *Procedure:* (1) The test slide is first treated with a specific **unlabeled** antiserum (primary combining reaction). It is allowed to react with the antigen and the nonantibody globulin is then washed off. (2) This is followed by treatment with a **fluorescent labeled** antiglobulin specific for the unlabeled antibody (second combining reaction). (3) The excess antibody is washed free and the preparation is cover-slipped and examined with the fluorescent microscope. (See Fig. 9-3.)

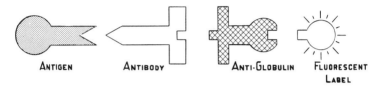

ANTIGEN   ANTIBODY   ANTI-GLOBULIN   FLUORESCENT
                                                LABEL

Figure 9-3.   Fluorescent antibody staining reaction — indirect method

STAINING PROCEDURE
(Sample Method*)

Use air-dried cryostat sections. Set up a series of Coplin jars.

1. Pour on saline buffered to pH of 7.0 to 7.2. Leave for **5 minutes.**
2. Repeat with fresh buffer solution for **5 minutes.**
3. Third change of fresh buffer solution for **5 minutes.**
4. Fix tissues in acetone (prechilled to 5°C. in refrigerator) for **30 seconds.**
5. Wash with buffered saline for **5 minutes.**
6. Repeat with buffered saline for **5 minutes.**
7. Repeat with buffered saline for **5 minutes.**

* From Seminar on Immunopathology, University of California San Francisco Medical Center, Program Chairman, John C. Lee, M.D., March 14–15, 1970. Workshop by D. Murrell Green.

8. To prevent evaporation prepare a moist chamber by completely moistening two paper towels and fold and place them very flat on the counter and cover with a moist inverted staining dish.

9. Remove excess buffer from the slides by wiping the slide dry except for the area of the section.

10. Place a drop of labeled antiserum on the tissue and place slide in the moist chamber for *30 minutes* at room temperature.

11. Rinse off antiserum with buffered saline and place slide in a fresh change for *5 minutes,* in a second fresh change for *5 minutes,* and in a third fresh change for *5 minutes.*

12. Coverslip slides from the last change of buffer, using clean coverslips. Mounting media consists of 9:1 glycerol and buffer. An acid pH could result in quenching of the fluorescence.

13. Examine under oil immersion with the light microscope or by dark-field microscopy with the fluorescent microscope.

Storage of Stained Slides

Slides may be stored in the refrigerator for as long as 2 months; however, they fade slightly on storage.

QUIZ

1. Define fluorescence.
2. List three advantages and three disadvantages of fluorescent antibody techniques.
3. Define antigen, antibody, antiserum, and conjugates.
4. List four fluorochromes.
5. What kind of tissue sections (method of processing) are used for FA techniques?
6. What is the "direct" method of tagging?
7. What is the "indirect" method of tagging?

REFERENCES

Barka, T., and Anderson, P. J.   *Histochemistry.* New York: Hoeber Med. Div., Harper & Row, 1965, p. 334.

Coons, A. H., Creech, H. J., Jones, R. N., and Berliner, E.   The demonstration of pneumococcal antigen in tissues by the use of fluorescent antibody. *J. Immunol.* 45:159–170, 1942.

Coons, A. H., Leduc, E. H., and Connolly, J. M.   Localization of antigen in tissue cells. II. Improvements in a method of the detection of antigen by means of fluorescent antibody. *J. Exp. Med.* 91:1–13, 1950.

Coons, A. H., Leduc, E. H., and Connolly, J. M.   Studies on antibody production. I. A method for the histochemical demonstration of specific antibody and its application to a study of the hyperimmune rabbit. *J. Exp. Med.* 102:49–60, 1955.

Coons, A. H., Leduc, E. H., and Kaplan, M. H.   Localization of antigen in tissue cells. VI. The fate of injected foreign proteins in the mouse. *J. Exp. Med.* 93:173–188, 1951.

Davidsohn, I., and Henry, J. B.   *Todd-Sanford Clinical Diagnosis by Laboratory Methods* (14th ed.). Philadelphia: Saunders, 1969, p. 810.

Lillie, R. D.   *Histopathologic Technique and Practical Histochemistry* (3d ed.). New York: McGraw-Hill, 1965, p. 266.

Lipp, W.   Use of gel filtration and polyethylene glycol in the preparation of fluorochrome labelled protein. *J. Histochem. Cytochem.* 9:458–459, 1961.

McClure, D. M.   The development of fluorescence microscopy for tubercle bacilli and its use as an adjunct to histological routine. *J. Clin. Path.* 6:273–281, 1953.

Pearse, A. G. E.   *Histochemistry, Theoretical and Applied.* Boston: Little, Brown, 1960, p. 137.

Riggs, et al.   Isothiocyanate compounds as fluorescent labeling agents for immune serum. *Amer. J. Path.* 34:1081–1097, 1958.

Seminar on Immunopathology, University of California San Francisco Medical Center, John C. Lee, M.D., Chairman, March 14, 1970.

Silver, H. and Sonnenwirth, A. C.   Modifications in the fluorescence microscopy technique as applied to identification of acid-fast bacilli in tissue and bacteriological material. *J. Clin. Path.* 19:583–588, 1966.

Truant, J. P.   Fluorescence microscopy of tubercle bacilli stained with auramine and rhodamine. *Henry Ford Hosp. Med. Bull.* 10:287–296, 1962.

10

Preparation of Bone Sections

Because of its hard nature bone requires special treatment. Before bone or any calcified tissue can be processed and sectioned on an ordinary microtome, it must have the lime salts removed. *This process is called decalcification.* Removal of the calcium is achieved chiefly with acids in which the calcium carbonate and phosphate salts of the bone are soluble. The time taken for complete decalcification is dependent on (1) thickness of the specimen, (2) compactness or density of the bone, (3) strength of the solutions used, and (4) the temperature at which it is decalcified. Higher than room temperature accelerates decalcification but impairs staining. Decalcification above 50°C. causes disintegration. Some workers recommend the use of a mechanical stirrer to speed up decalcification. Lillie's investigation did not confirm this hypothesis. There is no ideal method of decalcifying bone sections, since acids always produce distortion or alteration of the tissue, and diagnosis is of necessity delayed awaiting complete decalcification.

The bone specimen must be cut into fairly small pieces first (very dense or hard bone 2 to 5 mm. thick, softer tissue 4 to 6 mm. thick) to allow penetration of the decalcifying solution. A saw with a thin blade (band saw or jeweler's saw) should be used; it produces less tearing of the surrounding tissue. As soon as the small sections are obtained, the bone must be *fixed* to preserve and toughen the soft tissue and cellular structures attached to it. Buffered 10% neutral formalin is recommended for use as a fixative for bone because it penetrates well and renders the soft tissues resistant to the acids present in the decalcifying fluid. After fixation, the tissue must be washed thoroughly to remove the excess fixative. It is then ready for decalcification.

141

METHODS OF DECALCIFICATION

1. Acid method
2. Ion-exchange resins
3. Electrical ionization
4. Chelating method

ACID METHOD

The acid method is perhaps the most widely used for the routine processing of large amounts of bony tissue. Decalcification of the fixed, washed tissues should be carried out at room temperature in large jars with the decalcifying solutions added *generously.*

The agents most used for decalcification are *aqueous* solutions of nitric acid, formic acid, and trichloracetic acid. They may be used in combination with a neutralizer to prevent excessive tissue swelling. Alcoholic solutions for decalcification are used when glycogen is to be preserved but their use is infrequent otherwise, since the alcohol is said to suppress ionization.

Good histologic and cytologic detail cannot be expected if tissue is left too long in the decalcifying solution. The ideal length of time for decalcification of tissue is 24 to 48 hours. When possible it should not be prolonged beyond 4 days. However, some very dense bone blocks will take 14 days or longer for complete decalcification. Mallory recommended that the tissue be suspended in a piece of gauze in the upper part of the jar in order that the dissolved salts sink to the bottom. The acid solutions should be changed daily or even twice a day for better decalcification.

Acid Decalcifying Solutions

Both nitric and formic acid produce minimal distortion and act quickly, but nitric acid has the disadvantage of inhibiting a good nuclear stain.

NITRIC ACID. Decalcification is usually carried out in large quantities of 5% aqueous solution of nitric acid, changing the solutions every day or twice a day for 1 to 4 days. Nitric acid will decalcify bone more rapidly than formic acid, but it produces a marked decrease in the stainability of the tissue after 20 hours.

TRICHLORACETIC ACID. Stronger concentrations of trichloracetic acid are required for adequate decalcification, and it is generally used in a 10% aqueous solution, with decalcification carried out in large quantities of the solution.

FORMIC ACID. This is generally accepted as most suitable for decalcification of large pieces of bone from the standpoint of both decalcification and good preservation of stainability even if it has been necessary to leave bone in this acid for a prolonged time.

FORMIC ACID-HYDROCHLORIC ACID COMBINATION
(See page 148.)

FORMIC ACID DECALCIFICATION SOLUTIONS
(After Morse)

SOLUTION A		SOLUTION B	
(50% formic acid)		(20% sodium citrate)	
88% formic acid	500 ml.	Sodium citrate	200 gm.
Distilled water	500 ml.	Distilled water	1000 ml.

Make these as stock solutions. At time of use combine equal parts of the two solutions. The sodium citrate is used to counteract excessive swelling caused by the acid.

Washing Tissue

After tissues are decalcified, it is necessary that they be thoroughly washed in running water for 3 to 8 hours to remove the last traces of the decalcification solutions. Sections may also be neutralized after decalcification with acids by immersing in a weak solution (2%) of lithium carbonate for a similar period of time.

Staining

The routine hematoxylin and eosin stain gives satisfactory results after acid decalcification. Masson's hematoxylin-phloxine-safran and the Giemsa stain are also recommended. Failure to stain properly is most often *due to overtreatment in acid* decalcifying solutions or to insufficient washing out of the acid. Just before staining, the bone sections may be neutralized by placing the slides briefly in a 1% aqueous solution of lithium carbonate.

Sections of bone are quite likely to float off the slides during staining, particularly following treatment in acid alcohol. It is worthwhile to check the slides after they have been deparaffinized. If the bone sections show signs of loosening, it is best to collodionize the sections before proceeding with the staining technique (page 284).

PROPRIETARY DECALCIFYING SOLUTIONS

Commercially available decalcifying solutions of undisclosed content are available. They are rather expensive, but they do a remarkable job in the rapidity with which they decalcify. Such decalcifying solutions require handling different than the traditional acid solutions with which we are familiar. Manufacturer's instructions should be followed carefully. A composite of the findings of our laboratory, and those of John Budinger, M.D., Lawrence Hospital, Bronxville, N.Y., and A. Wu and L. Michaels (*Canad. J. Med. Tech.* 31:224, 1969) are listed below.

Considerations for RDO * Decal Solution

1. Great care must be taken not to overdecalcify. The action is rapid, in most cases occurring in 4 hours or less. *Overnight decalcification must be avoided.* If bone sections are left in RDO longer than needed, almost total digestion of the tissue occurs and histologic detail is ruined. At the end of the work day, if the tissues are not completely decalcified, remove from the RDO solution and place in 10% formalin

* RDO is available from Du Page Kinetic Laboratories, Downer's Grove, Ill. 60515.

overnight. In the morning, rinse the tissue free of the formalin and return it to the RDO solution. Check closely to determine the end point of decalcification.

2. RDO is best reserved for those sections not requiring more than 4 to 8 hours in the decalcifying solution, i.e., cancellous bone less than 1.0 cm. in thickness and dense cortical bone less than 0.5 cm. in thickness. Very small fragments of bone will decalcify in 1½ to 4 hours. Larger specimens require 6 to 8 or as long as 12 hours.

3. A peculiarity in the use of RDO is a hardening effect on the tissue which may erroneously suggest incomplete decalcification. This may falsify the end point of decalcification if for instance pliability were being used to make this determination. Read the manufacturer's instructions.

4. Avoid the use of metal containers. Use plastic capsules or paper embedding bags.

5. With RDO a brown sediment may appear on standing but can be filtered out without loss of strength. The solution is said to remain stable for at least 4 months.

6. RDO can be used following fixation, or bone may be simultaneously fixed and decalcified by placing it in a mixture of 9 parts of RDO to 1 part of concentrated full-strength formalin. Bone curettings may be fixed and decalcified simultaneously with the mixture described and will be ready for processing in 1½ hours.

7. The volume of the solution should be approximately 10 times the volume of the bone. A short period of washing following decalcification is suggested.

8. With proper usage, cellular detail is very well preserved.

ION-EXCHANGE-RESIN METHOD

The tissue must first be fixed and washed. It is then decalcified for 1 to 14 days with any one of the ion-exchange resins available commercially. Some of these resins are used in combination with formic acid, whereas others are used alone. Specific directions for processing will be found on the container.

Dotti, Paparo, and Clarke (*Amer. J. Clin. Path.* 21:475, 1951) combined an ion-exchange resin (WIN-3000* — an ammonium salt of a sulfonated resin) with aqueous dilutions of formic acid in graduated concentrations which they called RAF (*r*esin *a*nd *f*ormic acid). They reported the following advantages: (1) cellular detail was well preserved the superior to the standard formic acid–sodium citrate method; (2) decalcification was faster; (3) daily changing of solutions was eliminated. Cancellous bone (2–3 mm. thick) decalcified in 2 to 3 hours in 10% and 20% RAF. Cancellous bone (5–6 mm.) decalcified in 4 to 8 hours in the same strength solutions.

If speed is essential, a 40% RAF may be employed. Good preservation was maintained if tissues were not left in this strength solution for more than 8 days. Large pieces of dense bone may be placed in 40% RAF for 24 hours to soften, trimmed to 3 mm., and placed in 40% RAF for an additional 24 hours. If speed is not essential, it was found that tissue could be left in 10% RAF up to 20 days without distortion.

10% RAF SOLUTION. To 10 gm. of resin, add 80 ml. of a 10% aqueous solution of formic acid.

20% RAF SOLUTION. To 10 gm. of resin, add 80 ml. of a 20% aqueous solution of formic acid.

In the author's experience, this resin-formic acid combination offers one of the best methods of decalcifying bone. It is rapid in action and causes minimal damage to tissue. Good results in our laboratory have been obtained with the following formula.

10% RAF DECALCIFICATION SOLUTION

WIN-3000 (ion-exchange resin)	100 gm.
10% formic acid (aqueous)	800 ml.

(RAF 10% appears to be the strength of choice for all sections of cancellous bone.)

ELECTRICAL IONIZATION METHOD

Richmond et al. (*Arch. Path.* 44:92, 1947) described a method of rapidly removing calcium compounds from bone by electrolytic action.

---

* WIN-3000 may be obtained from Special Chemicals Department, Winthrop Laboratories, 90 Park Avenue, New York, N.Y. 10016.

Principle of Method

Insoluble calcium salts in the specimen are changed to ionizable salts by the action of the acids, and the electrical field between the electrodes causes the calcium to migrate rapidly from the specimen (anode +) to the carbon (cathode −). The negative ions (acid radicals) are rapidly driven from the carbon (cathode −) pole to the specimen (anode +), maintaining a high concentration of acid radicals around the specimen to speed the reaction.

Electrical ionization applies the principle of electrolysis to shorten the time required for decalcification of bone specimens for histologic sections. The decalcification process develops about three times faster with electric current than under normal conditions. In their investigation, Verdenius and Alma (*J. Clin. Path.* 11:229, 1958) assert that this acceleration is brought about equally by the influence of the electrical field and the rise in temperature. Lillie et al. (1951) in their study concluded that the increased speed of reaction resulted *solely* from the rise in temperature due to the passage of the electric current. With the electrolytic method there is the advantage that the bone requires a relatively short exposure to acids.

An apparatus is used employing an acid bath in a durable glass jar, in which the bone specimens are suspended. An electrode assembly immersed in the decalcifying solution and consisting of a heavy graphite cathode and a platinum-wire anode is arranged to maintain an electric field. The platinum electrode repels the positive calcium ions, and the graphite electrode attracts these ions. Current is supplied by a power unit. When current passes through a solution a rise in temperature occurs. Very high temperatures not only increase the speed of reaction but also cause disintegration. The temperature is regulated between 30° and 45°C. to avoid overheating (Fig. 10-1).

Blocks of cancellous bone, such as marrow, 3 to 5 mm. thick, will decalcify in 45 minutes or less in this apparatus. More compact bone may take 16 hours or longer. The bone should be removed just as soon as decalcification is complete. A disadvantage of the electrical ionization method is that only a limited number of specimens can be processed at one time. Also, electrically decalcified sections generally do not stain well.

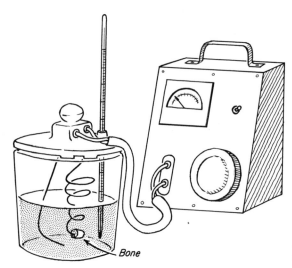

Figure 10-1. *Electri-cal decalcifying unit*

Method

Small bone sections are fixed, washed, and then decalcified in the electrolytic apparatus using a formic acid-hydrochloric acid bath for 1 to 4 hours. *Note:* This formula is an effective decalcifier without the use of the electrolytic apparatus but decalcification will take longer.

SOLUTIONS FOR ELECTROLYTIC DECALCIFICATION

88% formic acid	100 ml.
Hydrochloric acid	80 ml.
Distilled water to make	1000 ml.

Discarding solutions after 8 hours of use assures maximum speed of decalcification. Solutions should not be used for longer than 12 hours, since they lose their effectiveness.

Wash in running tap water for 3 to 6 hours. Dehydrate, clear, and embed in the usual manner.

CHELATING AGENTS

Organic chelating agents absorb metallic ions. The word chēlē comes from the Greek word for claw, which means to grab. EDTA combines with calcium to form a nonionized soluble complex. Disodium ethylenediamine tetraacetic acid (EDTA) is the chelating agent obtained commercially under such trade names as Versene,* Sequestrene,† and Questex. Most workers report optimum decalcification with a saturated (10%) solution of EDTA. It is recommended that for best results the solution be adjusted to a pH of 6.5 to 7.5, since alkaline solutions have a tendency to hydrolize protein to some degree. EDTA decalcifying works best on cancellous bone and is not nearly as effective as other agents for dense cortical bone. It will take 2 to 4 days to decalcify specimens 3 to 4 mm. thick, although a longer time in the decalcifying solution is not harmful.

Advantages

1. Preservation of histologic detail and staining qualities is excellent.
2. Careful washing following the decalcifying process is unnecessary.
3. Technique can be used with advantage on bone marrow curettings.
4. Glycogen in bone or cartilage is best preserved by the use of EDTA as the decalcifying agent, following fixation with acetic-alcohol formalin (Trott).

Disadvantages

1. Method is slower than other decalcifying solutions.
2. For optimum results the bone must be no thicker than 3 to 4 mm.

VERSENE METHOD

1. Fix tissue thoroughly in 10% buffered formalin. Wash tissues.
2. Place in a saturated aqueous solution (10%) of buffered Versene 20 times the volume of the tissue. Change solution daily.

---

* Versene can be obtained from Bersworth Chemical Co., Framingham, Mass.
† Sequestrene can be obtained from Alrose Chemical Co. Providence, Rhode Island.

3. When decalcification is complete, rinse in water briefly and transfer to 70% alcohol.

4. Tissue is ready to be processed on the Autotechnicon, as usual.

DETERMINING THE END POINT OF DECALCIFICATION

Ideally bone is left in the decalcifying solutions for the minimum time to ensure decalcification and removed immediately thereafter. If sections are left in these solutions longer than is absolutely necessary, the staining qualities will be impaired or the histologic details may be destroyed. Before leaving for the day, the technician should *make sure that no specimen is left in the decalcifying solutions overnight,* if it can at all be avoided.

The tissue may be tested to determine whether it is soft enough to be cut on the microtome by inserting a needle into it. If the needle enters the section easily, the bone is ready to be processed. This method of testing should be used sparingly, as it injures the tissue and produces artefacts. Decalcification may also be checked by the pliability of the tissue. If it bends easily and is flexible, it is decalcified. A third method and perhaps the best is by x-ray determination — a method not easily worked into the schedule of a routine histology laboratory. The specimen is x-rayed at intervals of 2, 4, and 6 hours and at 24-hour intervals thereafter.

The fourth method is by chemically testing the solution to determine calcium loss. After a period of decalcification, approximately 5 ml. of the decalcifying fluid is aspirated from the base of the jar containing the specimen. To this is added 5 ml. of 5% ammonium oxalate and 5 ml. of 5% ammonium hydroxide. Mix and allow to set for 10 to 30 minutes. If the solution is cloudy or turbid after the elapsed time, the decalcifying solution should be changed and the test made again after an additional period of decalcification. The specimen is considered properly decalcified when a clear solution is obtained.

QUIZ

1. Are tissues fixed before or after decalcification?
2. Why is it necessary to decalcify tissue?
3. List four methods of decalcification. Give technique in outline form. List advantages and disadvantages of each method.
4. Why must tissues be thoroughly washed after decalcification?
5. What stains are recommended after decalcification?
6. How do you determine whether or not the issue has been sufficiently decalcified?

REFERENCES

Birge, E. A., and Imhoff, C. E.   Versenate as a decalcifying agent for bone. *Amer. J. Clin. Path.* 22:192, 1952.

Dotti, L. B., Paparo, G. P., and Clark, B. E.   The use of ion exchange resin in decalcification of bone. *Amer. J. Clin. Path.* 21:475, 1951.

Handbook. *The Operation and Care of the Ionic Bone Decalcifier.*   Available from Martin Sweets Company, Louisville, Ky.

Lillie, R. D., Laskey, A., Greco, J., Jacquier Burtner, H., and Jones, P.   Decalcification of bone in relation to staining and phosphatase techniques. *Amer. J. Clin. Path.* 21:711, 1951.

Luna L. (Ed.) *Manual of Histologic Staining Methods of the Armed Forces Institute of Pathology* (3d ed.). New York: McGraw-Hill, 1968, p. 9.

Richman, I. M., Gelfand, M., and Hill, J. M.   Laboratory methods and technical notes: a method of decalcifying bone for histologic section. *Arch. Path.* 44:92, 1947.

Trott, J. R.   The presence of glycogen in the rat liver following in vitro processing in decalcifying agents. *J. Histochem. Cytochem.* 9:6, 1961.

Verdenius, H. H. W., and Alma, L.   A quantitative study of decalcification methods in histology. *Amer. J. Clin. Path.* 11:229, 1958.

Preparation of Bone Marrow

Bone marrow may be processed as a smear or touch preparation or as a biopsy specimen.

SMEARS. The tissue is spread out in a thin, even film across a clean slide or coverglass, ideally so that the cells are only one layer in thickness. The smear is then fixed and stained.

TOUCH PREPARATIONS. A touch preparation may be obtained by lightly touching a clean glass slide or coverglass to the freshly cut surface of the tissue. The cellular elements adhere to the slide. The touch preparation is then fixed and stained.

PROCESSING BONE-MARROW SMEARS AND TOUCH PREPARATIONS

Dry the smear by waving it in the air. When drying multiple smears, dry by fanning. Fix and stain by any of the standard methods used for blood smears, such as Wright's stain, Giemsa's stain, or the May-Grünwald-Giemsa stain. Reliable, ready-to-use staining solutions of any of the above stains may be purchased from laboratory supply houses.

Alcoholic stains fix the blood in the first step of the staining process. Before aqueous stains, films should be fixed in methyl alcohol for 3 to 7 minutes. This fixation should be done in a covered dish. The slide should then be taken out and allowed to dry before staining.

The staining reaction of the dyes is very sensitive to changes of pH. All reagents and the atmosphere of the laboratory should be free of acid. Fresh distilled water (pH 6 to 6.8) is necessary for good staining results. On standing, distilled water usually becomes unfit for use. Fresh buffer solutions may be used instead of distilled water.

Note. In the staining methods given below, the times given are approximate — the strength of the dyes varies with standing.

MAY-GRÜNWALD-GIEMSA STAIN FOR SMEARS

The May-Grünwald stain is a saturated solution of the eosinate of unpolychromed methylene blue in methyl alcohol. The Jenner stain is identical with the May-Grünwald stain and may be interchanged. Used alone, the May-Grünwald solution stains rather weakly. For this reason it is desirable to combine the staining properties of the Giemsa method with those of the May-Grünwald. The Giemsa stain contains azure II-eosin. The May-Grünwald contains methylene blue-eosin.

In this technique the May-Grünwald or Jenner stain is initially applied to the bone-marrow smears, which will be both fixed and weakly stained in this step. The smears are then restained with a dilute Giemsa solution.

Staining Solutions

MAY-GRÜNWALD STAIN

May-Grünwald dye *	1 gm.
Absolute methyl alcohol	500 ml.

Mix thoroughly and age for 1 week.

BUFFER SOLUTION pH 6.8

Harleco buffer salt mixture †	5 gm.
Distilled water	500 ml.

A one percent solution of the mixture yields the labeled pH.

* May-Greenwald dye — Harleco Company, Cat. #262.

† Buffer salt mixture pH 6.8 (sodium and potassium phosphates), Harleco Co., Cat. #4034.

GIEMSA STAINING SOLUTION

Buffer solution pH 6.8	30 ml.
Giemsa stain (ready-to-use) *	1 ml.

Make solution fresh. Do not reuse.

Staining Procedure

1. Fix the air-dried film by covering with the May-Grünwald stain for *3 minutes.*

2. Flood with an equal amount of the buffer solution and leave the diluted stain for an additional *5 minutes.* An irridescent scum is a proper reaction and is easily washed off.

3. Wash slide with buffer solution.

4. Flood slides with dilute Giemsa solution. Leave for *12 minutes.*

5. Rinse off stain with buffer solution.

6. Wipe back of slide clean.

7. Place slide in vertical position to air-dry. When completely dry, coverslip with Permount or Histoclad.

REFERENCES.

Jones, R. McClung. *Handbook of Microscopical Technique* (3d ed.). New York: Paul B. Hoeber, Inc., 1950, p. 224.

Strumia, M. M. *J. Lab. Clin. Med.* 21:930, 1936.

* Giemsa Blood Stain, Azure B Type Biological Staining Solution, Harleco Co., Cat. #619.

WRIGHT-GIEMSA STAIN

Solutions

WRIGHT STAIN (READY TO USE)

GIEMSA STAIN* (READY TO USE)

BUFFER (pH 6.8)
(See page 153.)

Staining Procedure

1. Prepare smears on coverglass and air-dry by fanning.

2. An inverted small paper cup makes a good receptacle for coverglasses during staining. Place coverglass blood side up on inverted cup.

3. Place 10 drops of Wright stain on coverglass. The Wright stain will fix the tissue in this step. Allow to act for *2 minutes.*

4. Dilute stain by adding 10 drops of buffer to the Wright stain on the coverglass. Leave stain on for an additional *2 minutes.* In this step the stain will be ionized and a staining reaction will take place. Move preparation gently to mix solutions.

5. Rinse off dye solution with fresh distilled water.

6. Dilute Giemsa stain (ready to use) 1 to 10 with buffer. Cover smear with this diluted Giemsa and let stain for *10 minutes.*

7. Rinse with fresh distilled water.

8. Allow smears to air-dry. If desired, mount coverglass on glass slide with Permount.

PREPARATION OF BONE-MARROW ASPIRATES IN SECTIONS

Aspirated bone marrow is usually obtained with a sternal puncture needle. Smears are made and the remainder is processed as a biopsy specimen.

* Giemsa tissue stain, Wolbach modification, Harleco item #6203.

Fixation

It has been my experience that the best bone marrow sections are those which are initially fixed in Zenker's fluid with acetic acid. In addition to fixing, the acetic acid in the Zenker's solution will decalcify the tiny spicules of bone which may be mixed with the blood clot, with consequent improvement in the appearance of the cut sections. Zenker-formol is most frequently recommended for the fixation of bone marrow because the acetic acid in the original Zenker formula lyses red blood cells. I find no disadvantage to this in its application to the study of marrow cells in a biopsy specimen. The chromate fixation with Zenker's or Helly's fluid permits optimum staining results with the stains most used for bone marrow sections, such as Wolbach's modification of the Giemsa stain, May-Grünwald Giemsa, Mallory's phloxine methylene blue, and Lillie's azure-eosinate method.

Bone marrow aspirates (usually $1 \times 1 \times 0.5$ cm. or smaller) are fixed in Zenker's with acetic acid or Zenker-formol for 3 to 6 hours. For very small fragments of marrow, 3 hours' fixation will be sufficient. If pigments (hemosiderin and hemoglobin) rather than cellular structure are of prime consideration, fix bone marrow in buffered neutral formalin.

Procedure Following Fixation

After fixation the tissue must be washed for 1 to 3 hours in running tap water. The marrow can then be processed on the Autotechnicon as usual and will give satisfactory results.

However, a better method for treating bone marrow but one which has the single disadvantage of taking more time is as follows. Very fine sections are obtained with this method. The oil of cedarwood treatment improves the cutting of the sections.

1. Fix bone marrow aspirate in Zenker's with acetic acid or Zenker-formol for *3 to 6 hours.*

2. Wash in running water for *1 to 3 hours.*

3. Dehydrate in 70%, 80%, 95%, and absolute alcohols for *1 hour each.*

4. Place in oil of cedarwood * and leave *overnight*.

5. Extract excess oil of cedarwood by placing tissue in xylene in the incubator at 56° to 58°C. for *15 to 30 minutes*.

6. Impregnate with 3 changes of paraffin of *1 hour each*.

7. Embed in paraffin and section on the rotary microtome at 4μ thick. Since the marrow is not always present throughout the clot, it is advisable to take three sections, each cut at a different level of the paraffin block.

8. Stain with hematoxylin and eosin, Wolbach's modification of the Giemsa stain (page 241), Mallory's phloxine methylene blue (page 252), or the May-Grünwald and Giemsa stain (page 355).

PREPARATION OF AUTOPSY BONE MARROW

If there is no question of metastatic disease in the bone, and if only the marrow is to be studied, far superior autopsy marrow sections are obtained by the following method.

Remove a plug of marrow and slice thin. Fix for 24 hours in Zenker's with acetic acid. If the marrow is cut thin enough and is free of hard bone, the acetic acid in the fixative will decalcify the cancellous bone during the 24-hour period. Wash sections in running water for 1 to 3 hours, and process as for bone-marrow aspirates.

If the bone is to be studied, after fixation and washing, place a small section of bone marrow with attached hard bone into the decalcifying agent (pages 143 and 146), for 24 to 48 hours. If the sections are left too long in acid decalcifying solutions, the cellular detail of the delicate marrow cells will be injured, if not destroyed.

Wash tissues thoroughly after decalcification. Dehydrate, clear, and infiltrate with paraffin as usual.

PREPARATION OF BONE-MARROW BIOPSY SPECIMENS (TREPHINE METHOD)

When the architectural features of both bone and marrow are important in diagnosis, or when for technical reasons or because of

---

* Terpineol may be substituted for the oil of cedarwood.

disease changes no marrow aspirate can be obtained with needles, surgical removal of a small cylindrical piece of bone and the contained marrow may provide material for diagnosis. Touch preparations of the marrow may be made before fixation. Tissue relationships and good cytologic details are both preserved if the trephine biopsy is promptly fixed, later sawed in half if necessary, efficiently *decalcified,* and processed as for aspirates (p. 156).

QUIZ

1. What is a "touch preparation"?
2. What fixatives are recommended for bone-marrow studies?
3. Give in outline form the complete method for processing bone-marrow aspirates.
4. Why is it recommended that three sections be taken at different levels of the block?
5. What stains are recommended for bone-marrow sections?
6. How does a trephine biopsy differ from a bone-marrow aspirate?

12

Exfoliative Cytology Techniques

   I. Cell Block
  II. Papanicolaou Smears
 III. Nuclepore Filter Membrane Method
 IV. Sex Chromatin Techniques

In the normal cycle of life, cells of the body are continually being renewed by cell division. In the process of growth, the bottom, newly formed layer pushes up, dislodging the surface layer of cells into surrounding body fluids. Cells shed into the fluid are representative of the nearby organ. Samples are taken from the patient, and after careful preparation they are microscopically examined. The size, shape, and staining qualities of the cells, or any minute abnormality will differentiate normal from diseased cells.

Exfoliative cytology is of proved value in the early detection of cancer; its use thus increases the probability of cure. The cells are exfoliated (shed) into body fluids and secretions, and these provide material for diagnosis. Three main techniques are used to process this material: *cell blocks, smear preparations,* and *membrane filter methods.* If the submitted specimen is sufficient in quantity, two of the techniques are performed on the same sample. If the amount of the specimen is scant, the material is processed as a Papanicolaou smear or by the membrane filter method, whichever is more suitable for the material to be studied. If the cytologic preparations suggest cancer, additional tests including *biopsy* (the removal of a piece of tissue from the area in question) can then be made to confirm the diagnosis.

I.   Cell Block

It is possible to prepare pleural, ascitic, or other body fluids or exudates and to section them on a rotary microtome, using the paraffin-embedding technique. The procedure is often used for diagnosis when cancer is suspected or to provide evidence of metastatic disease. If a delay in processing is anticipated, refrigerate the material to prevent decomposition. When possible it is recommended that the fluids be collected in an anticoagulant (e.g., potassium oxalate, heparin, and sodium citrate-citric acid) and processed in the fresh state promptly.

In our laboratory we have found it best to maintain our own supply of 500 ml., flat-sided medicine bottles with graduated measurements embossed on the glass. These are thoroughly washed and dried, the anticoagulant is added (according to the formula that follows), and the bottles are delivered to Central Supply where the bottles are placed directly on the paracentesis and thoracentesis trays, *before* the pack is sterilized. This step eliminates the necessity of calculating the amount and adding the anticoagulant at the time the fluid is drawn, and also provides some assurance of a better preserved specimen. An fluid exceeding the 500 ml. capacity of the bottle is collected separately in a special plastic drawstring bag with milliliter guide measurements printed on it. The total volume is delivered to the laboratory for documentation purposes.

ANTICOAGULANT FOR THORACENTESIS TRAYS

Sodium citrate	25.5 gm.
Citric acid	8.0 gm.
Distilled water	100.0 ml.

Directions: 2 ml. of the above are added for each 100 ml. of fluid, or 10 ml. are added to each 500 ml. size bottle.

Method of Processing

1. A record is made describing the general characteristics of the material and the volume received. Descriptive terms might include blood-tinged, clear, yellow, amber, frothy, mucinous, and so forth.

Any flecks or macroscopic fragments present in the specimen are removed, fixed, and processed as a biopsy specimen.

2. Agitate the fluid slightly, pour into three 50 ml. test tubes, and centrifuge at medium speed for 15 to 30 minutes. If the fluid is remarkably low in cellular content, it is advisable to decant and discard the supernatant, add more of the fluid, and centrifuge it once more to obtain a more representative sample. Some workers recommend adding an equal amount of 95% alcohol to the fluid before centrifuging. Our practice is *not* to add the alcohol. If Papanicolaou smears are to be done (following step 3), the alcohol, because it initiates fixation, will interfere with close adherence of the cells to the slides. It is strongly recommended that Papanicolaou smears always be prepared to accompany the cell block. A combination of the two techniques provides optimum diagnostic material.

3. After the fluid is spun down, pour off the supernatant; this will leave the cell sediment in the bottom of the test tube.

4. Make two smears from a portion of the sediment for the Papanicolaou technique (page 167).

5. Pour a small amount of fixative * directly into the test tube and let it stand for 15 to 30 minutes or longer, if possible. The fixative will cause the sediment on the bottom of the tube to coagulate into a soft mass and facilitate removal. Pour off fixative. If the sediment (button) does not fall out readily when the tube is inverted and tapped, remove with a wooden applicator stick.

6. To prevent loss of the specimen, wrap the recovered sediment in lens or cigarette paper and place in a tissue capsule. If there is a large amount of sediment to be processed, divide into smaller portions, each no wider than 1.5 cm. and no more than 2 mm. thick (size of a dime). This will ensure proper fixation.

7. The material should be fixed for 6 to 24 hours. If the amounts of sediment do not exceed the recommended size, 6 hours will be adequate for fixation.

8. After complete fixation, the material is ready to go through the routine processes of dehydration, clearing, and infiltration on the automatic tissue-processing machine. The cell block is embedded and then sectioned on a rotary microtome.

---

* Zenker-Formol solution.

9. If the quantity of material received is too small to spin down, make smears for the Papanicolaou technique (page 166) or process with the Nuclepore filter technique (page 172).

II.   *Papanicolaou Smears*

The method of preparing and evaluating exfoliated cells developed by Papanicolaou has become an important diagnostic adjunct in daily use in today's pathology laboratory. The primary purpose of examination of a Papanicolaou smear is for the cytologic diagnosis of cancer. However, this technique is also used to determine chromosomal sex, the effects of estrogen hormones, and the presence as well as sometimes the type of infection.

Smears are made from material collected from various regions, e.g., *vaginal, endocervical, and endometrial smears; prostatic smears; smears of urine sediment; sputum, gastric,* and *bronchial aspirates; pleural* and *peritoneal fluids.* Methods of obtaining the specimen include aspiration, swabs, abrasive techniques, and lavage.

In gynecology the simple procedure of collecting secretions and making smears is easily and conveniently done in the doctor's office. These smears provide a rapid although not always conclusive means of diagnosis. Diagnosis cannot be made by any one laboratory procedure alone. Cytology is not a substitute for biopsy, and positive results from a Papanicolaou smear examination are usually confirmed by surgical biopsy.

In interpreting smears the morphology and alterations of single cells are used. Proper methods of specimen collection, preparation, and careful labeling will greatly enhance the accuracy of evaluation of the smear. In addition an adequate number of cells must be present which are representative of the site under suspicion.

The percentage of accuracy which can be expected in recognizing uterine cancer by vaginal smears exceed 80 percent of cases examined by the most skilled cytologists. Bronchial secretions may show tumor cells in nearly the same percentage of lung cancers. Gastric secretions, urine, and other material are more difficult for many cytologists, but possibly 50 percent of cancers elsewhere may be recognized cytologically.

COLLECTION OF SPECIMEN

Prostatic and Gynecologic Material

Smears should be made on clean slides. The patient's name and age, the date that smear was obtained, and the type of smear should be written on a paper label with lead pencil and attached to the slide with an aluminum paper clip. When more than one slide on the same patient is placed in a jar, the paper clip will also serve to keep the slides separate, permitting the fixative to come in contact with the entire cell film. Smears that are not to be stained immediately can be preserved in 95% alcohol or in ether-alcohol solution for several days or even weeks without deterioration if the level of the fixing solution is kept above the smear. (See other fixation methods, page 167.)

Serous Fluids

Serous fluids (*gastric and bronchial washings, exudate, and peritoneal and pleural fluids*) are best processed in the fresh state as soon after collection as possible. It is recommended that an anticoagulant be added to bloody fluids immediately upon collection. If a delay in processing is anticipated, the specimen may be preserved by refrigeration or by the addition of an equal amount of 10% formalin. If specimens are received in large quantities, refrigeration serves the purpose better. These specimens are centrifuged in order to concentrate the cells before making smears or a cell block, or both.

GASTRIC WASHINGS. These are delivered to the laboratory in ice packs to prevent deterioration, and handled promptly, as cells of gastric fluid degenerate rapidly. Cell block and Papanicolaou smears are made from this material.

URINE. The first specimen voided in the morning is best, but it must be delivered to the laboratory immediately. Membrane filters salvage all of the cells and are a preferable method of processing (see page 172).

Sputum

For cytologic purposes sputum should reach the laboratory within 1 hour of expectoration, and should be smeared and fixed promptly to preserve cellular detail. An early morning specimen produced by deep coughing provides the best material. The specimen should be examined for any blood-flecked areas or particulate material. If present, smears are made from these areas. Sputum specimens in some laboratories are digested with enzymes (i.e., trypsin) to liquefy or dissolve out the mucus. The enzyme is added to the sputum, incubated or placed on a slightly heated magnetic stirrer until the mucus is dissolved, and then centrifuged to concentrate the cells. For best results digestion methods must be carefully controlled.

If a delay in delivering the sputum sample to the laboratory is anticipated, smears should be made at the doctor's office and promptly fixed. The remainder (if any) of the sample is preserved in 70% alcohol or 10% formalin. Both smears and sputum specimen are then delivered fixed to the laboratory.

SPUTUM CONCENTRATION METHOD

Discussion

The method described homogenizes and concentrates the sputum to provide a sediment that can be uniformly smeared in a thin distribution over the glass slide. Its main advantage is that the sample represents the entire specimen, rather than a random portion. A high-speed blendor is used to homogenize the specimen. The sample is then centrifuged to separate the cells from the mucus. This is followed by a brief second mixing. Smears are made from this material, air-dried and stained with the Papanicolaou staining technique.

Fixation is accomplished with 50% ethyl alcohol containing 2% polyethylene glycol (Carbowax 1540).* The 50% dilution should be

---

* Available from Union Carbide Co.

made from 95% alcohol, avoiding the use of absolute alcohol. The 50% strength prevents the mucoproteins from coagulating; they subsequently will go into solution with the blending. The blending mixes the mucus with the alcohol and disperses the cells throughout the liquid. Carbowax is added to the fixative to prevent the cells from shrinking, and its use allows the smears to be air-dried and held, if necessary, before staining. Before combining with the alcohol, the Carbowax must be liquefied by storage in the paraffin oven at 58°C.

Sᴘᴜᴛᴜᴍ Fɪxᴀᴛɪᴠᴇ

50% Ethyl alcohol (or isopropanol)	100 ml.
Melted Carbowax 1540	2 ml.

Collection. The deep cough sputum specimen is collected after the patient washes the mouth with water. The specimen is expectorated into a large-mouth bottle about half full with the alcohol-Carbowax fixative. The container is sealed and shaken. Multiple specimens can be collected in the same container. If not collected in this manner, the fresh specimen is placed in the fixative immediately on receipt at the laboratory. The specimen may remain in this fixative for days, if necessary, without detriment.

Technique for Fresh Sputum Specimens

1. Immediately on receipt add the alcohol-Carbowax mixture to the specimen to make a total aliquot of 50 to 100 ml. If the sputum is unusually abundant, the specimen may be diluted to 200 ml. volume. Fix specimen for a minimum of *1 hour.*

2. Place the specimen in a micro sample cup, attach to the Waring food blendor and blend at high speed (21,000 RPM) for *3 to 5 seconds.* If the specimen is not uniformly blended the agitation may be continued for another *5 seconds.* This homogenization has not been found to be injurious to the cells.

3. Transfer the sputum to round-bottom test tubes (15 x 50 mm. size) and centrifuge at 1000 to 1500 RPM for *10 minutes.*

4. Decant the supernatant fluid leaving a very small amount of this fluid to admix with the now granular, pale centrifugate. The second mixing of this material, which is best accomplished with an electric

shaker (i.e. Vortex mixer), will form a thick, granular, almost paste-like mixture within a *few seconds.*

5. Place 1 or 2 drops of the homogenized centrifugate (if thick) and 2 to 4 drops (if thin) on clean slides (no albumen necessary). Gently spread the material as evenly as possible by superimposing a clean slide and gently manipulating the material until it is dispersed between the two slides. The slides are then pulled apart by a sliding motion. Two to 4 slides are made from each centrifuged tube.

6. Allow the slides to air-dry completely. Because of the thin protective coating of the wax, smears may be left in this condition for months without ill effect.

7. If desired, wax may be removed by placing smears in tap water or 80% alcohol for *5 minutes.* Follow the Papanicolaou staining method.

MATERIALS.   Waring Blendor, Scientific Products Cat. No. 8350–2

Eberbach semi-micro stainless steel sampler, Scientific Products Cat. No. 8395–1

Centrifuge

Vortex mixer or any electric vibrator

NOTES.   1. The finished, stained slide reveals a fine uniform granular surface with excellent cell recovery.

2. The homogenized sediment does not, however, provide a good cell block.

3. Between the blending of each specimen, the micro-sampler should be decontaminated with 2% Amphyl, followed by a thorough wash with hot soapy water.

REFERENCE.   Saccomanno, G., Saunders, R. P., Ellis, H., Archer, V., Wood, B. G., and Beckler, P. A.   Concentration of carcinoma or atypical cells in sputum. *Acta Cytol.* (Balt.) 7:305–310, 1963.

PREPARATION OF CYTOLOGIC MATERIAL

The composition and properties of body fluids and secretions differ, and they must be handled accordingly. Secretions which are viscid in nature — e.g., *cervical, vaginal, nipple,* and *prostatic* — are smeared directly onto clean glass slides (no egg albumen) and placed in the fixative *immediately*. Smears made from specimens that are highly viscous adhere well to slides because of the mucus and/or protein in the material. Once fixed, they lose this adhesive quality. These are relatively high in cell content.

It is necessary to centrifuge some specimens — e.g., *urine, exudates,* and *bronchial, gastric,* and other *aspirates* and *washings* — before making smears. This type of specimen usually contains a lower concentration of cells suspended in a large quantity of fluid. The material is centrifuged, using three to four 50-ml. conical tubes, for approximately 15 to 30 minutes at medium speed or until a well-packed cellular sediment appears in the bottom of the tubes with a clear supernatant liquid above. The supernatant fluid is carefully decanted and discarded, and the sediment smeared uniformly onto glass slides that should first be *coated* with a thin film of *egg albumen* (or other commercial adhesive) to provide greater adhesion of cells. If sufficient sediment remains after making the smears, it is wise to process this as a biopsy specimen (cell block, see page 160).

The collected material for all smears is distributed *uniformly* over clean glass slides. The end edge of a second clean slide may be used to spread the material in a thin film, leaving a 1-inch allowance at one end of the slide for labeling.

FIXATION

To secure a good specimen, freshly prepared smears should be fixed *immediately,* as exfoliated cells decompose rapidly. Fixation of the smear before it dries is important. Cells exposed to drying before they are fixed will be poorly preserved and show marked distortion. If both cytologic and bacteriologic surveys are required of the specimen, it must be divided and a portion allocated to the bacteriology laboratory *before* fixation.

FIXING SOLUTIONS. The universally accepted fixative for Papanicolaou smears is *equal parts of 95% ethyl alcohol and ether*. Other solutions that have come into popular use are 95% ethyl or isopropyl alcohol and acetone. Whereas some types of smears will be fixed in

15 minutes, a minimum of 1 hour will permit more complete penetration of the cells. Also the preparation will adhere to the slide better if it is thoroughly fixed.

Commercial aerosol spray fixatives such as Cyto-Spray, Spray-Cyte, and Pro-Fixx have specific application in this area. These are alcohol-soluble and water-soluble fixatives designed for use in exfoliative cytology. They not only fix the cells but provide protection by coating the slide with a translucent film. Their composition is generally polyethylene glycols combined with isopropyl alcohol. They fix and preserve cellular elements in a one-step procedure. They are convenient and solve the problem of mailing the slides to the laboratory; postal regulations prohibit the mailing of inflammable fluids such as ether-alcohol or acetone. If the spray has been applied unevenly or with a too heavy hand, it may be necessary to remove the excess prior to staining, by immersing the slides in several changes of water or 80% alcohol.

Contamination of Smears

"In the process of staining, cells, cell clusters, or even small parts of the film of a smear ('floaters') may become detached from a slide and adhere to other slides stained in the same container. This is a rare occurrence yet it may lead to a false positive evaluation if positive 'floaters' adhere to a negative smear." (Papanicolaou, G. N. *Atlas of Exfoliative Cytology.* Cambridge: Harvard University Press, 1954, pp. 3–6.)

The following recommendations may help to reduce the chance of such contamination.

1. Agitate slides as little as possible. While processing slides, observe cautious handling.

2. Replace frequently all solutions used in the staining procedure. Wash staining dishes thoroughly.

3. Do not crowd slides within the staining dishes.

4. Stains, particularly the first stain used (hematoxylin), should be filtered before use.

5. Detachment of "floaters" occurs more frequently in exudates and urines. It is advisable, therefore, to stain such smears in separate jars and renew the solutions more frequently.

STAINING SMEARS

After fixation the slides may be stained routinely with hematoxylin and eosin or other stains, or they may be stained with the Papanicolaou method, which is to be preferred.

Papanicolaou Staining Method, Standard Technique

1. After fixation in equal parts of 95% alcohol and ether, hydrate the slides in 80%, 70%, and 50% alcohols (*6 dips* each).
2. Rinse in distilled water.
3. Stain in Harris's hematoxylin (without acetic acid, diluted with an equal amount of distilled water) for *6 minutes* or full strength hematoxylin for *1–3 minutes.*
4. Rinse in distilled water. (All rinsing should be very gentle to prevent smears from being washed from the slides.)
5. Dip in an 0.25% aqueous solution of hydrochloric acid *6 times* or 0.5% hydrochloric acid *3 times.*
6. Place in running tap water and wash for *6 minutes.* Slides may be checked visually with the microscope to see if the nuclei are adequately stained. Decolorize again in acid alcohol if they are overstained or return to the hematoxylin if they are pale.
7. Run through distilled water and 50%, 70%, 80%, and 95% alcohols, *6 dips* each.
8. Stain in OG-6 for *1½ minutes.*
9. Rinse in 95% alcohol, 3 changes, *6 dips* each.
10. Stain in EA-36 or EA-50 for *1½ minutes.*
11. Rinse in 95% alcohol, three changes. Dehydrate and clear by running through two changes of absolute alcohol and one change of a mixture of equal parts of absolute alcohol and xylene. Clear in three changes of xylene. Approximately *6 dips* each.
12. Mount in Permount or any other satisfactory neutral medium.

Note: To be certain that the specimen is adequately dehydrated and cleared, leave the smears in the solutions (alcohols and xylene) until the liquid runs off the slides in a smooth, clean sheet. If the slide is removed too soon, rivulets will show on the surface. Some very mucinous smears may require clearing in carbol-xylene (see page 50).

RESULTS.   Nuclei — blue

Cytoplasm — varying shades of pink, blue, green, yellow, and orange

STAINING SOLUTIONS

The Ortho Pharmaceutical Corporation (Raritan, New Jersey), supplies excellent ready-to-use dye solutions (EA-36, EA-50, EA-65, and OG-6) for this technique. In use, these stains are filtered and added to as they evaporate. The formulas are given for those who wish to make their own. To provide greater transparency, the EA-36 and OG-6 counterstains are made up with 95% alcoholic solutions of dyes. Orange G, light green, and Bismarck brown powdered stains are not readily soluble in 95% alcohol. For this reason the formulas below call for dissolving the dyes in an aqueous solution and then diluting with alcohol. (*A Manual of Cytotechnology,* published by the National Committee for Careers in Medical Technology; edited by Dr. J. W. Reagan; p. 11-5.)

HARRIS'S ALUM HEMATOXYLIN
(See page 227.)

OG-6 STAIN

1. Prepare a 10% aqueous solution of orange G, using distilled water. Allow to stand for several days.

2. Prepare the OG-6 staining solution as follows:

Orange G, 10% aqueous solution	50.0 ml.
95% ethyl alcohol	950.0 ml.
Phosphotungstic acid, C.P.	0.15 gm.

Store in a dark, well-stoppered bottle, and filter before using.

EA-36 STOCK STAINS

1. Prepare the following aqueous solutions, using distilled water:

2% light green, S.F., yellowish
10% Bismarck brown Y

Allow them to stand for several days.

2. Prepare alcoholic stock solutions:

(A) *0.1% Light Green*

2% aqueous light green	50 ml.
95% ethyl alcohol	950 ml.

(B) *0.5% Bismarck Brown*

10% aqueous Bismarck brown	10 ml.
95% ethyl alcohol	190 ml.

(C) *0.5% Eosin*

Eosin Y, water- and alcohol-soluble	5 gm.
95% ethyl alcohol	1000 ml.

EA-36 WORKING STAINING SOLUTION

Combine:

0.1% light green (stock solution A)	450 ml.
0.5% Bismarck brown (stock solution B)	100 ml.
0.5% eosin (stock solution C)	450 ml.
Phosphotungstic acid, C.P.	2 gm.
Lithium carbonate, C.P., saturated aqueous solution (1.25%)	10 drops

Mix well and store in a dark, well-stoppered bottle. Filter before using.

QUIZ

1. What is the purpose of a Papanicolaou smear?
2. What regions are the sources of material collected for making smears?
3. What methods are used to obtain material?
4. What are the fixing solutions for these smears?
5. How soon after preparing the smear should it be placed in the fixative?
6. What is a "safe" minimum time for fixation?
7. How are fluids that are low in cellular content and large in quantity processed? (For instance, gastric lavage.)
8. Give the complete Papanicolaou staining method in outline form.
9. How are smears best prepared for mailing or transporting to a laboratory?

REFERENCES

Fawcett, D. W., Vallee, B. L., and Soule, M. H.   Method for concentration and segregation of malignant cells from bloody, pleural, and peritoneal fluids. *Science* 111:34–36, 1950.

McGrew, E.   Concentration of cells from body fluids for cytologic study. *Amer. J. Clin. Path.* 24:1025–1029, 1954.

Sagi, E. S., and Mackenzie, L. L.   The use of acetone as a fixative in exfoliative cytological studies. *Amer. J. Obstet. Gynec.* 73:437–439, 1957.

Seal, S. H.   A method for concentrating cancer cells suspended in large quantities of fluid. *Cancer* 9:866–868, 1956.

RECOMMENDED READING

National Committee for Careers in Medical Technology: *A Manual of Cytotechnology,* edited by J. W. Reagan, 1962.

Papanicolaou, G. N.   *Atlas of Exfoliative Cytology.* Cambridge: Harvard University Press, 1954.

Staff of the Vincent Memorial Laboratory: *The Cytologic Diagnosis of Cancer.* Philadelphia: Saunders, 1950.

III.   Nuclepore Filter Membrane Technique

In addition to cell blocks and Papanicolaou smear techniques, membrane filters are being used increasingly in diagnostic cytology. The filters are designed to isolate or collect cells from body fluids in a concentrated area on a membrane. The membrane is then fixed, stained, and viewed microscopically.

Filter membrane technology provides a simple, rapid, and effective method of recovering exfoliated cancer cells from ascitic, pleural, bronchial, or cerebrospinal fluids, gastric washings, and urine. With or without vacuum pressure, *fresh unfixed* fluid is filtered through a membrane disc. A deposit of cells is retained on the filter (disc). Immediately *after* filtration the filter is placed in a fixative. Following fixation it is clipped to a slide, stained, dehydrated, and cleared. It is then mounted on a glass slide and coverslipped and is ready for examination.

Perhaps the chief advantage of this method is that small quantities of fluid, e.g., spinal fluid, containing too little sediment for either a cell block or a smear will provide adequate material for interpretation, since as little as 1 to 2 ml. can yield enough cells to make a diagnosis. It is recommended that the volume of very small samples be increased by the addition of an equal volume of normal saline prior to filtration.

The membrane filter technique eliminates the necessity of centrifuging in most instances. However, with large volumes of clear fluid of low cellular content, it would be advantageous to centrifuge the specimen prior to filtration so as to obtain a more concentrated specimen. It should be remembered that greater accuracy in diagnosing malignancies from sediments of serous fluids is possible when two methods, i.e., cell block and filter membrane, or Papanicolaou smear and cell block, are used.

There are several obvious disadvantages to the use of membrane filters — in particular, overcrowding or clumping of cells, unwanted staining of the filter matrix, distortion of morphology caused by suction, and difficulties encountered in mounting and storing because of the thickness of the filters. Many of these problems are reduced or eliminated by General Electric's Nuclepore filter. It is a clear, transparent membrane made of plastic (polycarbonate) film, available in disc or rectangular form. The film has randomly spaced uniform cylindrical holes or "pores" which act like a sieve, allowing the fluid and unwanted cellular material to flush through the pores while retaining the cells on the surface of the film. It is chemically nonreactive with the reagents most used in processing, practically indestructible, and retains a viewing field free of background staining, a common failing of the cross-hatched type filter.

ADVANTAGES OF MEMBRANE TECHNOLOGY

1. Close adherence of cells to the filter reduces the possibility of cells washing off, and consequently loss of tumor cells is minimized.

This close adherence of cells also reduces the hazard of cross contamination. Cells do not always adhere to the glass slides on smear preparations.

2. The filter membrane technique concentrates cells and furnishes a more clearly representative sample of cell types, even with large quantities of material of relatively low cellular content.

3. The technique permits direct collection of cells from fluid. Nearly all fluids may be readily filtered without the necessity of centrifugation.

4. The filter membrane technique is the preferred technique for recovering sufficient cells from small amounts of fluid. Its salvage ratio is greater.

SPECIMEN PREPARATION AND HANDLING

Practically all cytologic determinations are done with a 5μ ($\frac{5}{10}$ micrometer) or 8μ ($\frac{8}{10}$ micrometer) pore filter. To avoid the artefacts produced by vacuum and for simplicity, we recommend the use of a Swinnex-25, round, disposable, plastic filter holder with a silicone gasket. These are very inexpensive, perform well, and can be washed, autoclaved and reused if desired.

The material to be filtered should be processed immediately upon collection to avoid decomposition of cells and to preserve morphological integrity of the cell. It is necessary that the specimen be thoroughly mixed before filtering to ensure obtaining a representative and adequate cell sampling. Generally a 5 to 10 ml. aliquot provides a good sample. When the specimen has a high cell concentration, e.g., pleural fluids, it is best to use only 5 ml. or dilute with an equal volume of saline, or both, to avoid cell clumping or clogging of the filter. When the quantity of the specimen is small (1 to 2 ml.), 5 to 10 ml. of saline to wash out the container in which it is received and to increase the total volume is recommended. If the fluid is relatively clear or contains few cells in a large quantity of fluid, it is best to centrifuge this sample in order to concentrate the cells.

It is important to avoid fixation *before* filtration, because otherwise proteins precipitated by the fixative may clog the filter, absorb dyes, and obscure detail. With fresh samples the soluble proteins are flushed through the filter and leave the cells deposited on the membrane.

NUCLEPORE FILTER MEMBRANE TECHNIQUE

INDICATIONS. For cytodiagnosis on urines, spinal fluids, bronchial washings, or any body fluid received in very small amount or of low cellular content. May also be used for sex chromatin determinations on amniotic fluid.

MATERIALS.   25 mm. Swinnex filter holder (Millipore Filter Corp., Bedford, Mass. 01730, Cat. No. SX00 025 00, with silicone gaskets but less filters, non-sterile)

25 mm. Nuclepore filters (General Electric Co., Vallecitos Rd., Pleasanton, Cal. 94566)

12 cc. syringe (no needle necessary)

Normal saline

50% ethyl alcohol

95% ethyl alcohol

Small Petri dish

Fine forceps

Disposable pipettes or rubber dropper bulbs

Procedure

1. Describe specimen and document amount received.

2. Unscrew Swinnex-25 filter holder, insert Nuclepore shiny side down, place gasket on top of filter, and screw top back in place.

3. With eye dropper or pipette wash the filter by discharging several milliliters of normal physiologic saline through hole on top of filter holder.

4. Mix specimen thoroughly to suspend cells, and aspirate fluid from its container into a 12 cc. disposable syringe (no needle necessary). Aspirate approximately 5 to 10 ml.

5. Holding syringe and filter holder over a disposable paper cup, discharge syringe contents into filter holder, pushing as much fluid through as will pass easily. When pressure begins to build on the

plunger, enough cells have been collected. Hold filter holder level so that cells will collect evenly across its surface.

6. Detach syringe, and with eye dropper again wet filter with saline (same as step 4). The saline washes will eliminate proteinaceous and other unwanted material from the filter, leaving a clear field.

7. To fix cells to filter, wet with 5 to 10 ml. of 70% alcohol with eye dropper.

8. Unscrew top of filter holder and remove filter with forceps, keeping cell side (or top) upright.

9. To complete fixation, transfer filter to a prelabeled Petri dish (3.5 cm. in diameter) containing enough 95% alcohol to completely cover. Minimum fixation time is 30 minutes. Filter may stay in fixative until ready to stain.

Staining

Following fixation, filters may be stained in small Petri dishes or clipped to a glass slide and placed in a standard staining rack, hydrated in 70%, then 50% alcohol, and water, and stained in the usual manner. If they are to be stained attached to a slide, cytology membrane clips are used and the clips fastened to the edge of the membrane. Be sure that the cellular surface is faced away from the slide to allow full contact of solutions on the cells. At no time in the processing should the filter be allowed to dry. The filter may be stained with hematoxylin and eosin, the Papanicolaou stain, chromosome stains, Prussian blue technique, or other special stains with little or no modification of these techniques. Following staining, the membrane filters are dehydrated, cleared, and mounted in Permount in the usual manner.

Eliminating Pore Outline

The visible pores may prove a distraction for some observers. The following procedure is suggested to eliminate the pore outline. Chloroform will partially dissolve the filter and fill in the holes, consolidating it into a poreless transparent sheet.

1. After staining, dehydrating, and clearing, remove clips and place filter *cell side down* on a slide that has been wetted with xylene. Carefully raise and lower filter to the slide to avoid entrapment of air.

2. Position slide on a flat, even surface and gently blot the filter dry with smooth bibulous paper. The filter will dry out and lose its transparency.

3. When filter is completely dry, squirt 2 to 5 drops of chloroform from an eye dropper evenly over the surface of the filter, starting in the center and working in circles to the periphery of the disc. Take care not to jar filter during this step. Work away from drafts. Cover preparation with an inverted Petri dish that is slightly elevated with a wooden applicator stick to control the rate of evaporation, which will take 1 to 2 minutes. During evaporation the filter must be carefully watched. If the filter dries too rapidly or for too long, it will curl and become useless.

4. After the chloroform has evaporated and the filter is dry, the slide is returned to xylene and then mounted in Permount.

Note: If the filter becomes cloudy with this technique (seen after coverslipping), it is most likely caused by too rapid evaporation of the chloroform.

Another situation that may occur from the chloroform treatment is that the cells may run or scatter over the slide. To counteract this, avoid overcrowding the filter with cells, and always begin the application of chloroform at the center, working toward the outer edges.

If you encounter a precipitate following pore elimination procedures, McAlpine and Ellsworth suggest that shortly following application of the chloroform, the filter be blotted quickly and carefully with bibulous paper and then allowed to air dry. It is then rinsed well in xylene, drained and coverslipped with Permount.

QUIZ

1. What is the Nuclepore filter technique used for? What material is processed?
2. When is material fixed? In what solution?
3. Give in outline form the basic steps in processing a sample of serous fluid.
4. How are the filters stained? Name two recommended staining techniques for these.

REFERENCES

Application Handbook for Nuclepore Membrane Filters, available from General Electric Company, Vallecitos Rd., Pleasanton, California 94566.

McAlpine, L. W., and Ellsworth, B.   A modified membrane filter technique for cytodiagnosis. *Techn. Bull. Regist. Med. Techn.* 39:154–156, 1969.

Reynaud, A. J., and King, E. B.   A new filter for diagnostic cytology. *Acta Cytol.* (Balt.) 11:289–294, 1967.

Seal, S. H.   A sieve for the isolation of cancer cells and other large cells from the blood. *Cancer* 17:637–642, 1964.

IV.   Sex Chromatin Testing

In 1949 Barr and Bertram (*Nature* 163:676–677, 1949) demonstrated that there was a distinct morphologic difference between the cells of males and females, and they introduced a method of determining the sex chromatin pattern of an individual. The identification of true (genetic) sex is important in the diagnosis of congenital defects and in the treatment of children of ambiguous sex. Sex chromatin determinations are also done in the investigation of infertility, which may have as its cause a sex chromatin defect.

Barr showed that females have a distinct, elongated, intranuclear mass of chromatin (Barr body) which lies against the inner aspect of the nuclear membrane. It stains deeply, is round or planoconcave in shape, and measures 1μ or less in size. In the female pattern, a large percentage (as much as 50 percent in some instances) of the cell nuclei counted will show Barr bodies and be "Barr positive." Although all female cells probably have this, a 100 percent count is never possible because all nuclear membranes would not lie in the same plane of the microscopic field. In males, less than 4 percent of the nuclei will show the Barr body. The findings on a sex determination are reported as "chromatin positive" or "chromatin negative," rather than female or male.

Sex chromatin patterns can be determined by peripheral blood smear in which a "drumstick" appendage to the nucleus of polymorphonuclear neutrophils rather than the Barr body is the finding. Sex chromatin patterns can be determined by source material obtained from biopsy of the gonad, skin biopsy, or by buccal mucosal scrapings. In fact, evaluation can be made on any tissue which has cells with large vesicular nuclei. The basal epithelial cells of the buccal mucosa are easily accessible, and buccal smears are almost universally used for this purpose.

Amniotic fluid epithelial cells are also used for the prenatal detection of genetic diseases and to predict the sex of the unborn child. The cells that are shed in amniotic fluid are already somewhat degenerated and are more difficult to interpret. Use of filter membranes for collection, staining, and interpretation of these cells is preferred to smear techniques (pp. 172–177).

In human cytogenetics there are two methods of sex chromatin determination. The smear technique given here is a screening procedure, and abnormal findings shown by this method must always be confirmed by karyotyping, a more complex but effective method of chromosome analysis.

COLLECTION OF SPECIMEN FOR SMEARS

The inner surface of the oral mucosa of the cheek or upper lip is scraped with a wooden tongue depressor to provide the cells.

1. Have patient rinse mouth free of any excess mucus or food particles.

2. With a tongue depressor, scrape the buccal mucosa. Discard this initial sample. Scrape again, with fairly firm pressure in the same area to reach the deeper cells.

3. Spread collected material evenly on *three* clean, albuminized slides. If smears are not spread evenly, the cells will be difficult to evaluate.

4. Immerse slides in 95% ethyl alcohol immediately. Fix cells from 30 to 60 minutes.

Note: Make control slides in the same manner. Any female laboratory technician can provide control material.

Remove the first slide from the alcohol, cover smear with aceto-orcein staining solution from an eye dropper, allow to set for 15 to 30 seconds, rinse with distilled water, coverslip, and check under the microscope. The quick wet mount is used solely to determine if the specimen of the buccal mucosa has an adequate sampling of proper cells. If the wet mount is promising, proceed with permanent sections, using either Guard's stain or the standard aceto-orcein technique. If the material collected is unsatisfactory, repeat collection procedure as described.

STAINING

The hematoxylin in the routine hematoxylin and eosin stain (in fact all of the basic dyes) will stain the Barr body, but many screeners have a preference for what they consider to be more selective stains, i.e., Feulgen stain, cresyl violet, thionine, Papanicolaou technique, aceto-orcein, or Guard's stain.

ACETO-ORCEIN STAIN

INDICATIONS.   For sex chromatin interpretation

FIXATION.   Fix immediately on collection in 95% ethyl alcohol for a minimum of 30 minutes.

TECHNIQUE.   Buccal scrapings. Run a control (known positive) with test smear.

Staining Solutions:

ACETO-ORCEIN STAIN
(After Lillie)

Orcein	4 gm.
Hot glacial acetic acid	180 ml.
Distilled water	220 ml.

Heat acid to 80°C. in pyrex flask placed in a beaker containing water. Remove flask from heat and add orcein while shaking or stirring rapidly (or use a mechanical stirrer). Gradually add distilled water while continuing to stir or shake. Stopper flask and bathe under cold running water. When the stain has cooled, filter and store in a brown bottle. The stain keeps very well. In fact it improves on aging.

FAST GREEN STAIN

Fast green	0.06 gm.
95% ethyl alcohol	200.00 ml.

Add fast green to the alcohol, and stir or shake to dissolve. Stable solution.

Staining Procedure

1. Hydrate slides in 70% alcohol for *2 minutes.*

2. Stain in acetic orcein stain for *5 minutes.*

3. Wash in distilled water for *10 seconds.*

4. Dehydrate in 70%, 80%, and 95% ethyl alcohol about *5 dips each.*

5. Stain in fast green solution for *1 minute.*

6. Wash in 95% alcohol.

7. Dehydrate in absolute ethyl alcohol, two changes *5 dips each.*

8. Clear in xylene 2 to 3 changes and leave in last xylene for *5 minutes.*

9. Coverslip with Permount or Histoclad.

RESULTS.   Sex chromatin body — red

Cytoplasm and other nuclear chromatin — green

GUARD'S SEX CHROMATIN STAIN
(Modified by R. D. Otis and M. M. Shea)

INDICATIONS.   For sex chromatin interpretation

FIXATION.   Fix immediately in 95% ethyl alcohol for a minimum of 30 minutes.

TECHNIQUE.   Buccal smears or amniotic fluid processed with a membrane filter.

Run a control (known positive) through with test smear.

DISCUSSION. The Biebrich scarlet dye is differentiated out of or displaced from all nuclear chromatin with the exception of the mass of sex chromatin by the counterstain fast green. This differentiation is controlled by checking with the microscope until all but the Barr bodies are stained green.

Some workers recommend collodionization (see page 284) immediately following fixation to prevent loss of cells.

Staining Solutions

BIEBRICH SCARLET STOCK SOLUTION

Biebrich scarlet, water soluble	4.0 gm.
Phosphotungstic acid	1.2 gm.
Glacial acetic acid	20.0 ml.
Distilled water	200.0 ml.

Dissolve the Biebrich scarlet in 10 to 20 ml. of distilled water. Mix well to form a paste. Slowly add remainder of water, being certain that the dye is completely dissolved. Add phosphotungstic acid. Add glacial acetic acid. Pour solution into storage container and label it as a stock solution. This stain improves on standing. Results are more predictable if the stock preparation is 4 to 6 months old. Store in the dark at room temperature.

BIEBRICH SCARLET WORKING SOLUTION

Biebrich scarlet stock solution	50 ml.
Absolute ethyl alcohol	50 ml.

Combine *just before use.*

FAST GREEN SOLUTION

Fast green, F.C.F.	1.0 gm.
Phosphomolybdic acid	0.6 gm.
Phosphotungstic acid	0.6 gm.
Glacial acetic acid	10.0 ml.
50% ethyl alcohol to make	200.0 ml.

Dissolve the fast green in 10 ml. of 50% alcohol. Add the acids in the order given. Slowly add remainder of the 50% alcohol to yield 200 ml. Store at room temperature in a dark place.

Staining Procedure

1. Hydrate the alcohol-fixed smears in 70% alcohol for **2 minutes.**
2. Stain in the Biebrich scarlet working solution for **3 minutes.**
3. Rinse slides in 50% ethyl alcohol.
4. Counterstain slides in fast green. Check slides for differentiating action in the fast green **after 15 minutes.** Cytoplasm and nucleus should be green, with only the sex chromatin body staining red. Continue for an additional 5 to 15 minutes, if necessary. Pyknotic nuclei will not differentiate and will remain red.
5. Dip several times in ethyl alcohol rinses of 50%, 70%, 95%, and absolute alcohol.
6. Rinse in an additional change of absolute alcohol and blot with bibulous paper to remove excess alcohol.
7. Clear slides in xylene, 2 changes, for **5 minutes each.**
8. Mount in Permount.

RESULTS. Sex chromatin (Barr body) — red
Background — green
Nuclei — green
Pyknotic nuclei — red

REFERENCE. Otis, R. D., and Shea, M. M. A rapid staining modification of Guard's sex chromatin technic. *Amer. J. Clin. Path.* 49:137–139, 1968.

QUIZ

1. Describe the Barr body.
2. For what purpose do we perform sex chromatin testing?
3. What is the source of material used for smears?
4. In outline, give method of collection of cells for this procedure.
5. List two or more stains used for sex chromatin determinations.

REFERENCES

Barr, M. L., and Bertram, E. G. A morphological distinction between neurones of the male and female and the behavior of the nucleolar satellite during accelerated nuclear protein synthesis. *Nature* 163:676–677, 1949.

Barr, M. L., and Carr, D. H. Sex chromatin, sex chromosomes and sex anomalies. *Canad. Med. Ass. J.* 83:979, 1960.

Guard, H. R. A new technic for differential staining of the sex chromatin and the determination of its incidence in exfoliated vaginal epithelial cells. *Amer. J. Clin. Path.* 32:145–151, 1959.

Parsons, L., and Sommers, S. C. *Gynecology.* Philadelphia: Saunders, 1968, p. 77.

13

Histology

Histology is the study of the microscopic structure of tissue. Some knowledge of it is necessary if the histologic technician is to identify properly the tissue with which she is working.

Tissue consists of minute elements (*cells*) more or less regular in appearance, definitely grouped and arranged, held together by intercellular cement, and performing a definite function. The cells of a tissue may be arranged to form an organ or merely a supporting structure.

There are four kinds of tissue including *epithelial, connective, muscle,* and *nerve* tissue. In common usage the term "tissue" is also applied to any specimen of biologic material.

CELLS

A cell is a small mass of *protoplasm* containing a *nucleus.* The nucleus is usually a globular, dark-staining body having a sharp outline and occupying a central position. It will respond to nuclear stains such as hematoxylin and basic aniline dyes.

A *nucleolus* is a small body found within the nucleus. It is not always present, but in some cells more than one nucleolus may be found within the nucleus.

The *cell wall* is the membrane which limits the cell (Fig. 13–1).

TYPES OF TISSUE

Cells differ greatly in form and size. The nucleus of the cell conforms somewhat to the shape of the cell.

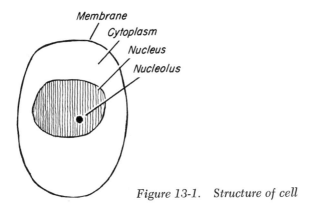

Figure 13-1.   Structure of cell

Epithelial Tissue

In epithelial tissue — tissue lining surfaces — cells predominate, and so we see many cells that vary in size, shape, and arrangement (Fig. 13–2).

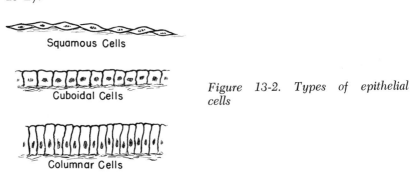

Figure 13-2. Types of epithelial cells

Connective Tissue

Connective tissues are the supporting tissues of the body (Fig. 13–3). They are characterized by a predominance of intercellular rather than cellular substance.

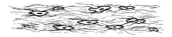

Figure 13-3.   Connective tissue cells

CONNECTIVE TISSUE

Connective tissue incorporates collagen, elastic fibers, fibrils, reticulin, adipose tissue, cartilage, and bone.

Collagen

Collagenous connective tissue is made up of hundreds of minute fibers, more or less parallel in arrangement, that present a wavy appearance (Fig. 13–4). The fibrils may be separated or united into

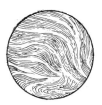

Figure 13-4. Collagen

thin or coarse strands, or they may be fused into homogeneous masses. STAINING PROPERTIES: Collagen is very permeable to dyes. It stains strongly with acid aniline dyes following pretreatment in acid solutions, such as phosphomolybdic, phosphotungstic, acetic, or picric acids. Stains for collagen are the Masson trichrome, Verhoeff-van Gieson, Mallory's aniline blue, and the Mallory-Heidenhain (AZAN) stain.

Ground Substance

In connective tissue, ground substance is a viscous, gelatinous cement, rich in carbohydrates (mostly neutral and acid polysaccharides) which supports structures like reticulin, collagen, and elastin. STAINING PROPERTIES: Ground substance of connective tissue will be stained by alcian blue-PAS or the Müller-Mowry colloidal iron-PAS. It will also stain metachromatically. Formalin fixation is recommended for ground substance.

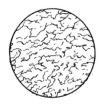

Figure 13-5.   Reticulin

Reticulin

Reticulin is a fine connective tissue consisting of delicate bundles of fibrils which form a network (Fig. 13–5). Electron microscopy has provided some evidence to support the contention that reticulin is young collagen or small bundle collagen. STAINING PROPERTIES: To study reticulin, it is necessary to employ a special stain, usually involving silver. Formalin fixation is recommended for most silver reticulin methods, but some techniques specify Helly's or Bouin's fixation. Because of its carbohydrate component (embedded as it is in a matrix of ground substance), it will be colored by the PAS method. However, the very delicate fibers will stain more selectively with one of the silver nitrate techniques.

Elastic Fibers

Elastic tissue is a type of connective tissue. It is homogeneous and is without obvious fibrils. Elastic fibers are slender, straight, branched, and connected, forming a network that is interfelted with collagenous fibers (Fig. 13–6). They are commonly found in skin, lung, and the tunica intima and media of arteries and large veins. STAINING PROPERTIES: With routine hematoxylin and eosin staining, elastic fibers take up the acid dye (eosin) and are not readily identified. After special pretreatment with oxidizers (i.e., ferric salts) they will stain selectively with basic dyes (i.e., basic fuchsin) and be readily visible. The dye

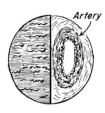

Artery   *Figure 13-6.   Elastic fibers*

orcein combined with hydrochloric acid in alcoholic solution has an affinity for elastic tissue. Staining techniques specific for elastic fibers are Verhoeff's elastic tissue stain, resorcin fuchsin, aldehyde fuchsin, and acid orcein.

Adipose Tissue

When adipose tissue is studied after ordinary preparation (paraffin embedding), merely a network of fibers and cell boundaries is seen, and the fat is represented only by empty spaces or vacuoles (Fig. 13–7). This is because the fat has been removed by the alcohols and other fat solvents used to dehydrate and clear in the processing, leaving just the white fibrous connective tissue and membranes that enclose the

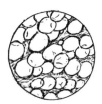

Figure 13-7. Adipose tissue

cells. Special techniques (frozen sections and Carbowax sections) that avoid the use of these fat solvents are employed when the presence of fat is to be documented. For the same reason, frozen sections for fat staining are *always* mounted in aqueous mounting media. Classifying all fats under adipose tissue is a simplification, for while the different lipids have the common characteristic of being soluble in organic solvents (i.e., lipid solvents), they are very diversified in their staining properties. In addition to simple fats there are complex lipids, probably bound to protein, that require specific staining for identification. GENERAL STAINING PROPERTIES: Osmic acid will stain fats. It is soluble in and forms a black compound with them. Staining techniques most frequently employed include Oil red O, Sudan black B, Sudan brown, and Luxol fast blue for myelin. All dyes for staining fat must be dissolved in a medium (alcohol, acetone, pyridine) in which the dye is less soluble than it is in the fat.

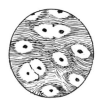

Figure 13-8.   Cartilage

Cartilage

Cartilage (Fig. 13–8) is characterized by a solid, intercellular substance resembling mucus in staining properties, called chondromucoid (chondro = cartilage). Chondromucin stains brilliantly with alcian blue-PAS and the Müller-Mowry colloidal iron method. Cartilage will stain yellow with the Masson hematoxylin-phloxine-safran (HPS) stain.

Bone

There are two kinds of bone tissue, cancellous or spongy bone, and compact or solid bone (Fig. 13–9). Bone is very dense in character.

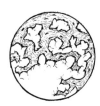

Figure 13-9.   Bone

It is composed of inorganic (66 percent) and organic (34 percent) materials. The inorganic calcium salts are soluble in acids. In order to cut bone sections, it is necessary to remove these salts. The lime salts are removed chiefly with acids in which the calcium carbonate and phosphate salts of the bone are soluble. STAINING PROPERTIES: Both the routine hematoxylin and eosin and the Giemsa stains give good morphological detail of bone sections. The Masson hematoxylin-phloxine-safran (HPS) stain is also recommended.

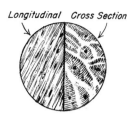

Figure 13-10.   Muscle tissue

MUSCLE TISSUE

Muscle

In muscle tissue the fibers are collected into definite groups. All fibers are parallel and grouped into small bundles. Muscle tissue is either smooth, with longitudinal striping, or striated, with cross markings that show when cut lengthwise (Fig. 13–10). STAINING PROPERTIES: Skeletal muscle striations will stain selectively blue with Mallory's PTAH. The alcian blue-PAS method will stain ground substance of muscle. Muscle will stain pink to red in the Masson Trichrome and red to orange with the Mallory-Heidenhain AZAN stain.

NERVE TISSUE

Nerve tissue is composed of neurons (nerve cells) and supporting cells located in both gray and white matter which are special connective tissue cells of the central nervous system called glial cells (Fig. 13–11). A common type of glial cell is the astrocyte. Actually there is a feltwork of fine fibers in which are contained the nerve cells, glial cells, and their processes. The larger peripheral nerves are coated

Figure 13-11.   Nerve tissue

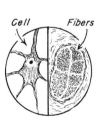

with a special fatty substance called myelin. STAINING PROPERTIES: Nerve fibers and sheaths stain rather weakly except with special stains. The fibers stand out clearly with silver nitrate techniques and with the PTAH stain of Mallory. Myelin, because it is a lipoprotein, stains distinctively with Luxol fast blue. It is a common practice to combine these special stains (Luxol fast blue-PTAH, Luxol fast blue-silver nitrate, and Luxol fast blue-PAS) to obtain a complete picture. Marchi's method for degenerated myelin requires a dichromate mordant which oxidizes normal myelin and blocks it from picking up the subsequent staining with osmium tetroxide. Degenerated myelin does not oxidize completely, and so it takes up the osmium tetroxide and becomes blackened.

Nissl Substance

Nissl substance or "tigroid" forms particulate clumps of material found in the cytoplasm of nerve cells. An absence of Nissl substance is an indication of degeneration of the nerve cells. Nissl substance will stain deeply with gallocyanin, thionine, toluidine blue, and methylene blue.

STAINS FOR NERVE TISSUE

Nerve fibers: will stain with Bodian's silver nitrate method
Nissl substance: Einarson's gallocyanin
Myelin: Luxol fast blue
Degenerated myelin: Marchi's method
Glial cells: Holzer's stain
Astrocytes: Cajal's gold sublimate method
General morphologic stain for central nervous system tissue is hematoxylin and eosin.

COMPONENTS OF CELLS OR TISSUE

Ameba

It is a one-celled protozoan animal. One type, parasitic in man, causes amebic dysentery. STAINING PROPERTIES: Amebae can be stained selectively with iron hematoxylin (Heidenhain's), phosphotungstic acid hematoxylin (PTAH), Best's carmine, and the PAS stain; the last two stain because of the glycogen content present in amebae.

Amyloid

Amyloid is an extracellular, abnormal protein complex deposited in various tissues, particularly in and around blood vessels, in certain disease states. Its name derives from the starchlike staining with iodine. The organs affected vary with the disease. The composition is uncertain and may vary from case to case.

When staining for amyloid, cut sections at 10 to 12μ, particularly if the quantity of material to be examined is small. STAINING PROPERTIES: (1) In the fresh state both glycogen and amyloid will stain mahogany-brown with iodine solutions. With amyloid this brown color turns blue if the material is subsequently treated with sulfuric acid. (2) Amyloid is metachromatic, presumably owing to the presence of acid mucopolysaccharides. It will show a metachromatic reaction with methyl violet, crystal violet, or methyl green. (3) Amyloid has an affinity for the dye Congo red and for cotton textile dyes. (4) Amyloid is both birefringent and dichroic, i.e., two colors or a change of color is evident under polarized light. If, after staining with Congo red, there remains a question as to the identity of the Congo red-stained material, the section should be examined under polarized light where it will produce a green, crumpled tinfoil appearance. (5) Amyloid will fluoresce a bright silvery blue to yellow when stained with the fluorochrome Thioflavin T.

Bacteria

ACID FAST. Most bacteria when placed in carbol fuchsin for a sufficient time will stain deeply. However, nearly all bacteria except tuberculosis and leprosy bacilli lose their color when treated immediately thereafter with an acid. *Mycobacteria tuberculosis* and *M. leprae* are thus often termed "acid fast." While it is a controversial subject, acid-fastness is most often attributed to the fatty capsule which surrounds these mycobacteria. STAINING PROPERTIES: The organisms will stain specifically with Ziehl-Neelsen, Kinyoun's and Fite's carbol fuchsin methods, and Truant's fluorochrome method, using auramine-rhodamine.

GRAM-POSITIVE AND GRAM-NEGATIVE BACTERIA.   The staining of bacteria falls into two groups, "Gram-positive" and "Gram-negative." In the Gram staining techniques an iodine solution is used to alter methyl or crystal violet so that the dye is retained by certain bacteria. Those bacteria retaining the dye are said to be Gram-positive. A Gram-positive organism is one stained with a basic aniline dye that *will not* be extracted from this iodine-dye-protein complex by alcohol. STAINING PROPERTIES: In addition to the Gram staining mentioned, bacteria will also be stained by the azure-eosin dye combinations, such as the Giemsa, May-Grünwald, and Mallory's phloxine methylene blue methods. Gram stains include the Brown and Brenn and Weigert-Gram techniques.

Bone Marrow

The azure-eosin staining techniques are widely used for the study of the morphology of all hematopoietic tissues (blood, spleen, and bone marrow cells). These include May-Grünwald, Mallory's phloxine methylene blue (PMB), Wolbach's modification of the Giemsa stain, and Lillie's azure A-eosin B techniques. Bone and bone marrow will stain nicely with a routine hematoxylin and eosin stain, but the methods listed provide more definitive staining of mast cells, basophil leukocyte granules, lymphocytes, and plasma cells.

Chromaffin

Chromaffin cells are found in the gastrointestinal tract, adrenal medulla, and retroperitoneal tissues. The variety found in the gastrointestinal tract is termed enterochromaffin cells. The substances found in these cells are called chromaffin because they are stained brown following oxidation by chromate solutions. In the natural or unfixed state they are colorless but will turn deep brown following chromate fixation. This is the Henle "chromaffin reaction." All chromaffin cells are argentaffin (have the capacity of reducing ammoniacal silver nitrate to black metallic silver without the addition of a reducing agent). STAINING PROPERTIES: Chromaffin will stain green-blue with Schmorl's azure eosin stain, is positive with the Schmorl ferricyanide reduction reaction, will stain bright purplish red in the Azan stain, is often PAS-positive, and, because it is argentaffin, will be stained black with the Fontana-Masson silver nitrate technique.

Fibrin

This is a specific fibrous protein derived from fibrinogen of the blood and it occurs in clots and certain acute inflammatory states. STAINING PROPERTIES: It stains pink and is not readily identifiable with the routine hematoxylin and eosin or the azure-eosin staining techniques. Although acidophilic in staining property, fibrin will stain selectively with hematoxylin in Mallory's phosphotungstic acid-hematoxylin stain, is PAS-positive, and will stain deep blue to black in the Weigert-Gram stain for fibrin.

Fungi

These masses comprise a group of living organisms resembling yeasts or molds, some of which are pathogenic in man. STAINING PROPERTIES: Most fungi will stain with hematoxylin on a routine H and E stain. The fungal capsules and walls are rich in polysaccharides, which explains why they are selectively stained with the Gridley, Bauer, alcian blue-PAS and McManus periodic acid-Schiff methods. Grocott's method will stain fungi and the azure-eosin techniques will also stain some species of fungi.

STAINS FOR FUNGI

Grocott, Bauer, and Gridley methods: will stain mycelial fungi and yeasts

Wolbach's Giemsa and the phloxine methylene blue of Mallory: will stain cryptococcus, actinomyces, and *Histoplasma capsulatum*

Brown and Brenn: will stain filaments of Nocardia and actinomyces

Ziehl-Neelsen and Kinyoun's stains: will stain *Nocardia asteroides* and *Nocardia brasiliensis*

Mayer's mucicarmine: will stain cryptococcus

Glycogen

Glycogen is a colorless carbohydrate cell product related to starch and dextrin commonly found in liver cells. It is water-soluble unless bound with protein complexes. It is a *neutral* polysaccharide. STAINING PROPERTIES: In the fresh state, glycogen will stain mahogany-brown with iodine solution. It is strongly PAS-positive. It stains positively with Best's carmine stain. Glycogen can be digested out of a tissue section with malt diastase (page 265) or with the ptyalin in sputum. Use of the enzyme to remove the glycogen from the sections serves as a control. Amebae will be stained by Best's carmine method because of their glycogen content.

Mast Cells

These cells occur individually in connective tissues and smooth muscle. They resemble monocytes with hematoxylin and eosin, but with special stains such as the Giemsa, the cytoplasm is seen to be filled with prominent granules. Mast cells produce or store histamine, heparin, and protein-digesting enzymes, which on discharge affect inflammatory reactions. STAINING PROPERTIES: Mast cells, presumably because of their heparin content, will be stained by any stain specific for acid polysaccharides, and for the same reason will stain metachromatically with the thiazine group and other basic dyes. Some metachromasia is alcohol labile, i.e., the dyes will be leached out by alcoholic dehydration. Metachromasia can be preserved by air-drying sections prior to clearing and coverslipping. An alternate to air-drying is the use of acetone for dehydration, avoiding the loss of stain due to the alcohols.

Mucin

Mucin is a carbohydrate. It can be either an acid or neutral mucopolysaccharide or a mucoprotein. It is found in many secretions, such as saliva and sputum, in gastric and intestinal contents, in the colonic lining layer, and in cervical and vaginal fluid. It occurs in benign and malignant tumors, such as in certain adenocarcinomas which are mucin-producing. Connective tissue mucin is practically the same as ground substance (page 187). Thus, some mucin will be colored by stains for connective tissue ground substance and epithelial mucin by Mayer's mucicarmine stain. Epithelial mucins will also be stained by the PAS method. Alcian blue will stain connective tissue chondroitin and mucoitin sulfuric acid mucins.

Plasma Cell

A plasma cell is a modified lymphoid cell present in the blood only in certain diseases, being more commonly found in connective tissue. The cell has a strongly basophilic cytoplasm with a heavy chromatin pattern radially placed like the spokes of a wheel. STAINING PROPERTIES: It will stain specifically with the azure-eosin stains like Wolbach's modification of the Giemsa stain or Mallory's methylene blue. Methyl green pyronin will also stain the plasma cell.

PIGMENTS

Calcium

Small calcific deposits in tissue are frequently present in placenta, thyroid, ovary, cysts, and prostatic curettings. STAINING PROPERTIES: Calcium salts will stain deep blue with alum hematoxylin and are readily identified on the routine H and E stain. Two special stains used to identify small or equivocal deposits as calcium are Alizarin red S, (which like hematoxylin forms a dye lake with the calcium) and the von Kossa silver nitrate stain, which actually demonstrates the presence of phosphates or carbonates, rather than calcium, which are reduced to metallic silver.

The use of fixatives containing calcium carbonate, calcium acetate, or calcium chloride may produce pseudocalcium crystals which could be misleading.

Carbon

An exogenous pigment, it can be found in lungs and axillary and mediastinal lymph nodes. It is black and cannot be bleached out or dissolved with any known solvents. When found increased in the areas above the condition is termed anthracosis.

Ceroid

Yellow globules which give off a natural green-yellow fluorescence, ceroid is PAS-positive, stains with acid-fast stains, and is sudanophilic.

Hemofuscin

A hematogenous pigment occurring as light yellow granules, it *will not* react positively to iron-staining reaction (Prussian blue).

Hemosiderin

A hematogenous pigment occurring as bright yellowish brown granules and masses, it *will* react positively to iron-staining reaction. For maximum preservation fix tissue in 10% buffered formalin.

Lipofuscin

A pigment found in heart, liver, and other cells of older people, it is called wear-and-tear pigment. Lipofuscin will generally stain PAS-positive. Some lipofuscins are sudanophilic. They are insoluble in dilute acids and alcohols.

Melanin

A dark brown natural pigment that is found in cells (skin, hair, choroid, and iris of eye) as brown or black granules, the pigment is very difficult to extract but will bleach slowly in strong oxidizers like hydrogen peroxide and potassium permanganate. STAINING PROPERTIES: Melanin is both argentaffin and argyrophilic (page 384). Melanin-producing cells contain the enzyme dopa oxidase, which can be localized histochemically. Melanins will also chelate ferrous iron. Melanin can be demonstrated by the Fontana-Masson method, the Schmorl reduction test, and the ferrous iron method. When possible, a known control should be run with the test section.

Silica

Silica crystals are readily detected in routine paraffin sections when they are examined by polarized light. They have a distinctive needle or broken-glass configuration.

Urates

Sodium urate is a clinical finding in gout, particularly in masses called tophi. Urates have the ability to reduce silver nitrate (Gomori silver methenamine method) and blacken the urate crystals. Urates can be distinguished from carbonates and phosphates by their solubility in dilute lithium carbonate. Recommended fixative is absolute alcohol, for the crystals are slightly soluble in water.

Staining

The object of staining is to identify different tissue components by their color reactions.

The staining techniques presented on the following pages represent a compilation of methods that have proved to give consistently reliable results. They are the stains most often required in a routine pathology laboratory. For registration examinations as well as for general purposes, it is necessary to know the constituents, procedures, and results of these staining methods. If possible, the student should execute each stain several times to become thoroughly familiar with it. The appendix of the book contains more advanced staining techniques and stains which are required less often.

For practical purposes, the paraffin method is regarded as the predominant procedure in microtechnique. Other methods are of special application only. For this reason most of the techniques quoted are for paraffin-embedded sections.

STAINING REACTIONS, METHODS, AND TYPES

Staining Reactions

Staining reactions in histologic studies may be accomplished by:

ABSORPTION OR DIRECT STAINING. The tissue is soaked in and becomes *penetrated* by the dye solution. The tissue becomes colored but is otherwise unchanged.

INDIRECT STAINING. The staining reaction is dependent on the use of intermediary treatment with a *mordant,* usually a heavy metal.

PHYSICAL STAINING. This is simple solubility of the dye in the elements of the cell. For instance, dyes for fat stains are more soluble in the fat than they are in the solvents used for their preparation.

CHEMICAL STAINING. A new substance is formed which is usually irreversible. Examples are the Prussian blue reaction and the periodic acid-Schiff reaction.

ADSORPTION PHENOMENA. Adsorption is accumulation on the surface of the component. Staining is brought about or influenced by the affinity of acids to bases and bases to acids (electrical attraction), so that (predictably) certain ions will be adsorbed by some substances much more readily than by others. This is perhaps the explanation of much of our differential staining.

The mechanism of staining is accomplished by both physical and chemical reactions and may be brought about by only one of the factors mentioned or may be the result of a combination of penetration, adsorption, and chemical influence. Proportionately there are limited chemical staining reactions that are irreversible.

Staining Methods

Staining methods may be grouped as follows:

1. Vital staining
2. Routine staining
3. Special staining

VITAL STAINING. Vital stains are stains applied to living tissue. This is accomplished by injecting the staining solutions into some part of an animal body or by mixing the stain with living cells. This method of staining is primarily used for research purposes.

ROUTINE STAINING. A routine stain is one that stains the various tissue elements with little differentiation except between nucleus and cytoplasm. General relationships among cells, tissues, and organs are demonstrated. *Example:* Hematoxylin and eosin stain.

SPECIAL STAINING. Special or selective staining methods are of a more limited range. They demonstrate special features of the tissue such as bacteria, fungi, particular cell products, and microscopic intracellular and intercellular structures. *Example:* Feulgen stain for desoxyribonucleic acid.

Types of Staining

REGRESSIVE STAINING. In a regressive stain, the tissue is first over-stained and then partially decolorized. Differentiation is usually controlled visually by examination with a microscope. When regressive staining is employed, a sharper degree of differentiation is obtained than with progressive staining (page 209).

PROGRESSIVE STAINING. In progressive staining, once the dye is taken up by the tissue it is not removed. Differentiation in progressive staining relies solely on the selective affinity of dyes for different tissue elements. The tissue is left in the dye solution only until it retains the desired amount of coloration.

GENERAL STAINING INFORMATION

Staining is generally accomplished by soaking the tissue in a solution of a dye. Certain tissue components combine with the colored ions of the dye and become colored. In general the acidic (negatively charged) elements attract the cationic dyes, and the basic (positively charged) elements attract the anionic dyes. Ordinarily acid dyes stain the cytoplasmic components of tissue, and basic dyes stain the nuclei of cells. To provide a complete histologic picture, a combination of the dyes used sequentially is employed to define in contrasting colors both the acidophilic and basophilic constituents. Although basic dyes stain chromatin and acid dyes stain cytoplasm, cytoplasm frequently contains basophilic material which accepts a certain degree of basic dyes, otherwise differentiation would be unnecessary. Cytoplasmic basophilia is very marked in pancreatic cells, certain tumor cells, and embryonic tissue.

The depth of coloration will be influenced by chemical affinity, density of the component, and permeability of the component by the dye. Staining reactions are also strongly influenced by pH of reagents, by method of fixation, and by other procedures such as oxidation and reduction, which alter the molecular structure of the tissue protein. Commonly used oxidizers are ferric salts, sodium iodate, mercuric oxide, potassium permanganate, and chromic and picric acids. It is a rule of thumb not to save and reuse oxidizers.

Length of time required for staining tissues varies with the particular staining technique from a few seconds to 24 or more hours. Methods of fixation, processing, and the very nature of the tissue itself influence staining reactions so that in most cases absolute time factors cannot be given. In addition the strength of the dyes varies on standing, and dye lots may differ one from another. However, with a little experimenting, the individual laboratory will find the optimum time of staining with its particular method of processing tissue.

With most stains, if the slides appear insufficiently colored after staining and rinsing, they may be returned to the dye solution and restained. With some stains it will be wiser to decolorize the section completely and start over. Personal experience will provide the knowledge on which to base the decision.

Washing and Dehydration

The washing or rinsing of tissue sections following staining is a necessary part of most staining techniques. Excess dye, mordants, or other reagents may react unfavorably or precipitate when placed in the fluid employed in the next step of the technique. Rinsing also eliminates the carrying over of one dye solution into the next. It also forestalls dilution or alteration of a reusable stock stain.

Whereas ethyl alcohol and its dilutions are generally employed for dehydrating, methyl alcohol, isopropyl alcohol, tertiary butyl alcohol, and acetone are preferable in some selected staining techniques. The thiazine dyes (such as toluidine blue, thionine, and methylene blue) are dissolved or leached out of the sections if ethyl alcohol is employed as the dehydrant. When an *alcoholic dye solution* is used, one may have to overstain the tissue deliberately before dehydrating in alcohols, or dehydrate in acetone in order to retain the dye. Occasionally a technique may recommend blotting the tissue section dry immediately after staining, and placing it directly into absolute alcohol, avoiding the differentiating action of the 95% concentration.

Dye Solvents

Solvents of dyes are nearly always water and dilutions of *ethyl* alcohol. The majority of dyes are more soluble in water than in alcohol. Unless there are directions to the contrary, always make up aqueous solutions with distilled water. Although isopropanol may be substituted for ethyl alcohol in the dehydrating procedures prior to infiltration, it should not be used for preparation of alcoholic dye solutions or in making up acid alcohol.

In addition to the dye and its solvent, staining solutions often contain additives to preserve or stabilize the stain. Examples of preservatives are thymol, alcohol, and sodium salicylate. Glycerine is frequently added to retard oxidation and to stabilize the stain.

Counterstaining

A *counterstain* is the application to the original stain (usually a nuclear stain) of one or more additional stains that by contrast will bring out the differences between the various cell and tissue elements. These background stains are usually acidophilic solutions that color diffusely. It is advantageous to use dilute solutions for counterstaining or to shorten the staining time. A heavy or quick-acting counterstain can mask or cover up the nuclear detail unless staining is carefully controlled by dipping the sections rapidly, rinsing, and checking the results visually by examination with the microscope. For very exacting results, it is often preferable to eliminate counterstaining so as not to mask the very component to be isolated.

Storage and Reuse of Stains

Unless there are specific instructions to the contrary, most stains can be saved and reused until they show signs of losing their staining capability. Before placing sections in stains that are to be reused, rinse slides with distilled water and drain. Once a staining solution begins to show a precipitate or gives poor staining results, it should be discarded and replaced with a fresh solution. All bottles of staining solutions should be clearly labeled and dated at time of preparation. All ripened solutions of hematoxylin should be stored in brown bottles in the dark to prevent further oxidation.

Some stains require a "ripening" period before they reach peak performance. If spontaneous ripening of solutions is preferred over chemical means, it will be necessary to anticipate the need by several weeks or months (as in the PTAH stain), and keep a supply ahead. Other stains that improve on standing are Guard's stain and the aceto-orcein stain, both of which are used for sex chromatin determinations, and toluidine blue and thionine. In our laboratory we make up 1000 ml. of Mallory's phosphotungstic acid-hematoxylin stain (PTAH) and allow it to ripen spontaneously for 4 to 6 months. If you are starting a new batch of PTAH, you can accelerate the ripening by adding a small aliquot of a fully oxidized PTAH solution. When the solution is a rich purple, we remove 100 ml. to a separate container. The remainder (or stock solution) is stored in the dark. As the solution is used, a mark is placed on the label. After the solution has been used 10 to 15 times, we discard the 100 ml. aliquot. We then wash and dry the container and remove and filter into it an additional 100 ml. from the stock storage bottle. In this way we avoid dilution of the original solution. The same method of control may be used for any reusable stock solution so as to maintain its potency.

Most staining solutions are stored at room temperature. Solutions that require refrigeration are Schiff's reagent, Best's carmine, aldehyde fuchsin, methyl green, azocarmine, and the stock methenamine-silver nitrate solution of Gomori and Grocott. It is best to allow these refrigerated solutions to come to room temperature before immersing the slides in them.

Factors Influencing Staining Reactions

1. The components of the fixative used (reaction is intensified with formulas containing picric acid and potassium dichromate, as in Bouin's, Helly's, and Zenker's fluid)
2. pH of fixative
3. pH of solutions

4. Mordants

5. Chemicals or reagents which produce oxidation or reduction

Basic Staining Rules

1. Keep stains and solutions covered when not in use.

2. Filter stains before use.

3. After slides are removed from the drying oven, allow them to come to room temperature before placing in xylene.

4. Once the slides have been placed in the first xylene to remove the paraffin, do not allow them to dry out.

5. Make certain that the level of any solution used in staining completely covers the tissue on the slides.

6. Renew water baths after each rack of slides that has been processed.

7. Drain all slides (tilt rack over the solution, then blot bottom of tray with paper toweling) before moving on to the next solution.

8. Use the microscope. There is no quality control without one.

Coating Paraffin Sections with Celloidin (Collodionization)

Tissue sections which are inadequately fixed or torn or which have developed air bubbles beneath them are likely to float from the slides during staining. These sections may be more firmly attached to the slide by coating the slide with an 0.5% solution of celloidin (see "How To" chapter, page 284).

Alkaline reagents dissolve albumen, and sections may loosen or become detached from the slide while in the staining or dehydrating solutions. Therefore it is advisable to coat paraffin sections with a thin film of celloidin before treating with any of the alkaline silver methods to promote greater adhesion of the tissue to the slide. In our laboratory we process a duplicate on all sections to be stained with silver nitrate solutions, one with and one without the collodionization. Following staining and microscopic examination, we select the better slide and submit this to the pathologist. Some investigators (Pearse) recommend that sections that are to be stained for the purpose of demonstrating glycogen should also be collodionized. Bone sections which look as if they may become dislodged from the slide should also be treated with the celloidin solution.

Restaining

Fairly often a technician is required to restain a section that has been stained, coverslipped, and dried. See specific instructions in "How To" chapter, page 282.

Control Slides

Controls are very necessary for certain stains in order to establish a check on the staining solution or staining technique. To maintain such controls, secure a block of a known positive (e.g., a severe tuberculosis case). Cut a few slides and stain them to be certain that they are "positive." If the organisms are present, cut as many slides as possible from the block, recognizing that at some point in the series the control is likely to become "negative." Dry, label, and store these slides in covered boxes identified as to the content. Process a control with the patient slide in question.

Screen the control and mark the positive area with a felt marking pen or a dot of India ink before presenting the slides to the pathologist. The laboratory should maintain a set of control slides on the following: acid-fast bacilli, iron pigment (Fe control), amyloid, glycogen, bacteria, fungi, and if possible, spirochetes and coccidioides. A section of colon may be used as a mucin control. A section of duodenum or a cross section (with tunica muscularis) of appendix will serve as control material for PAS-staining.

Avoiding Stains on the Skin

Dye stains on the hands are to be avoided. In addition to the obvious stigma of poor technique, there is a health hazard. Dyes are slowly absorbed by the skin and may eventually produce injurious effects. The prompt local application of 0.5% acid alcohol followed by flushing with running tap water will usually be effective in removing most dyes.

Clorox will remove some stubborn stains. As a preventive measure, wear disposable plastic gloves when handling dye solutions and slides.

Maintaining a File of Staining Information

Save reference information on all stains or techniques on cards or in a notebook. An index card filing system is a convenient and rapid reference file. Each card should bear the following information: title of the technique or stain; author's name; and title, volume number, date, and pages of the journal or book from which the stain was taken.

A typewritten Procedure Manual should be maintained and updated on all procedures routinely performed in the laboratory.

DIFFICULTIES IN STAINING

Tissues may be difficult to stain for the following reasons:

1. The staining solution may have deteriorated and needs replacing.
2. The staining solution may not be "ripe." This is particularly true in dye solutions employing hematoxylin.
3. The decalcifying solution or the fixative, may not have been washed out thoroughly. For instance, picric acid and potassium dichromate solutions stain (or color) tissues.
4. The tissue may be inadequately fixed, allowing autolysis to take place and impairing staining.
5. Tissues that have been stored for long periods in 70% alcohol or 10% formalin do not accept the dye solutions readily; consequently they frequently require special handling (see "How To" chapter, pages 276 and 283).

STAINING TERMINOLOGY

MORDANT. A mordant links the dye more strongly to the tissue. The mordant may be applied to the tissue before the stain (as in chromate, mercurial, or picric acid fixation), or it may be included as part of the staining technique or in the dye solution itself. Mercury, chromium, aluminum, iron, and in fact salts of most metals are employed as mordants. The reaction or compound that results in the combination of the mordant and dye is known as a "lake." Some tissues require a mordant in order to accept the dye at all (Fig 14-1). In other instances, the mordant is used to ensure a specific staining reaction (page 389).

A.
DIRECT STAINING

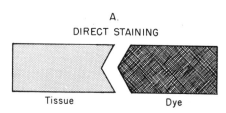

Tissue   Dye

Figure 14-1.   Mordanting process

B.
INDIRECT STAINING

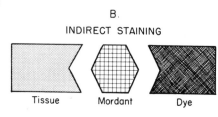

Tissue   Mordant   Dye

DECOLORIZATION.   Decolorization is the partial or the complete removal of the stain from tissue sections. When the color is removed selectively (usually with microscopic control) it is called *differentiation*. When sections are to be restained with a technique different from the original, they are completely decolorized. Alcohol made slightly acid by the addition of hydrochloric acid (0.5% and 1.0% solutions) is perhaps the most used agent for extraction of excess color. (See "How To" chapter, pages 282–283.)

DIFFERENTIATION.   In *regressive staining,* differentiation is the removal or washing out of excess stain until the color is retained only by the tissue components that are to be studied. This is generally accomplished with acid alcohol, ethyl alcohol, or dilutions of the mordant previously applied to the tissue. When one differentiates in the mordant originally used to bind the dye to the tissues, the dye is gradually drawn from the tissue to combine with the free mordant in solution.

Also, basic dyes may be differentiated by a weakly acid medium and acid dyes by a weakly basic one.

Whatever the solution, the slide is immersed in the differentiator, withdrawn into the atmosphere, and reimmersed in the solution. Exposure to the air may oxidize and improve the differentiation. The slide is kept in constant motion so that decolorization will be even. Both differentiation and depth of coloration are visually controlled by examination with a microscope.

Following differentiation of some stains, it will be necessary to run the slides very rapidly through the alcohols to prevent loss of the stain. Dehydration with acetone, tertiary butyl alcohol, clove oil, aniline, or equal parts of absolute alcohol and xylene is recommended in some staining procedures to avoid this loss.

BASOPHILIC.   Substances so described are stainable with basic dyes and are substances which are usually acid in nature.

ACIDOPHILIC.   Substances so described are stainable with acid dyes and are substances that are usually basic in nature.

SUDANOPHILIC.   Substances so described are stainable with oil soluble dyes such as Sudan III, Sudan IV, Sudan Black B, and Oil red O.

ARGYROPHILIC.   Substances so described are stainable with silver nitrate solutions (see Glossary, page 384).

ARGENTAFFIN.   Substances so described are stainable with silver nitrate solutions *without* chemical reduction procedures (see Glossary, page 384).

METACHROMATIC.   Substances so described will stain in a color or hue different from that of the staining solution itself. For instance, mast cell granules will stain selectively red-violet to red when stained with toluidine blue. The primary group of substances which shows metachromasia is acid mucopolysaccharides.

DYES

Dyes are ordinarily divided into classes, **natural** and **synthetic,** and categorized by their affinity for certain tissue components, **acidic** and *basic.* They may be further classified by their chemical composition (e.g., thiazine, azo, rosaniline, and so on) or according to their main application (oil-soluble dyes or fluorescent dyes). Synthetic dyes usually have greater staining power and permit a broader spectrum of color than natural dyes. The nomenclature of biological stains is confusing because many different names apply to the same dye or stain. For instance, crystal violet is synonymous with gentian and methyl violet. The Harleco Company * has tried to eliminate some of this confusion by listing their catalogue of dyes under the most common name and cross referencing them under their synonyms.

A further aid in exactly identifying a biological stain or dye is by the use of its color index number. This is indicated by the initials *C.I.* followed by a series of numerals, e.g., *Eosin Y, C.I. 45380.* The Biological Stain Commission has done much to standardize the variance in dyes. They assay batches of dyes and stains for chemical and optical properties. Those tested and approved by the Commission bear the label *Certified* and give the user some assurance of the quality and performance of the particular dye lot. The handbook *Biological Stains* (Conn, H.J., Williams & Wilkins, Baltimore, 1969) presents a comprehensive syllabus of dyes and their properties, and the student is referred to this text for more complete study.

Dyes should be bought only in a quantity that is likely to be used up within the year. It is good practice to date all bottles of dye on receipt and store in a cool dark place.

Natural Dyes

Natural dyes are few in number, the most important being hematoxylin and carmine. Hematoxylin is derived from the core of the logwood tree. Carmine (carminic acid) is a scarlet dye made from the ground bodies of cochineal beetles. Both are nuclear (basic) stains. Hematoxylin is not a true dye until partially oxidized (ripened) either by exposure to air or by chemical means. Both hematoxylin and carmine are usually combined with aluminum or iron salts (mordants) when employed for histologic staining. When hematoxylin is com-

* Biological Stains, Harleco, 60th and Woodland Avenue, Philadelphia, Pa. 19143.

bined with alum, a blue color lake results. When combined with ferric salts the dye solution is black.

Orcein and saffron also are natural dyes. Orcein is made from lichens and requires oxidation to develop its blue-violet color. Orcein combined with weak hydrochloric acid is used for staining elastic tissue. Saffron is obtained from the dried stigmas of a species of crocus and is yellow-red to yellow in its dry orthochromatic state and yellow in solution. With the exception of hematoxylin, all of these natural dyes have synthetic counterparts.

Aniline and Other Synthetic Dyes

Aniline is a colorless coal-tar derivative. It is the base from which many brilliant synthetic dyes are made. Aniline dyes offer a wide range in both color and action. The chemical composition of the dyes may be basic (cationic), acid (anionic), or neutral (amphoteric). The effect of acid dyes will be intensified in a solution the reaction of which is acid, and basic dyes stain more intensely in alkaline solutions. The staining persuasion of the amphoteric dyes can easily be shifted by the pH of the fluid in which they are placed.

BASIC STAIN. In a basic stain, it is the base of the dye that contains the coloring substance. Basic colors stain nuclei, basophil granules, and bacteria. The acidic components in tissue attract basic dyes.

ACID STAIN. In an acid stain, it is the acid component or anion that contains the coloring matter. Acid dyes stain cytoplasm diffusely and have an affinity for acidophil granules. The acid stains provide effective contrast to the nuclear stain. The basic components in tissue attract acid dyes.

METACHROMATIC DYES. Certain dyes have the valuable property of staining a variety of tissue components in hues or colors different from that of the staining solution itself. *For example,* thionine which is blue in its orthochromatic state will stain different tissue constituents with colors ranging from blue to red-violet. Nearly all metachromatic dyes are basic.

POLYCHROMATIC DYES. These are compound dyes or dye mixtures that contain the components of different colors. *For example,* the

Acid Dyes
(usually cytoplasmic)

Acid fuchsin
Aniline blue
Biebrich scarlet R
Congo red
Eosin B
Eosin Y
Fast green FCF
Light green, SF yellowish
Metanil yellow
Methyl blue
Orange G
Phloxine B
Picric acid
Ponceau S

Basic Dyes
(usually nuclear)

Alcian blue
Azure A
Azure C
Basic fuchsin
Bismarck brown
Carmine (carminic acid)
Celestin blue B
Cresyl violet
Crystal violet
Gallocyanine
Janus green B
Luxol fast blue
Malachite green
Methyl green
Methyl violet
Methylene blue
Neutral red
Nile blue sulfate
Pyronin (weakly basic)
Orcein
Safranine O
Thionine
Toluidine blue O

Fluorescent Dyes
(fluorochromes)

Acridine orange
Auramine O
Fluorescein
Rhodamine B
Sulforhodamine B
Thioflavin T

Metachromatic Dyes
(all basic)

Azure A
Azure B
Azure C
Basic fuchsin
Bismarck brown
Crystal violet
Methyl violet
Methylene blue
Thionine
Toluidine blue

Fat-Soluble Dyes

Sudan black B
Nile blue A
Oil red O
Scarlet B
Sudan III
Sudan IV

Giemsa stain is a combination of blue and red dyes of the thiazine and eosin groups.

FAT-SOLUBLE DYES.   These dyes are more readily soluble in the fats than they are in the solution in which they are used. The staining reaction is the simple absorption of the dye by the tissue lipids.

FLUORESCENT DYES.   A limited number of dyes (both acid and basic) have the property of fluorescing with ultraviolet light. They function as "tracers" in immunopathologic studies. Their use requires special treatment and equipment.

A partial list of numerous artificial dyes, classified according to their use, is given on p. 213.

METALLIC STAINS AND IMPREGNATIONS

A few metals can be used for staining specific tissue elements which do not stain readily with other methods. The salts are reduced to an opaque insoluble residue as a metal or metallic hydroxide in certain tissue elements or spaces. Thus the terms "impregnation" and "reduction" would be perhaps more accurate than "stain," for the coloring matter is held physically either as a precipitate or as a reduction product in certain tissue components. Although salts of osmium, mercury, lead, and uranium are sometimes used, the most valuable metal for this purpose is silver in the form of silver nitrate. The selectivity of silver nitrate for neurological staining, reticulum, spirochetes, fungi, melanin, urates, and argentaffin cells makes possible the staining of components not easily identified by other staining methods.

The ammoniacal silver nitrate solutions are most commonly employed. They are used for the impregnation of reticulum, central nervous system tissues, and argentaffin cells. However, silver nitrate is frequently combined with methenamine (after Gomori) in a variety of silvering procedures that are used for staining fungi, urates, and basement membranes. Simple aqueous silver nitrate solutions are used to demonstrate spirochetes and calcium salts. These solutions require *developing* with special reagents or strong light.

Although there are multiple formulas for the reticulum-staining solutions (diammine silver), they are nearly all either silver oxide or silver carbonate preparations. The silver is precipitated from the silver nitrate solution with sodium or potassium hydroxide (*silver oxide*) or with lithium carbonate (*silver carbonate*), and then the precipitate is dissolved with ammonia water. The minimum ammonia used to form the diammine silver radical is the ideal amount. Regardless of the method of preparation of the solution, the results are similar.

Silver Nitrate Solution Generalities

With all silver nitrate techniques, the following will apply:

1. Glassware must be chemically clean. Use the formula given on page 27 or clean glassware with concentrated nitric acid followed by several rinses in distilled water.
2. Triple distilled water should be used throughout.
3. The atmosphere should be dust-free.
4. Avoid the use of metal containers or forceps.
5. Only reagent grade silver nitrate should be used.
6. Because of high alkalinity of ammoniacal silver solutions, paraffin sections may loosen from the slides.
7. In the preparation of ammoniacal silver solutions it is better to leave a few granules of silver nitrate precipitate undissolved or have the solution faintly turbid or opalescent than have it completely clear. If the solution is absolutely clear, add a few more drops of the silver nitrate until the solution shows a faint turbidity.

Time Factors

1. Staining solutions range in strength from 1% (Foot's) to 10% (Laidlaw's), so that the time necessary for impregnation will vary with the technique used, from 1 minute to 2 hours or longer.
2. Incubating at higher than room temperature shortens the impregnation time.
3. Leaving the sections in the solution for too long will reduce their specificity. Different tissue components require different time intervals for impregnation, e.g., nerve endings will require much longer staining time than reticulum. Davenport recommends that the technician who

is working with a substance with which she is unfamiliar take three slides and impregnate at different time intervals.

4. With some silver techniques a yellow to brown coloration of the tissue will be evident after a period of time in the silver solution, alerting the technician that impregnation has taken place. With other silvering methods the section will show no color change until it is placed in the developer.

Specificity

1. Too much ammonia will inhibit proper impregnation. The more ammonia used, the lighter the staining result.

2. Insufficient rinsing after immersion in silver nitrate solutions leaves sections too dark. Sections should be carefully rinsed.

3. Leaving sections in the solution longer than necessary for a particular component will produce overstaining and reduce specificity.

Fixation

Most techniques stipulate formalin fixation, although Laidlaw specified Bouin's fluid for his reticulum method, and Foot recommended Zenker's solution.

Oxidizers and Sensitizers

Nearly all reticulum methods employ oxidizers or sensitizers prior to impregnation with silver nitrate. These are potassium permanganate, ammonioferric alum, sodium iodate, potassium dichromate, and uranium nitrate. Following impregnation, nearly all reticulum methods reduce the silver nitrate with a dilution of formalin. Some cell components (argentaffin) have the inherent ability to reduce the silver, and these require no chemical reduction.

Gold Toning

Nearly all silvering techniques are followed by supplementary treatment in gold chloride. The gold chloride "tones" the silver, turning it gray. The gold chloride eliminates the yellow background, gives greater transparency, and improves differentiation. Tissue sections should be carefully washed before placing them in the gold chloride solution and need be left in it not longer than 5 minutes.

Sodium Thiosulfate

All methods remove unreduced silver with sodium thiosulfate (hypo). A bath of 1 to 2 minutes is probably completely adequate for this step. Lillie doubts that any considerable amount of reducible silver remains but concedes that it is traditional with silver nitrate techniques.

STAINING PROCEDURE

While the steps of the various staining methods differ somewhat, they may be roughly arranged in the following order:

1. Deparaffinization (with paraffin-embedded sections)
2. Staining
3. Decolorizing and differentiating
4. Dehydrating
5. Clearing
6. Mounting (coverslipping)

Deparaffinization

The following steps are required before staining cut sections of paraffin-embedded tissues. Once the paraffin has been removed from the sections, the slides must never be allowed to dry.

1. Pass slides through two changes of xylene to remove paraffin (2½ minutes in each).
2. Pass slides through two changes of absolute alcohol to remove xylene (2½ minutes in each).
3. Rinse sections in one or two changes of 95% alcohol (few dips).
4. If sections have been fixed in Zenker's fluid or any other fixative

containing mercuric chloride, place sections in an 0.5% solution of iodine in 80% alcohol for 5 to 10 minutes to remove the mercuric deposits. Iodine may be reused until it becomes light (page 28).

5. Rinse in 80% alcohol (few dips).

6. Remove iodine by treating the sections with a 5% aqueous solution of sodium thiosulfate (hypo) for 2 to 5 minutes or until the sections are bleached.

7. Wash the slides carefully but thoroughly in running tap water to remove hypo (2 to 5 minutes). The sections are now ready to be stained.

EQUIPMENT FOR STAINING

Unlike the procedure followed in the celloidin method, paraffin sections are mounted and stained on the slide. Paraffin sections are usually stained in slotted glass dishes or in metal or glass staining racks.

The slotted glass dishes hold from 5 to 19 slides, over which the different solutions are poured. The slides are placed on end singly or in staggered fashion in the dishes (Fig. 14-2).

Metal or glass staining racks or carriers that hold from 10 to 30 slides upright are transferred to appropriate-sized glass dishes containing solutions necessary for the staining procedure. These are very convenient for the technician who must process large numbers of slides.

Slides may be stained by employing a series of Coplin jars filled with the various reagents. These slotted jars hold from 5 to 9 slides. The slides are individually passed through the series, differentiation being controlled with the microscope. The use of Coplin jars is desirable for special stains.

COVERSLIPPING

The purpose of a coverglass is to preserve the mounted tissue section and to provide a transparent surface through which it can be examined under the microscope. The coverglass is cemented to the

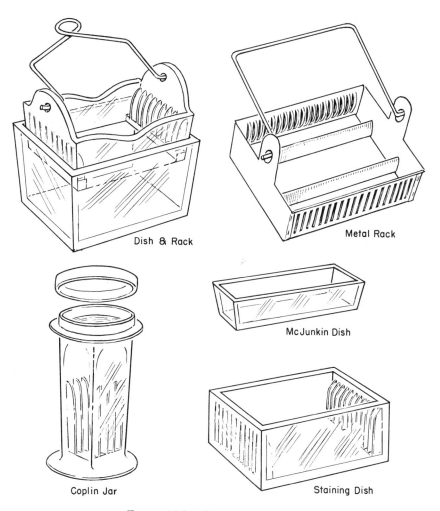

Dish & Rack

Metal Rack

McJunkin Dish

Coplin Jar

Staining Dish

Figure 14-2.   Staining equipment

slide with a mounting reagent. The size of the coverslip is dependent on the size of the tissue section to be covered. It should be large enough to leave a margin of several millimeters around the tissue.

Regardless of the technique used for coverslipping, some general rules apply to all methods.

1. Work on a clean, flat surface, such as a lint-free, white, folded towel. The coverglasses should be clean and loose on the towel.

2. The mounting medium should be of good spreading consistency — not too thick, nor too thin. It should drop readily off the rod. If the media is too thin the solvent will evaporate, leaving air spaces. If it is too thick it will not spread evenly. *Note:* To thicken, remove cover and allow some of the solvent to evaporate. To thin, dilute with a few drops of xylene.

3. The size of the drop of mounting media must be sufficient to occupy the entire space between the coverglass and slide and will vary slightly with the size of the coverglass used. Experience is necessary to obtain a complete film without excess.

4. After the slide is removed from the last clearing solution (xylene), wipe extra sections that will not fit under the coverglass from the slide with a clean piece of gauze. At the same time wipe the underside of the slide to remove any adherent particles of tissue or stain. Reimmerse in xylene.

5. Following application of the coverslip, excess mounting media must be cleaned from the slide. The coverglass will not move as much if a few minutes' drying time has elapsed. Clean coverglass edges if necessary with a camel's-hair brush moistened with xylene, or cover fingernail of index finger with gauze moistened with xylene and gently wipe edges. A light touch is necessary so as not to disturb the coverglass.

6. Do not allow tissue to dry out at any time during coverslipping or it may later become opaque.

Method A

1. Place a small round drop of the mounting reagent in the center of the lower extreme edge of a clean *coverglass* (Fig. 14-3).

2. Rinse slide in xylene, drain, and bring the slide up to the edge of the coverslip. Invert the slide so that the mounting reagent just touches it. Gently complete the inversion. The coverslip should cover the entire section. If possible, mount so that on completion the top edge of the coverslip is aligned with the top edge of the slide. Any air bubbles that may be present must be gently eased out from beneath the coverslip. If bubbles cannot be easily removed, place the slide back into the xylene until the coverslip drops off, rinse, and remount.

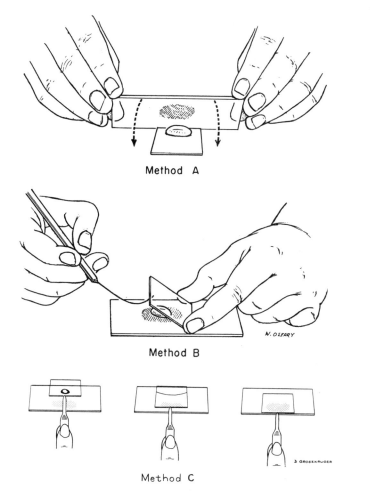

Method A

Method B

Method C

Figure 14-3. *Coverglass technique*

Method B

1. Place the slide flat on the towel. Place a round drop of mounting reagent over the center of the tissue section. With the aid of a histologist's pick, lower a clean coverglass so that it completely covers the tissue section. Lower the left side of the coverglass first with the right side following.

Method C

1. Position the slide with the labeling or frosted end to the left. Place a drop of Permount just above the tissue section.

2. With a fine forceps, pick up coverslip by its extreme lower edge (centrally) and line up top edge of coverslip to the globule of mounting medium.

3. Draw coverslip down, lower it at the same time, and draw the mounting media down to and position it evenly over the tissue section. Media and coverglass are both brought flush to the lower edge of the slide.

4. Check for air bubbles. If necessary, clean as described.

MOUNTING REAGENTS

In order for tissue to be preserved and studied under the microscope, it must be mounted in a suitable medium. The mounting medium permeates the tissue spaces, improving the index of refraction. Resins, natural or synthetic, are dissolved in a solvent that will be miscible with the clearing agent (xylene). As the slide dries, most of the solvent from the mounting medium evaporates, leaving the sections enclosed in an almost solid substance. A good mounting reagent will dry quickly, will have a suitable index of refraction, and will not discolor or fade tissue sections. Setting of the mounting medium can be accelerated by placing the slides flat in the paraffin oven or incubator or on a hot plate at temperatures not exceeding 45°C.

Mounting Reagents for Permanent Mounts

Permanent mounting reagents can be used only if slides have been dehydrated and cleared in xylene prior to mounting. These mounting reagents may be purchased ready to use, or the dry resins or crystals may be purchased, and solutions prepared to the consistency preferred. The resin or crystals are dissolved in xylene, toluene, or benzene in excess. The solution is then filtered through fine gauze and allowed to evaporate to the proper consistency under dust-free conditions.

NATURAL RESINS. (Canada balsam, gum dammar). Natural resins are rarely used, for they are acid, and yellow or darken with age. The ideal mounting medium is neutral. An acid mounting medium will cause fading of basic dyes, and basic mounting media will fade acid dyes.

SYNTHETIC RESINS. (Pro-Texx, Permount, Histoclad, Harleco Synthetic Resin). Synthetic resins are neutral and do not darken or become acidic with age. They will not affect stains, are less viscous, and dry faster. The high melting point of the synthetic mounting media makes them preferable for microprojection, with no fear of melting or creating bubbles.

Water-Soluble Mounting Reagents for Specific Purposes (Syrup Mounts)

Frozen sections mounted directly from water, or paraffin sections which must not be dehydrated or cleared in the usual manner (e.g., Lieb crystal violet stain) require special mounting reagents, such as glycerin, gum syrup, Brun's fluid, or commercially available water-soluble mountants such as Paragon, Aquamount, Abopon, and Clearcol (page 92). These reagents are miscible with water, hold the coverslip in position, and improve the refractive index. They are not permanent preparations but may be preserved for varying periods of time by sealing the edges of the coverslip with nail polish.

HOW TO APPROACH A NEW STAINING TECHNIQUE

1. Read over technique, being mindful that some staining solutions require aging or extended periods of oxidation before they are useful.

2. If possible, obtain the original article in which the technique was published and read it through, for it may provide you with additional insight into the method.

3. Do not be intimidated by instructions that say "stain for 30 minutes to 3 hours." The instruction is probably valid insofar as the author is concerned, for in the case of dyes, all lots are not necessarily

identical and methods of fixing and processing alter staining affinity. Recognize that there are no absolutes and nearly all staining techniques will require some minor modification in your particular laboratory.

4. Obtain a tissue block of the appropriate material from the pathologist and cut at least 10 to 20 slides of the tissue.

5. Make up solutions exactly to technique specifications. On first trial make no substitutions in percentages, reagents, or time intervals.

6. Process one slide following the directions exactly. Compare your results with those cited in the technique. If you have not obtained comparative results, do not discount the technique as being unworkable or unreliable.

7. If time interval instructions range from 1 to 2 hours or more, spot check at 15-minute intervals.

8. Compare modifications of the staining method which may have been made by investigators other than the originator.

9. To determine the problem, attack only one step at a time until it is resolved.

Problems and Possible Solutions

1. If the material was not initially fixed in accord with recommendations of the author, postmordant the cut section in the proper fixative.

2. If there is *loss of a dye* counterstain, you will have to determine where or why the dye was lost. Process one or more slides, watching for the point at which the color is lost. Try to correct the deficiency by lengthening or shortening the time in one solution, or dilute the strength of the differentiator if you are losing color too fast at this stage. *Example:* If the solution in which the color is removed is 80% alcohol, substitute 95% alcohol to eliminate the water content as the problem. If this is unsuccessful perhaps it is the alcohol that is extracting the dye and you may need to dehydrate in acetone. Occasionally the dye is preserved by blotting the section with filter paper and transferring directly to absolute alcohol, eliminating intermediary strengths.

3. If on the other hand your material is *overstained,* you may need to shorten the staining time or dilute the strength of a certain dye solution. If your staining is too intense with the recommended strength

solution, dilute the dye solution with the appropriate solvent, e.g., if the stain is a 2.5% solution in 50% ethyl alcohol, try staining with a 1.5% strength in 50% ethyl alcohol. Or, you might increase the strength of the differentiator.

4. Keep notes on what has occurred and rewrite the procedure to fit your laboratory requirement.

Q U I Z

Staining

1. What is the purpose of staining?
2. What are meant by absorption staining, chemical staining, adsorption staining, and indirect staining?
3. a. Define a "routine" stain. b. Define a "special" stain.
4. How are sections deparaffinized prior to staining?
5. List two natural dyes and eight artificial dyes.
6. Name two metals which are used for metallic stains and impregnations.
7. a. Define a "basic" dye. b. Define an "acid" dye.
8. a. What is regressive staining?
   b. What is progressive staining?
9. Define a mordant.
10. What is a counterstain?
11. What is collodionization? For what purpose is it used?
12. What are "controls"? How are they used?
13. List several precautions in the use of silver nitrate solutions.
14. a. What stain would you employ for the following?
    b. What colors would result?

acid-fast bacilli	fibrils
amyloid	fungi
bone marrow	glycogen
connective tissue	hemosiderin
elastic tissue	nuclear stain
fat	reticulum

Mounting Reagents

1. What is the purpose of a mounting reagent?
2. What are the properties of a good mounting reagent?
3. List:
   a. Two natural-resin mounting mediums.
   b. Two synthetic-resin mounting mediums.
   c. Two water-soluble mounting reagents for frozen-section mounts.

ROUTINE HEMATOXYLIN STAINING

Hematoxylin, a natural dye, is perhaps the most used and most valuable staining reagent in histologic work today. Hematoxylin is used in combination with various metals, e.g., aluminum, iron, chromium, copper, and tungsten. Used alone, hematoxylin is a nonspecific stain; its selective staining power is dependent upon the metals with which it is combined.

The active coloring agent in most hematoxylin stains is *hematein.* Hematein is formed by means of oxidation, a process which takes a number of days or weeks and is spoken of as "ripening." This ripening can be accomplished rapidly by the use of certain oxidizing reagents such as potassium permanganate, sodium iodate, and mercuric oxide. Spontaneous ripening can be accomplished by exposure to light, air, and heat. Excessive oxidation (overripening) will render the stain useless.

There are several hematoxylin formulas — Harris's, Delafield's, Mayer's, and Weigert's, to name a few. Hematoxylin combined with aluminum salts will stain blue. Hematoxylin combined with ferric salts will stain blue-black. Those most commonly used employ aluminum as the metal component. Of these, Harris's hematoxylin is perhaps most in general use today.

The principle of the staining methods with the various solutions of alum hematoxylin are essentially the same. The time element depends primarily on the ripeness of the solution and on the fixative used. Generally, it will take from 1 to 15 minutes to stain the nuclei.

Hematoxylin may be applied as a progressive or as a regressive stain. When staining progressively, the slides are left in the hematoxylin only long enough to stain the nuclei blue. More often hematoxylin is used as a regressive stain; that is, the tissues are first overstained and then decolorized to remove the excess color. A dilute acid alcohol is usually employed to decolorize these sections. After the tissues have been decolorized they must be washed thoroughly to stop the acid action. From the wash they are blued in plain running tap water for several minutes, a saturated solution of lithium carbonate, or water that has been slightly alkalinized by the adding of a few drops of concentrated ammonium hydroxide. Method of blueing is optional.

Following blueing with either lithium carbonate or ammonia water, sections must be thoroughly washed. Any alkaline solution remaining on the sections will inhibit the acid (eosin) stain and produce fading on storage. Also, lithium carbonate crystals will form on the tissue if it is not washed free.

For routine studies eosin is usually the selected counterstain for hematoxylin.

Hematoxylin Staining Solutions

HARRIS'S ALUM HEMATOXYLIN

Hematoxylin	5.0 gm.
Absolute alcohol	50.0 ml.
Aluminum ammonium sulfate	100.0 gm.
Distilled water	1000.0 ml.
Mercuric oxide	2.5 gm.

Dissolve the hematoxylin in the alcohol with the aid of gentle heat. Dissolve the alum in the water by the aid of heat. When each is completely dissolved, combine the two solutions together in a large Pyrex Erlenmeyer flask (2000-ml. capacity). Bring the mixture to a boil as rapidly as possible. Turn off the flame. While moderate bubbling continues, add the mercuric oxide, *slowly* to prevent frothing or boiling over. The solution at once assumes a dark purple color. As soon as this occurs, cool the solution by plunging the flask at once into a tub of cold water. Allow cold water to run continuously from the tap into the tub. Rotate the flask in the cold water until the solution is cooled evenly throughout. As soon as it is cool the solution is ready for staining, but improves if it is allowed to stand for 2 to 3 days. To encourage ripening, stopper the flask lightly with a gauze square and leave flask where it will be exposed to light.

It is sometimes recommended that 5 ml. of glacial acetic acid be added to each 100 ml. of hematoxylin to increase the nuclear clarity. However, overstaining with hematoxylin, followed by partial decolorization in an acid bath (0.5% hydrochloric acid), will yield the same results. A disadvantage in the use of acetic acid in stock hematoxylin solutions is that it decreases the stability and shortens the life of the solution.

Ripened stock solutions of hematoxylin should be stored in airtight bottles away from the light to prevent further oxidation and deterioration of the stain. The dish of hematoxylin in the staining series can be replenished as needed by adding filtered stock solution to the dish.

Staining time: formalin fixation — approximately 1 to 6 minutes.
Helly or Zenker fixation — 15 seconds to 2 minutes.

TEST FOR STAINING POWER OF HEMATOXYLIN. According to McClung's text you may test the staining power of hematoxylin by adding a few drops of it to 50 ml. of tap water. If the hematoxylin is good, the water will turn a bright, clear purple or blue-violet color. Exhausted solutions will not be clear and bright, and the color will be rusty or green.

MAYER'S HEMATOXYLIN

(Progressive stain)

Hematoxylin	1.0 gm.
Distilled water	1000.0 ml.
Sodium iodate	0.2 gm.
Ammonium or potassium alum	50.0 gm.
Citric acid	1.0 gm.
Chloral hydrate *	50.0 gm.

Dissolve the hematoxylin in water with the aid of gentle heat. Add the sodium iodate and then the alum. Shake occasionally until the alum is dissolved, and then add the citric acid and the chloral hydrate. The color of the stain will be red-violet.

This solution keeps well.

Staining time: *3 to 5 minutes.* Wash thoroughly in tap water to blue. Before the wash, Mayer's hematoxylin will appear understained but the blueing in water deepens the coloration considerably. Allow for this by washing a minimum of 10 minutes.

* This is a hypnotic and may be obtained through the pharmacy or from Sigma Chemical Co., P.O. Box 14508, St. Louis, Mo. 63178, chloral hydrate crystals "for laboratory use."

WEIGERT'S IRON HEMATOXYLIN
(Progressive stain)

SOLUTION A

Hematoxylin	1 gm.
Alcohol, 95% ethyl	100 ml.

SOLUTION B

Ferric chloride (29% aqueous solution)	4 ml.
Distilled water	95 ml.
Hydrochloric acid, concentrated	1 ml.

Note: Lillie simplified the aqueous portion (Solution B) by using

Ferric chloride ($FeCl_3 \cdot 6H_2O$)	2.5 gm.
OR	
Ferric chloride ($FeCl_3$) anhydrous	1.5 gm.
and	
Distilled water	99.0 ml.
Hydrochloric acid, concentrated	1.0 ml.

Weigert's is a very popular and versatile nuclear stain. It is used in combination with many special staining techniques. Stock solutions of Solution A and Solution B may be prepared and stored separately at room temperature. They will keep well.

Just before use combine equal parts of Solution A and Solution B. Ferric salts oxidize hematoxylin immediately and the mixture will turn a deep black.

Staining time: 2 to 10 minutes, or until nuclei are black and distinct. Rinse slides in distilled water and check stain with microscope. If tissue is very chromatic and absorbs the dye solution so rapidly that it becomes overstained, the excess dye may be removed by differentiating the section in a dilution of the ferric chloride (approximately 2% solution).

LILLIE'S HEMATOXYLIN

Hematoxylin	5.0 gm.
Aluminum ammonium sulfate	50.0 gm.
Glycerol	300.0 ml.
Distilled water	700.0 ml.
Sodium iodate	0.5 gm.

Dissolve hematoxylin and ammonium alum in the distilled water. Add glycerol and ripening agent. Stain is ready for immediate use. Dilute the hematoxylin with distilled water, half and half, and filter before use.

EOSIN

Eosin, an acid synthetic dye, stains cytoplasm with different degrees of intensity. It stains readily and brilliantly after Zenker fixation. The reason for this is that heavy metals such as mercuric salts combine with acid groups and therefore increase acidophilia. A longer time is required to stain formalin-fixed tissue.

Eosin is one of the most valuable counterstains known. Besides its widespread use as a counterstain for hematoxylin and other basic (nuclear) dyes, it is used in a large number of blood stains, e.g., Giemsa, Jenner, and Wright stains.

Eosin is used in both aqueous and alcoholic solutions. It is usually employed in 0.5% and 1.0% solutions. However, when eosin (or phloxine) is applied before an aniline dye such as methylene blue, a strong 2.5% to 5% solution must be used. Overstaining is necessary here, since the subsequent treatment in methylene blue extracts much of the acid stain.

Some of the eosin stain is removed from the tissues rather rapidly when they are dehydrated in 95% ethyl alcohol and more slowly by absolute alcohol. Therefore, you must allow for this by slightly overstaining the sections and rapidly dehydrating them in the 95% alcohol and the absolute alcohol.

If sections become overstained with eosin and it cannot be readily removed in 95% alcohol, place sections in a dilute alkaline solution (0.1% ammonia water in 95% alcohol).

The selection of an eosin formula is largely a matter of preference. Eosin Y will give a pink-yellow coloration. Eosin B will give a deeper pink-blue coloration. Picric acid added to the eosin will intensify connective tissue staining in the cytoplasm and add color dimension. Other eosin dye solutions which incorporate acid fuchsin and orange G develop a variety of color zones. In our laboratory we modify a picro-eosin with an eosin solution found in the U.S. Navy Manual of Histologic Techniques, to give maximum cytoplasmic differentiation with a single staining solution.

0.5% Aqueous Eosin

Eosin Y, water-soluble	5 gm.
Distilled water	1000 ml.

Dissolve the eosin in water. If a deeper tone is desired, add 0.5 ml. of glacial acetic acid per 100 ml. of staining solution.

Staining time: 15 seconds to 2 minutes. Cytoplasm should stain a bright, transparent pink.

1% Alcoholic Eosin

Eosin Y, water- and alcohol-soluble	10 gm.
Distilled water	50 ml.

Dissolve the eosin thoroughly in the water and then add

95% ethyl alcohol	940 ml.

This eosin may be used as a stock solution and diluted with an equal part of 95% ethyl alcohol for use, or it may be used in the 1% strength.

Staining time: 0.5% solution — *15 seconds to 2 minutes*
1.0% solution — *few dips to few seconds*

The cytoplasm should stain a bright, transparent pink.

When staining solution weakens, add enough from the stock bottle to the staining dish to obtain good staining results.

Picro-Eosin

Eosin Y	16 gm.
80% ethyl alcohol	1440 ml.
Saturated aqueous picric acid (about 1.22%)	160 ml.

Dissolve eosin in alcohol and add the picric acid solution. Mix well and filter. This is ready for immediate use.

Navy Manual Alcoholic Eosin
Stock Solution

Eosin Y	10.0 gm.	
Orange G	2.5 gm.	
Acid fuchsin	1.26 gm.	
Distilled water	300.0 ml.	$\Big\}$ = 70% ethyl
Absolute alcohol	700.0 ml.	alcohol
Glacial acetic acid	0.5 ml.	

Mix dyes until dissolved with the water. Add alcohol. Then add acetic acid. If you are making a 70% alcoholic dilution from 95% ethyl alcohol, reserve the water portion for dissolving dyes before adding the alcohol. This solution is stable indefinitely.

WORKING SOLUTION

Dilute stock stain 1:3 with 70% ethyl alcohol, i.e.

Stock eosin solution	100 ml.
70% ethyl alcohol	300 ml.

Note: We find this working solution a little heavy and so use a small aliquot of the stock solution to augment and add color range to our picro-eosin.

We near fill the 500 ml. capacity staining dish with picro-eosin, and then add 10 to 20 ml. of the stock (undiluted) solution of the Navy eosin. The combination may be varied to suit fixation and processing methods. The amounts given are suitable for Helly fixation, with a larger aliquot of the Navy eosin added to produce the same results with formalin-fixed tissues.

GENERAL NOTES ON HEMATOXYLIN AND EOSIN STAINING

1. The routine hematoxylin and eosin stain is often referred to as a general "oversight" stain. This is a gross misnomer, for perhaps as much as 90 percent of all histologic diagnoses are made on this preparation. It remains the responsibility of the histologic technician to produce the very best possible H and E stains. The slides should be differentiated microscopically and not left to the capricious effect of "dips" and time intervals, which are actually only baseline guides. Following staining in hematoxylin and decolorization in acid alcohol, the slides should be examined under the microscope. Those which are understained should be returned to the hematoxylin. Those which are overstained should be decolorized further. The various tissues accept the dye differently, for instance lymphoid tissue stains deeply whereas adrenal gland or liver stain lightly. The counterstain eosin is of no less importance. Slides should be spot checked from the absolute alcohol rinse, returned to the eosin solution if too pale, or im-

Table 14-1. *Routine heamtoxylin and eosin staining procedure*

Step	Solution	Time	Function
(1) Deparaffinization	Xylene	2½ minutes	Remove paraffin
	Xylene	2½ minutes	Remove paraffin
	Absolute alcohol	2½ minutes	Remove xylene
	Absolute alcohol	2½ minutes	Remove xylene
	95% alcohol	Few dips (in and out)	Hydrate
(2) De-Zenkerization (for sections fixed in solutions containing mercuric chloride)	Alcoholic iodine	5 to 10 minutes (5 minimum)	Remove mercuric chloride deposits
(3) Rinsing	80% alcohol	Few dips (in and out)	Rinse iodine from slides
(4) Bleaching out iodine	Hypo (sodium thiosulfate)	2 minutes	Remove iodine from sections
(5) Washing	Tap water (at sink)	Several changes (wash thoroughly)	Remove hypo
(6) Staining	Hematoxylin	1 to 5 minutes (depends on strength of hematoxylin). Tissue will be overstained	Stain nuclei
(7) Rinsing	Tap water (at sink)	Few changes	Rinse slides of stain
(8) Decolorization	Acid alcohol 0.5%	1 to 3 rapid dips	Decolorize sections
(9) Rinsing	Tap water, running	1 minute	Stop acid action
(10) Blueing	Lithium carbonate	30 to 60 seconds	Blue nuclei
(11) Washing	Tap water, running	Several changes	Remove alkaline solution. If not removed it will inhibit acid (eosin) stain
(12) Check staining results with microscope. Nuclei should be bright clear blue, background light or colorless. Restain or decolorize if necessary			
(13) Counterstaining	Picro-eosin	Few dips to 1 minute, depending on fixation	Stain cytoplasm
(14) Dehydration	95% alcohol	Several dips	Dehydrate. Also removes excess eosin
	Absolute alcohol	Several dips to 1 minute	Dehydrate
	Absolute alcohol	Several dips to 1 minute	Dehydrate
	Absolute alcohol	Several dips to 1 minute	Dehydrate
(15) Clearing	Xylene	Several minutes	Clear out alcohol
	Xylene	Several minutes	Clear out alcohol
	Xylene	Several minutes	Clear out alcohol
(16) Mount in Permount			

Results: Nuclei – bright clear blue. Cytoplasm – pink.

mersed in 95 percent alcohol to remove excess color if overstained.

2. Preserve the integrity of solutions in your series by draining the basket of slides and blotting excess solution on folded paper toweling (held in the free hand) before transferring basket to next solution.

3. Active alum hematoxylin solutions develop a fluorescent sheen on the surface of the solution. Unless removed, sheets or clumps of the dye particles will be seen on the finished slide, obscuring detail. Between filterings or staining, this sheen can be removed by drawing paper toweling or filter paper across the surface of the staining dish.

4. Hematoxylin that has been used too long will require longer periods of immersion to produce nuclear staining. This additional staining time will also color the cytoplasm an unwanted blue-gray. When the eosin is applied, an overlay of pink on blue with a muddy cytoplasmic staining results. The minimum time in hematoxylin is best controlled by using the dye solution at the peak of its performance. When you have to lengthen staining time and you see that the cytoplasm is no longer light or colorless, discard the solution and replace with a fresh dish of stock hematoxylin.

5. Following dehydration in absolute alcohol, spot check the depth of coloration of the eosin-stained sections by holding one or more slides momentarily in front of white paper toweling. The white background will give a truer picture of staining intensity. The pink color will deepen slightly when transferred to xylene.

6. In so far as possible, arrange the microscope so that it approximates the lighting and the density of blue filter that the pathologist uses. Check your slides from time to time with his microscope so that you can see how the stains appear to him.

Routine and Special Staining Procedures

BENHOLD'S CONGO RED
(Puchtler, Sweat, and Levine Modification)

INDICATIONS. To demonstrate amyloid in tissue. (See also page 193).

FIXATION. Carnoy's fluid or absolute alcohol best for amyloid preservation. 10% formalin or Zenker-formol may be used.

TECHNIQUE. Paraffin. Cut 1 section at 6μ and 1 section at 10μ. Process with control slide.

DISCUSSION. This is a simple and reliable stain. Its main advantage in comparison with the crystal or methyl violet methods of staining amyloid is that the stained section can be kept indefinitely, since it is dehydrated and mounted in a permanent mounting medium. The modification given here has the additional advantage that no differentiation is required.

The pretreatment with alkaline alcohol-sodium chloride solution in step 5 of the staining procedure (page 236) increases the intensity of the staining significantly.

Staining Solutions

MAYER'S HEMATOXYLIN
(See page 228.)

1% SODIUM HYDROXIDE

Sodium hydroxide	1 gm.
Distilled water	100 ml.

SATURATED SODIUM CHLORIDE IN 80% ETHANOL
(SOLUTION A)

80% ethanol	100 ml.
Sodium chloride	1 gm.

This is a stock stable solution.

ALKALINE ALCOHOL-SODIUM CHLORIDE
(SOLUTION B)

80% ethanol-sodium chloride solution (Solution A)	50.0 ml.
Sodium hydroxide, 1% aqueous solution	0.5 ml.*

Combine *just before use* and filter.

* Note: With Zenker-formol fixation we found it necessary to reduce the amount of sodium hydroxide to five drops (rather than 0.5 ml.) in Solution B and in Working Congo Red solution in order to eliminate nonspecific staining.

STOCK CONGO RED ALKALINE SOLUTION

80% ethanol-sodium chloride solution (Solution A)   300.0 ml.
Congo red C.I. No. 22120   0.5 gm.

Stir thoroughly at intervals until solution is reasonably complete. This is a saturated solution of Congo red in ethanol-salt mixture. Let solution stand for 24 hours before use. Filter and keep in a tightly stoppered container. The stock solution will be stable for several months.

WORKING CONGO RED SOLUTION

Stock Congo red   50.0 ml.
1% sodium hydroxide   0.5 ml.*

Filter and use solution within 15 minutes.

Staining Procedure:

1. Deparaffinize sections through distilled water. *Use Control Section.*

2. Stain nuclei with Mayer's hematoxylin for *10 minutes.*

3. Blue in warm running water for *5 to 10 minutes.*

4. Rinse in distilled water, three changes.

5. Treat with alkaline alcohol-sodium chloride (Solution B) for *20 minutes.*

6. Transfer and stain in Congo red working solution for *20 minutes.*

7. Dehydrate rapidly in three changes of absolute alcohol, clear in three changes of xylene, and mount in Permount or Histoclad.

RESULTS.   Amyloid — deep pink to red
           Nuclei — blue
           Elastica — stains weakly with Congo red

REFERENCE.   Puchtler, H., Sweat, F., and Levine, M.   *J. Histochem. Cytochem.* 10:355, 1962.

* Note: With Zenker-formol fixation we found it necessary to reduce the amount of sodium hydroxide to five drops (rather than 0.5 ml.) in Solution B and in Working Congo Red solution in order to eliminate nonspecific staining.

BEST'S CARMINE STAIN FOR GLYCOGEN

INDICATIONS.   Identifying glycogen in tissues.

FIXATION.   Aqueous-based fixatives cannot be relied upon *after* 24 to 48 hours to demonstrate the maximum amount of glycogen in tissue (Trott, J. R.   *J. Histochem. Cytochem.* 9:703, 1961). Glycogen is best preserved in Gendre's solution, acetic alcohol formalin, Bouin's solution, and 10% alcoholic formalin. Optimal results are obtained if ice-cold fixation is carried out (page 264).

TECHNIQUE.   Paraffin sections coated with a thin celloidin film. The film of celloidin helps to prevent the loss of glycogen into the aqueous solutions.

Staining Solutions

CARMINE STOCK SOLUTION

Carmine	2 gm.
Potassium carbonate	1 gm.
Potassium chloride	5 gm.
Water, distilled	60 ml.

Combine and boil gently and cautiously in a 200 ml. flask for several minutes. When cool add:

Ammonium hydroxide, 58%	20 ml.

Ripen for 24 hours at room temperature. Keep this stock solution in the refrigerator in dark bottle. It will be stable for several weeks.

CARMINE WORKING SOLUTION

Stock carmine solution, freshly filtered	20 ml.
Ammonium hydroxide, 58%	30 ml.
Methyl alcohol	30 ml.

Use this dilute solution only once; do not save.

DIFFERENTIATING SOLUTION

Absolute alcohol	40 ml.
Methyl alcohol	20 ml.
Distilled water	50 ml.

Staining Procedure

Process a control slide with the other slides.

1. Deparaffinize sections in two changes of xylene, followed by two changes of absolute alcohol.

2. Directly from the absolute alcohol, coat slides in a thin solution of celloidin (page 284).

3. Harden celloidin in 80% alcohol for a *few minutes* and transfer sections to distilled water.

4. Stain sections deeply in Harris's hematoxylin for *3 to 5 minutes* or longer. Rinse in water.

5. Decolorize sections in acid alcohol (0.5% or 1%), leaving the nuclei a little dark. The ammonia in staining solutions decolorizes nuclei slightly.

6. Wash quickly in tap water.

7. Immerse in carmine working solution for *15 to 30 minutes.* Check control slide.

8. Place in differentiating solution for a *few seconds* only.

9. Wash quickly in 80% alcohol.

10. Dehydrate in 95% alcohol, two rapid changes.

11. Dehydrate in absolute alcohol, two or three changes.

12. Clear in xylene, two or three changes, and mount in any neutral mounting medium.

RESULTS   Glycogen — pink to red
              Nuclei — blue
              Amebae — red, due to their glycogen content

REFERENCE. Mallory, F. B. *Pathological Technique.* Philadelphia: Saunders, 1938, p. 126.

FOOT'S MODIFICATION OF HORTEGA'S SILVER CARBONATE METHOD FOR RETICULUM

The silver carbonate solution of Hortega is obtained by precipitating the silver from the silver nitrate solution with lithium carbonate and then redissolving that precipitate with ammonia. After treatment in this solution, the silver in the tissues is reduced in formalin.

Since there is a chance that the sections may become loosened from the slide in this alkaline solution, the slides may be coated with a thin celloidin solution to secure them (page 284).

INDICATIONS.   Staining reticulum in sections

FIXATION.   Zenker's fixative, Helly's fluid, or 10% formalin

TECHNIQUE.   Paraffin

Staining Solutions

SILVER NITRATE SOLUTION
(Foot's Modification of Silver Ammonium Carbonate Solution)

All glassware should be chemically clean. For optimum results, use only purest reagents available. This solution must always be freshly prepared.

Place 10 ml. of a *10% aqueous solution of silver nitrate* in a 100 ml. capacity graduated glass cylinder. *Add 10 ml. of a saturated (1.25%) aqueous solution of lithium carbonate.* Wash the white precipitate three or more times with *distilled water.* To do this, simply add approximately 30 to 40 ml. of distilled water to the silver carbonate mixture in the cylinder. Stretch Parawax over top of cylinder and shake cylinder vigorously. Allow precipitate to settle to bottom. Carefully decant the supernatant fluid. Do this and let settle three to five times or more. When completely washed, the precipitate will settle in a small compact mound of fine particles of a slightly green-gray color. Add *25 ml. of distilled water* to the cylinder. Almost dissolve the precipitate with *28% ammonia water,* added drop by drop (approximately 6 to 15 drops) while shaking the container vigorously. Avoid adding too much ammonia water; it is better to leave a few grains of precipitate than to add too much. The solution is then made up to 100 ml. with *95% ethyl alcohol.* Pour solution into a small flask (250 ml. capacity) for easier handling. A precipitate is again formed which is dissolved by a few more drops of ammonia water. This alcoholic solution is filtered, covered, and then warmed for 20 minutes in a paraffin oven at 56° to 58°C. Or, place solution in a screw-cap Coplin jar in the hot water flotation bath, warmed to 43°C., for 20 to 30 minutes.

Note: 28% ammonia water is same strength as 58% ammonium hydroxide.

0.25% POTASSIUM PERMANGANATE

Potassium permanganate	0.25 gm.
Distilled water	100.00 ml.

5% OXALIC ACID SOLUTION

Oxalic acid	5 gm.
Distilled water	100 ml.

20% NEUTRAL FORMALIN

Neutral formalin	20 ml.
Distilled water	80 ml.

0.2% GOLD CHLORIDE SOLUTION
(See also page 28)

Gold chloride	1 gm.
Distilled water	500 ml.

Staining Procedure

1. Deparaffinize sections as usual. If sections are Zenker-fixed, treat with iodine followed by hypo as usual.

2. Wash thoroughly in tap water.

3. Oxidize in 0.25% solution of potassium permanganate for *5 minutes.*

4. Rinse in tap water.

5. Bleach in 5% solution of oxalic acid for *10 minutes.*

6. Wash well in tap water, followed by distilled water.

7. Place in warm silver ammonium carbonate solution in the incubator or hot water bath at 37° to 43°C. for *10 to 30 minutes.* Tissues will show a yellow to brown coloration when impregnated. Remove from water bath and allow to cool briefly.

8. Rinse in distilled water.

9. Reduce in 20% solution of neutral formalin for *5 minutes.* Tissue will become amber in color.

10. Wash well in tap water.

11. Tone in 0.2% gold chloride solution for *5 minutes.* Sections will be grayed in this solution.

12. Wash well in tap water.

13. Fix in a 5% aqueous solution of sodium thiosulfate for **2 *minutes*.** The thiosulfate will remove all unreduced silver.

14. Wash well in tap water.

15. Counterstain if desired with alum hematoxylin and van Gieson's stain for nuclei and collagen. The counterstain is usually unnecessary in a well-stained slide, for the coarser connective tissue will be brownish-pink and well differentiated from the fine black reticulum.

16. Dehydrate in two changes of 95% alcohol followed by two or three changes of absolute alcohol.

17. Clear in two or three changes of xylene and mount.

RESULTS.   Coarse connective tissue fibers — brown-pink
                Reticulum — black to dark violet
                Nuclei — black

REFERENCE.   Jones, R. McClung. *Handbook of Microscopical Technique* (3d ed.). New York: Paul B. Hoeber, Inc., 1950, p. 258.

GIEMSA STAIN
(Wolbach's Modification)

INDICATIONS.   Delicate stain, very fine nuclear detail.
                Preferred stain for bone marrow and other hematopoietic tissue.
                Stain for inclusion bodies and for *Rickettsia*.
                Stain for mast cells and for bacteria.
                Will stain actinomyces, cryptococcus, and *Histoplasma capsulatum*.

FIXATION.   For best results, tissue should be fixed in Zenker's with acetic acid. If tissues were not originally fixed in Zenker's, slides may be deparaffinized and mordanted in:

          Stock Zenker's fluid   95 ml.
          Glacial acetic acid   5 ml.

Leave the slides in this solution for 15 to 30 minutes.

TECHNIQUE.   Paraffin sections cut at 4μ.

DISCUSSION. Note for step 4, page 243. The strength of the colophony (rosin) used for differentiating will have to be varied according to the fixative used. As high as a 50:50 concentration (colophony: 95% ethyl alcohol) may be required. Begin with a 25:75 ratio and if differentiation is proceeding at too slow a pace, add more rosin solution to the 95% alcohol.

Staining Solutions

GIEMSA STAIN (STOCK SOLUTION)

Azure II-eosin	3.0 gm.
Azure II	0.8 gm.
Alcohol, methyl	375.0 ml.
Glycerin	125.0 ml.

Combine reagents and filter. Stable solution. (Very fine solutions of stock Giemsa stain * can be purchased ready to use from laboratory-supply houses.)

GIEMSA STAIN (WORKING SOLUTION)

Giemsa stain (stock solution)	2.5 ml.
Alcohol, methyl	3.0 ml.
Distilled water (to which has been added 2 to 4 drops of 0.5% aqueous solution of sodium bicarbonate)	100.0 ml.

Prepare just before use.

10% COLOPHONY (ROSIN) SOLUTION
(See page 30.)

Staining Procedure

1. Deparaffinize and treat as for Zenker-fixed tissue. Wash thoroughly in tap water. Place sections in distilled water.

2. Immediately after mixing it, pour Giemsa working solution over slides. Stain should be changed twice during the first hour. Leave sections overnight in the third change of the staining solution.

---

* Giemsa tissue stain (Wolbach's modification), item #6203, Harleco Co.

3. Pour off stain. Place sections in distilled water. Sections will appear a homogeneous deep blue.

4. Differentiate each slide individually in 95% ethyl alcohol to which 10 to 25 ml. of a 10% solution of colophony (rosin) has been added. Keep slide in constant motion so that decolorization will be uniform. A series of Coplin jars is convenient for differentiation.

5. Control differentiation by rinsing slide in 95% alcohol and checking visually with microscope from time to time. Stop decolorization when the nuclei are bright blue and the cytoplasm is soft pink.

6. Dehydrate in two or three changes of absolute alcohol.

7. Clear in two or three changes of xylene, and mount in Permount or any neutral mounting medium.

RESULTS.   Nuclei — blue

Cytoplasm — pink

Inclusion bodies — blue or lavender

REFERENCE.   Mallory, F. B.   *Pathological Technique.* Philadelphia: Saunders, 1938, p. 195.

MODIFICATION OF THE GIEMSA STAIN FOR RAPID STAINING (RAPID GIEMSA)

1. Make up stain as for regular Giemsa working solution, or dilute 1 ml. of ready-to-use Giemsa stain with 10 ml. of distilled water. Preheat stain in 58° to 60°C. oven.

2. Deparaffinize sections. If not originally fixed in Zenker's with acetic acid, slides may be mordanted in Zenker's for *1 hour* at room temperature or for *30 minutes* in a 58° to 60°C. oven.

3. Wash sections thoroughly and treat with iodine followed by hypo. Wash thoroughly in tap water and rinse with distilled water.

4. Place sections in preheated stain in 58°C. oven, and stain for ½ *hour to 3 hours.* No second or third change is necessary. Without washing, slides may be checked with the microscope after ½ *hour.*

5. Differentiate as for standard Giemsa stain.

6. Dehydrate, clear and mount as usual.

RESULTS.   Essentially the same as with longer method

GOMORI'S IRON REACTION

In this reaction the loosely bound ferric iron in the tissue combines with potassium ferrocyanide to form ferric-ferrocyanide which has a bright blue color (Prussian blue). This is strictly a chemical reaction and the Prussian blue precipitate is insoluble. Because of the stability of the reaction, it can be combined (followed by) other special staining methods. To provide accurate results, be sure that iron-contaminated glassware and iron-containing chemicals are avoided.

INDICATIONS.   Demonstrating iron pigments in tissue

FIXATION.   Buffered neutral formalin (10%) or alcohol fixation preferred

TECHNIQUE.   Paraffin
Process with control slide

Staining Solutions

20% HYDROCHLORIC ACID

Hydrochloric acid, concentrated	20 ml.
Distilled water	80 ml.

10% POTASSIUM FERROCYANIDE

Potassium ferrocyanide	10 gm.
Distilled water	100 ml.

0.15% BASIC FUCHSIN

Basic fuchsin	0.15 gm.
50% ethyl alcohol	100.00 ml.

Staining Procedure

Process a control slide with the sections.

1. Deparaffinize sections through two changes of xylene, absolute and 95% alcohols down to distilled water.

2. Place slides in **equal parts** of 20% hydrochloric acid and 10% potassium ferrocyanide combined immediately before use. Reaction may take **20 to 30 minutes.** Check control slide. Iron pigments will be bright blue. Positive reaction will generally occur promptly (within 5 minutes). When amount of pigment is small and does not react grossly, leave for 30 minutes before considering it a negative result.

3. Wash thoroughly in distilled water.

4. Counterstain with a few dips of 0.15% basic fuchsin in 50% alcohol or counterstain in nuclear fast red (page 378). Basic fuchsin will stain the pigment hemofuchsin red. Rinse and check with microscope. Nuclei should be red, cytoplasm pink.

5. Rinse with **distilled** water.

6. Dehydrate with two changes of 95% alcohol, two or three changes of absolute alcohol.

7. Clear in two to three changes of xylene and mount in any neutral mounting medium.

RESULTS.   Iron pigments — bright blue
              Nuclei — red
              Cytoplasm — pink
              Hemofuchsin — pink to red if basic fuchsin is used

REFERENCE.   Mallory, F. B. *Pathological Technique*. Philadelphia: Saunders, 1938, p. 137.

GRAM-WEIGERT METHOD OF STAINING BACTERIA

INDICATIONS.   Staining bacteria in sections
               Will also stain most fungi

FIXATION.   Zenker's fluid or 10% formalin

TECHNIQUE.   Paraffin

Staining Solutions

2.5% PHLOXINE

Phloxine	2.5 gm.
Distilled water	100.0 ml.

This is a stable solution.

STIRLING'S CRYSTAL VIOLET

Crystal violet	5 gm.
Absolute alcohol	10 ml.
Aniline	2 ml.
Distilled water	88 ml.

This is a stable solution.

GRAM'S IODINE

Iodine	1 gm.
Potassium iodide	2 gm.
Distilled water	300 ml.

Staining Procedure

1. Deparaffinize sections as usual. Treat with iodine and hypo, if necessary.

2. Wash thoroughly in water and transfer sections to distilled water.

3. Stain nuclei lightly in alum hematoxylin (progressive stain).

4. Wash in several changes of tap water to blue nuclei.

5. Place in 2.5% phloxine solution for *5 to 15 minutes* in the paraffin oven at 56° to 58°C.

6. Rinse briefly in water.

7. Stain in aniline crystal violet (Stirling's solution) for *15 minutes* at room temperature.

8. Wash in distilled water.

9. Treat with Gram's iodine for *1 to 2 minutes.*

10. Wash in distilled water.

11. Blot with filter paper to dry. Decolorize and clear in several changes of aniline. Decolorize until blue color clouds cease to wash out and section is pink. Aniline and xylene in equal parts may be used instead of pure aniline for decolorizing organisms that stain delicately. Avoid inhaling aniline.

12. Rinse thoroughly in several changes of xylene to clear. Mount in Permount.

RESULTS. Gram-positive organisms — deep violet
Gram-negative organisms — unstained (or rose)

Nuclei — blue to violet
Connective tissue — rose
Mycelia — blue; conidia — red

REFERENCE. Mallory, F. B. *Pathological Technique.* Philadelphia:
Saunders, 1938, p. 272.

GRIDLEY'S STAIN FOR FUNGI

FIXATION. Any well-fixed tissue

TECHNIQUE. Cut paraffin sections at 6μ

Staining Solutions

CHROMIC ACID SOLUTION

Chromium trioxide	4 gm.
Distilled water	100 ml.

COLEMAN'S FEULGEN (SCHIFF'S) REAGENT[*]

Bring 200 ml. of distilled water to a boil, remove from flame and
add 1 gm. basic fuchsin. When fuchsin is dissolved, cool and filter.
Add 2 gm. sodium metabisulfite and 10 ml. of normal hydrochloric
acid. Let bleach for 24 hours, and then add 0.5 gm. activated carbon
(Norit), shake for about 1 minute, and filter through coarse paper.
The filtrate should be colorless. Repeat filtration if necessary. Store in
refrigerator.

NORMAL HYDROCHLORIC ACID

Hydrochloric acid, sp. gr. 1.19	83.5 ml.
Distilled water	916.5 ml.

SODIUM METABISULFITE SOLUTION

Sodium metabisulfite	10 gm.
Distilled water	100 ml.

[*] Schiff's reagents are interchangeable and any variant may be substituted,
providing it is of equal strength, or providing the time interval is lengthened or
shortened appropriately.

Sulfurous Rinse

Sodium metabisulfite, 10%	6 ml.
Normal hydrochloric acid	5 ml.
Distilled water	100 ml.

Aldehyde-Fuchsin Solution

Basic fuchsin	1 gm.
Alcohol, 70%, ethyl	200 ml.
Paraldehyde	2 ml.
Hydrochloric acid, concentrated	2 ml.

Let stand at room temperature for 3 days until solution turns deep blue-purple. Keep in refrigerator. Filter and allow to come to room temperature before using.

Metanil Yellow Solution

Metanil yellow	0.25 gm.
Distilled water	100.00 ml.
Glacial acetic acid	2 drops

Staining Procedure

1. Xylene, absolute and 95% alcohols to distilled water.
2. Place in 4% chromic acid for *1 hour* (oxidizer).
3. Wash in running water for *5 minutes.*
4. Place in Schiff's reagent for *15 minutes.*
5. Rinse in three changes of sulfurous acid rinse.
6. Wash for *15 minutes* in running tap water to develop red color.
7. Rinse in two changes of 70% alcohol and place slides in aldehyde-fuchsin solution for *15 to 30 minutes.*
8. Rinse off excess stain with 95% alcohol.
9. Rinse in water.
10. Counterstain lightly with metanil yellow solution for *1 minute.*
11. Rinse in water.
12. Dehydrate through 95% and absolute alcohols.
13. Clear in xylene and mount in Permount.

RESULTS. Mycelia — deep blue

Conidia — deep rose to purple

Background — yellow
Elastic tissue and mucin also stain deep blue

REFERENCES. Gridley, M. F. *Amer. J. Clin. Path.* 23:303, 1953.
*Armed Forces Institute of Pathology Manual of His-
tologic and Special Staining Technics,* 1957 edition.

KINYOUN'S ACID-FAST STAIN

INDICATIONS. Demonstrating acid-fast bacilli.

FIXATION. Formalin-fixed tissue preferred; others may be used.

TECHNIQUE. Paraffin. Use control slide.*

Staining Solutions

KINYOUN'S CARBOL FUCHSIN

Basic fuchsin	4 gm.
Phenol crystals, melted	8 ml.
95% alcohol, ethyl	20 ml.
Distilled water	100 ml.

Combine, leave in 37°C. oven overnight. Cool and filter.
Always filter stain just before use. Solution may be saved and reused. It is stable for several weeks.

ACID ALCOHOL 1%

Hydrochloric acid, concentrated	1 ml.
Alcohol, 95% or 70% ethyl	99 ml.

LIGHT GREEN 0.5%

Light green, SF yellowish	0.5 gm.
Distilled water	100.0 ml.
Glacial acetic acid	0.2 ml.

---

* If a positive tissue control is not available, tuberculosis organisms cultured
in the bacteriology laboratory can provide control material. Observing the necessary precautions, the cultured mycobacteria are transferred to gel foam and the gel
foam is fixed in formalin for 6 hours and processed on the Autotechnicon. After
casting, the block is sectioned and used as control material.

DILUTE LIGHT GREEN SOLUTION

Light green (stock 0.5%)	5 ml.
Distilled water	45 ml.

Staining Procedure

Process a control slide with the sections to be stained.*

1. Deparaffinize sections. If Zenker-fixed, treat as usual.
2. Wash thoroughly in tap water. Transfer to distilled water.
3. Stain in newly filtered Kinyoun's carbol fuchsin for *1 hour* at room temperature or in 37°C. incubator or in the hot water flotation bath at 43°C.
4. Wash well in tap water.
5. Decolorize in two changes of acid alcohol, until tissue is pale pink (approximately *10 to 20 seconds*). Decolorize in acid alcohol the minimum time to remove background coloration.
6. Wash well in tap water.
7. Counterstain by dipping lightly in 0.5% light green (or even the more dilute solution) for a *few seconds to 1 minute.* Rinse in water and check stain with microscope. Counterstain should be light so as not to mask bacilli. Depth of color should be checked after the 95% alcohol rinse. The cytoplasm should be a clear, even, light green. If sections become overstained with light green, remove excess color in running water or in water made slightly alkaline with lithium carbonate or ammonia water (see page 26).
8. Dehydrate in several changes of 95% alcohol and several changes of absolute alcohol.
9. Clear in at least two changes of xylene and mount in any neutral mounting medium.

RESULTS.   Acid-fast bacteria — bright red
Ceroid substances — bright red
Background — pale green

REFERENCE.   Kinyoun, J. J.   *Amer. J. Public Health* 5:867, 1915.

* If a positive tissue control is not available, tuberculosis organisms cultured in the bacteriology laboratory can provide control material. Observing the necessary precautions, the cultured mycobacteria are transferred to gel foam and the gel foam is fixed in formalin for six hours and processed on the Autotechnicon. After casting, the block is sectioned and used as control material.

MALLORY'S ANILINE BLUE STAIN

Differential staining is accomplished in part by the action of the phosphotungstic acid which has the property of extracting the acid fuchsin from collagen, leaving it in the muscle tissue and nuclei.

INDICATIONS. For staining connective tissue (collagen).

FIXATION. Zenker fixation preferred. Others may be used. If tissues were not originally fixed in Zenker's, slides may be deparaffinized and mordanted in:

Stock Zenker's fluid	95 ml.
Glacial acetic acid	5 ml.

Leave slides in this solution for 15 to 30 minutes.

TECHNIQUE. Paraffin

Solutions

0.5% ACID FUCHSIN

Acid fuchsin	0.5 gm.
Distilled water	100.0 ml.

ANILINE BLUE-ORANGE G SOLUTION

Aniline blue, water-soluble	0.5 gm.
Orange G	2.0 gm.
Phosphotungstic acid	1.0 gm.
Distilled water	100.0 ml.

Staining Procedure

1. Deparaffinize sections. Treat with iodine and hypo as usual. Wash thoroughly in tap water.
2. Rinse in distilled water.
3. Stain in 0.5% acid fuchsin solution for *1 to 5 minutes.* The longer staining time is usually necessary. If it is desirable to demonstrate collagenous fibers sharply, prestaining with fuchsin may be omitted.
4. Transfer directly to aniline blue-orange G solution without wash-

ing and stain for **20 minutes to 1 hour.** (Twenty minutes is usually sufficient time.) Stain may be saved and reused.

5. Transfer directly to 95% ethyl alcohol, several changes, to remove the excess stain.

6. Dehydrate with two or three changes of absolute alcohol.

7. Clear with two or three changes of xylene and mount in any neutral mounting medium.

RESULTS. Nuclei — red (if fuchsin is used)
Collagen fibrils — blue

REFERENCE. Mallory, F. B. *Pathological Technique.* Philadelphia: Saunders, 1938, p. 153.

MALLORY'S PHLOXINE AND METHYLENE BLUE STAIN (PMB)

INDICATIONS. Fine nuclear stain
Good stain for bone marrow and other hematopoietic tissue
Good stain for mast cells
Will stain inclusion bodies, Rickettsiae, and bacteria

FIXATION. For best results use Zenker's with acetic acid. If tissues were not originally fixed in Zenker's, slides may be deparaffinized and mordanted in:

Stock Zenker's fluid	95 ml.
Glacial acetic acid	5 ml.

Leave in this solution for 15 to 30 minutes.

TECHNIQUE. Paraffin

DISCUSSION. Note for step 6: See remarks under "Discussion" on page 242.

Staining Solutions

2.5% PHLOXINE

Phloxine B	2.5 gm.
Distilled water	100.0 ml.

1% Methylene Blue Solution

Methylene blue	1 gm.
Borax (sodium borate, tetra)	1 gm.
Distilled water	100 ml.

1% Azure II Solution

Azure II	1 gm.
Distilled water	100 ml.

Mallory's Methylene Blue-Azure II (Working Solution)

Methylene blue solution	5 ml.
Azure II solution	5 ml.
Distilled water	90 ml.

Colophony (Rosin) Solution 10%

Colophony	10 gm.
Absolute alcohol	100 ml.

Staining Procedure

1. Deparaffinize sections in the usual manner. Treat with iodine followed by hypo. Wash thoroughly in tap water. Place in distilled water.

2. Stain deeply in 2.5% phloxine solution for *30 minutes* at room temperature or *15 minutes* in a 58° to 60°C. oven.

3. Rinse lightly in water.

4. Stain in methylene blue-azure II working solution for *5 or 6 minutes.*

5. Place in distilled water.

6. Decolorize sections individually in 95% ethyl alcohol. Use Coplin jar containing 30 ml. of 95% alcohol to which has been added 20 ml. of colophony solution. The colophony aids in differentiating the nuclei. Keep the slide in constant motion so that decolorization will be uniform. If differentiation progresses too slowly increase amount of colophony.

7. Rinse slide in 95% alcohol and check with the microscope from

time to time. When the pink color has returned to the sections and the nuclei are deep blue and clear, dehydrate rapidly with several changes of absolute alcohol.

8. Clear in two or three changes of xylene, and mount in Permount.

RESULTS.   Nuclei and bacteria — blue
Collagen and other tissue elements — bright rose
Mast cell granules — purple
Rickettsiae — blue to violet

REFERENCE.   Mallory, F. B. *Pathological Technique.* Philadelphia: Saunders, 1938, p. 86.

MALLORY'S PHOSPHOTUNGSTIC ACID HEMATOXYLIN (PTAH STAIN)

INDICATIONS.   Stain for fibrils and fibrin
Stain for mitotic figures
Excellent nuclear stain
Stain for striated muscle
Stain for astrocytes
Stain for amebae

FIXATION.   For best results, Zenker's with acetic acid. If tissues have not been fixed in Zenker's fluid, slides should be deparaffinized and mordanted in:

Stock Zenker's fluid	95 ml.
Glacial acetic acid	5 ml.

Leave in this solution for 15 to 30 minutes.

TECHNIQUE.   Paraffin

Staining Solutions

PHOSPHOTUNGSTIC ACID HEMATOXYLIN (PTAH STAIN)

Hematoxylin	1 gm.
Phosphotungstic acid	20 gm.
Distilled water	1000 ml.

Dissolve the solid ingredients in separate portions of the water, the hematoxylin with the aid of gentle heat. When cool combine. Since this stain employs hematoxylin, the solution must be ripened before use. Mallory's text states that this ripening can be accomplished at once by adding 0.177 gm. of potassium permanganate to the staining solution. I have found that the best hematoxylin solutions for this particular stain are obtained by spontaneous ripening, even if it takes several weeks or months. When properly ripened the stain will have a rich purple color and will be opaque. It is advisable to prepare this stain well in advance (4 months) and store away from direct light. This is a stable, reusable stain (see additional information on page 205).

0.25% Potassium Permanganate

Potassium permanganate	0.25 gm.
Distilled water	100.00 ml.

5% Oxalic Acid

Oxalic acid	5 gm.
Distilled water	100 ml.

Staining Procedure

1. Deparaffinize sections and treat in usual way for Zenker-fixed tissue. Rinse thoroughly in distilled water.

2. Oxidize in 0.25% aqueous solution of potassium permangante for *5 to 10 minutes.* Discard solution.

3. Wash in water.

4. Bleach in 5% oxalic acid aqueous solution for *5 minutes* or just until sections are colorless.

5. Wash thoroughly in several changes of tap water. Rinse in distilled water.

6. Stain in phosphotungstic acid hematoxylin *overnight* or for *12 to 24 hours.* Stain may be saved and reused.

7. From the stain, transfer directly to 95% ethyl alcohol, followed by several changes of absolute alcohol. *Dehydrate quickly,* as alcohol readily extracts the red part of the stain.

8. Clear in several changes of xylene, and mount in Permount.

RESULTS. Nuclei and all fibrils — blue

Cytoplasm — yellow-pink to brown-red

Collagen — brown-pink
Fibrin — blue
Coarse elastic fibrils — purple tint
Mitotic figures — blue
Mitochondria — blue
Striated muscle fibers — blue
Astrocytes — blue
Ameba — blue

REFERENCE. Mallory, F. B. *Pathological Technique.* Philadelphia: Saunders, 1938, p. 76.

RAPID PTAH
(Phosphotungstic Acid Hematoxylin Stain Modified by S. P. Hicks)

FIXATION. If tissue was originally formalin-fixed, treat slide with Bouin's fixative for about 30 minutes. Wash out excess Bouin's fluid in running water. If tissue is Zenker- or Bouin-fixed, omit this step.

TECHNIQUE. Paraffin

Staining Solutions

STANDARD PTAH STAIN
(See page 254)

OR

RAPID PTAH STAIN

Dissolve *20 gm. of phosphotungstic acid in 900 ml. of hot distilled water.* Dissolve *1 gm. of hematoxylin in 10 ml. of absolute alcohol,* and mix with the phosphotungstic solution. Add *100 ml. of 0.25% potassium permanganate* (0.25 gm. potassium permanganate in 100 ml. of distilled water) and mix. Stain is ready to use.

5% IRON ALUM

Ferric ammonium sulfate (iron alum)	5 gm.
Distilled water	100 ml.

Staining Procedure

1. Deparaffinize sections as usual. Treat with iodine and hypo if mercuric chloride was present in fixative. Wash thoroughly in tap water.

2. If tissue has been formalin-fixed, mordant slides in Bouin's solution (page 38) for *30 minutes.*

3. Wash in running tap water for *3 to 5 minutes* to remove excess Bouin's solution.

4. Transfer to 5% iron alum for *15 minutes.*

5. Rinse and place in 5% oxalic acid for *5 to 10 minutes.*

6. Wash thoroughly in tap water followed by distilled water.

7. Place in PTAH stain for *30 minutes to 3 hours* in a 58°C. oven. Without washing, slide may be checked with microscope after 30 minutes.

8. When nuclei are bright blue and clear, transfer sections directly from stain (no washing) to 95% ethyl alcohol. Dehydrate quickly in 95% alcohol, followed by two or three changes of absolute alcohol.

9. Clear in several changes of xylene, and mount in Permount.

RESULTS.   Essentially the same as for the standard PTAH stain.

MASSON TRICHROME STAIN
(Goldner-Foot Modification)

The Goldner modification uses dilute solutions of the Masson stains to prevent overstaining and to increase the transparency of the sections, which consequently increases the histologic detail. It eliminates piling up of the light green in connective tissue or mucus, hence no obscuring of connective tissue detail.

INDICATION.   Stain for connective tissue

FIXATION.   Bouin's fluid, Zenker's fluid, or 10% formalin

TECHNIQUE.   Paraffin

Staining Solutions

WEIGERT'S HEMATOXYLIN
(See page 229.)

ACETIC ACID WATER 0.2%

Glacial acetic acid	2 ml.
Distilled water	1000 ml.

MASSON FUCHSIN-PONCEAU-ORANGE G
(STOCK SOLUTION)

Ponceau de xylidine (ponceau 2R)	2 gm.
Acid fuchsin	1 gm.
Orange G	2 gm.
Acetic acid water 0.2%	300 ml.

MASSON FUCHSIN-PONCEAU-ORANGE G
(WORKING SOLUTION)

Stock fuchsin-ponceau-orange G solution	10 ml.
Acetic acid water 0.2%	90 ml.

LIGHT GREEN SOLUTION 0.1%

Light green	0.1 gm.
Acetic acid water 0.2%	100.0 ml.

5% PHOSPHOTUNGSTIC ACID

Phosphotungstic acid	5 gm.
Distilled water	100 ml.

Staining Procedure

1. Deparaffinize sections as usual. Treat with iodine followed by hypo, if necessary. Wash well in tap water. Place in distilled water.

2. Stain in Weigert's hematoxylin for *3 to 5 minutes* or longer. Rinse in distilled water and check stain with microscope. Leave nuclei a little dark, since some of the hematoxylin will be removed during some of the following steps.

3. Rinse with distilled water.

4. Stain the sections in the filtered working solution of fuchsin-ponceau-orange G for *5 to 30 minutes.*

5. Rinse in acetic acid water.

6. Mordant in 5% phosphotungstic acid solution for *3 to 5 minutes.*

7. Rinse in acetic acid water for few minutes to eliminate the phosphotungstic acid and differentiate the color tones.

8. Stain in light green solution for *5 to 20 minutes.*

9. Treat with acetic acid water for *5 minutes.*

10. Dehydrate in two changes of 95% alcohol, followed by two or three changes of absolute alcohol.

11. Clear in two or three changes of xylene and mount.

RESULTS. Nuclei — black
Cytoplasm — red
Collagen — green
Mucin — green
Erythrocytes — yellow to orange

REFERENCE. Jones, R. McClung. *Handbook of Microscopical Technique* (3d ed.). New York: Paul B. Hoeber, Inc., 1950, p. 249.

OIL RED O (METHOD I)

Staining fat is accomplished by using dyes that are soluble in fat or lipoid material. For this reason, a fat stain is termed a physical stain. Fats and lipoids are chemically related substances. They are soluble in ether, chloroform, alcohol, xylene, acetone, and benzene. Since dehydrating and clearing agents for paraffin and celloidin are fat solvents, fat stains are done on frozen sections or on tissue processed with water-soluble wax (Carbowax).

INDICATIONS. Staining neutral fat in sections

TECHNIQUE. Free floating frozen sections

Staining Solutions

Oil Red O Stain (Stock Saturated Solution)

Oil red O	0.5 gm.
99% isopropanol	100.0 ml.
(isopropyl alcohol)	

This is a stock saturated solution. It is stable.

Oil Red O Stain (Working Solution)

Oil red O stock solution	6 ml.
Distilled water	4 ml.

Combine just before use.

Staining Procedure

1. Prepare the working solution of oil red O. Let stand for *5 to 10 minutes* and then filter. The filtrate can be used for several hours.

2. Stain thin frozen sections for *10 to 15 minutes.*

3. Wash in water.

4. Stain nuclei briefly (*10 to 30 seconds*) in Harris's hematoxylin. Blue in water.

5. Float out sections on water. Mount on slides.

6. Drain slide and coverslip section with gum syrup, glycerol, Brun's solution, or any commercially available water-soluble mountant. These are not permanent sections.

RESULTS. Fat — red
          Nuclei — blue

REFERENCE. Lillie, R. D. *Histopathologic Technic and Practical Histochemistry* (2d ed.). New York: McGraw-Hill, 1954, p. 303.

OIL RED O (METHOD II)

DISCUSSION. Propylene glycol is a recommended solvent for oil red O and other oil soluble dyes. Its use permits some control of differentiation. Because of this differentiation, cryostat sections mounted on glass slides stain more uniformly with the propylene glycol solution.

Oil Red O-Propylene Glycol

Dissolve 0.7 gm. of oil red O, a small amount at a time, in 100 ml. of absolute propylene glycol, stirring constantly. Heat to 100° to 110°C. and stir for 10 minutes. Filter hot through Whatman paper #2. Filtering is slow and can be expedited somewhat by filtering the dye solution in the paraffin oven. Cool to room temperature. Filter through a fritted glass filter of medium porosity, using suction. The solution may be stored in a 60°C. oven almost indefinitely.

TECHNIQUE. Cryostat sections, mounted on slide

Staining Procedure

1. Mount cryostat-cut sections on clean slide.
2. Fix the section in 10% formalin for *10 minutes.*
3. Wash sections in several changes of distilled water for *2 to 5 minutes* to remove excess formalin.
4. Dehydrate in 2 changes of propylene glycol for *3 to 5 minutes,* moving slides occasionally.
5. Stain in oil red O solution for *5 to 7 minutes* at 60°C., moving slides occasionally.
6. Differentiate and hydrate in 85% propylene glycol, moving slides back and forth for *3 minutes.*
7. Transfer slides to distilled water and counterstain with hematoxylin.
8. Wash in tap water and mount in glycerin or some other aqueous mountant.

RESULTS. Fat — red

Nuclei — blue

REFERENCE. Chifelle, T. L., and Putt. F. A. *Stain Techn.* 26:51, 1951.

PERIODIC ACID-SCHIFF REACTION
(McManus)

Schiff's reagent is essentially a decolorized basic fuchsin, with the specificity for aldehydes dependent upon the decolorization brought about by sulfurous acid. Materials colored by the periodic acid-Schiff reaction are said to be PAS-positive.

INDICATIONS. To demonstrate in tissue any of the following: glycogen, mucin, reticulum, basement membranes, and pituitary basophil granules.

FIXATION.   10% formalin, Zenker's fluid, or Helly's fluid

TECHNIQUE.   Paraffin

DISCUSSION. There are many formulas for Schiff's reagent, and these variants may be used interchangeably if the strength of the solution is the same or if the time interval is lengthened or shortened appropriately.

See complete discussion of PAS method, p. 309.

A section of duodenum or cross-section of appendix can be used as a "control."

Staining Solutions

0.5% PERIODIC ACID SOLUTION

Periodic acid crystals	0.5 gm.
Distilled water	100.0 ml.

SCHIFF'S REAGENT

Bring to a boil *200 ml. of distilled water.* Remove from heat and add *1 gm. of basic fuchsin* and stir to dissolve. Cool to 50°C. Filter and add *20 ml. of normal hydrochloric acid. Shake vigorously.* Cool to 25°C. and *add 1 gm. of sodium bisulfite. Shake vigorously.* Keep in the dark. The fluid may take 18 to 24 hours to become straw-colored. It is then ready for use. (Shaking with a few grains of activated charcoal will decolorize the solution immediately. Filter and use.) Store in refrigerator in tightly stoppered brown bottle. Discard when pink color appears. Solution will last from 2 to 4 months, depending on use. Schiff's reagents precipitate a white crystalline substance after varying periods of cold storage. Reconstitution is impractical.

NORMAL HYDROCHLORIC ACID

Hydrochloric acid, concentrated, specific gravity 1.19	83.5 ml.
Distilled water	916.5 ml.

S U L F U R O U S   A C I D   R I N S E

Sodium metabisulfite,
    10% aqueous   6 ml.
Normal hydrochloric acid   5 ml.
Distilled water   100 ml.

Make this solution up just before use.

Staining Procedure

1. Deparaffinize the sections. If Zenker-fixed, treat as usual. Wash thoroughly.

2. Rinse in distilled water.

3. Oxidize in periodic acid solution for *5 minutes.*

4. Rinse in distilled water and drain.

5. Place in Schiff's reagent for *15 minutes* in covered Coplin jar. Schiff's reagent should be brought to room temperature before use and tissue stained at room temperature.

6. Place in two changes of sulfurous acid rinse for *2 minutes* each.

7. Wash in running tap water for *5 to 10 minutes* to develop pink color.

8. Stain sections very lightly in Harris's hematoxylin (progressive stain) for *10 seconds to 2 minutes,* depending on the strength of the hematoxylin. Wash in water for a few minutes in order to blue hematoxylin. *Optional:* Overstain in hematoxylin and decolorize in acid alcohol, blue in lithium carbonate, and wash in running water.

9. Dehydrate in several changes of 95% alcohol and several changes of absolute alcohol.

10. Clear in two or three changes of xylene. Mount in any neutral mounting medium.

RESULTS.   The following stain rose to purple-red: glycogen, mucin, reticulum, basement membranes, and pituitary and thyroid colloid.

Nuclei — blue

REFERENCE.   McManus, J. F. A. *Stain Techn.* 23:99, 1948.

PERIODIC ACID-SCHIFF REACTION
WITH DIASTASE FOR GLYCOGEN TEST

FIXATION. There is still no one opinion as to the best method of fixing glycogen. Alcohol or alcoholic mixtures are generally recommended on the basis that glycogen is insoluble in them, while it is soluble in most aqueous fixatives. Theoretically, as applied to pure glycogen, this is true. However, in tissues where glycogen is embedded or bound in a complex mixture of proteins and lipids the situation is different. Most staining techniques recommend fixation in Gendre's solution, acetic-alcohol-formalin, Bouin's solution, and 10% alcoholic formalin. Generally, cold solutions are preferable, with refrigerator temperatures maintained during entire fixation period. Ice-cold alcohol (95% or absolute) may be used, but it causes polarization (streaming to one corner of the cell) and tends to cause glycogen to appear as large, coarse granules.

ENZYME DIGESTION AS A CONTROL. One of the oldest methods for differentiation of glycogen is the saliva test. It is based on the fact that saliva contains a diastatic enzyme which will dissolve out glycogen and starch but not mucin, amyloid, and other related substances. Consequently, it is accepted that if a substance stains positively without pretreatment but fails to do so after an exposure to saliva of 30 to 60 minutes, it must be glycogen or starch. On the other hand, if it persists in staining after the saliva test, it cannot be glycogen. At present a number of highly active diastase preparations are available which are efficient and more appealing than the time-honored saliva test.

TECHNIQUE. Celloidin-coated paraffin sections are recommended by some authorities. "When sections are being stained with the periodic acid-Schiff technique specifically for the demonstration of glycogen, they should be celloidin-coated. Periodic acid removes a large amount of glycogen from unprotected sections" (Pearse). However, diastase will not diffuse through celloidin; therefore, if celloidin-coated sections are to be used, do not coat sections until after they have been treated and washed free of the diastase solution.

Digestion with Diastase

Cut a duplicate (control) section. One section is to be treated with diastase before staining, the other stained without pretreatment.

1. Deparaffinize sections.

2. Reserve duplicate slide in 80% alcohol and place other section in 0.5% diastase solution at room temperature or in a 37°C. oven for *1 hour.*

DIASTASE SOLUTION

U.S.P. malt diastase	0.5 gm.
Distilled water	100.0 ml.

3. Wash section in running water for *10 to 15 minutes.*

4. Dehydrate treated section and section which has been reserved through two changes of 95% and absolute alcohols.

5. Coat sections with thin celloidin solution (page 284).

6. After coating sections in Coplin jar, stand slides on edge to drain for approximately *30 seconds to 1 minute* or until sections begin to whiten around edges.

7. Harden celloidin by placing slides in 80% alcohol for *2 to 5 minutes.*

8. Follow directions for periodic acid-Schiff test (page 263), steps 2 to 10 inclusive.

RESULTS. If the cell product in question is glycogen, it will be stained purple-red in the standard PAS-stained slide and will be unstained in the PAS-stained slide that has been treated with diastase.

REFERENCE. Gomori, G. L. *Microscopic Histochemistry.* Chicago: University of Chicago, 1952, p. 66.

TOLUIDINE BLUE STAIN FOR METACHROMASIA

INDICATIONS. To identify tissue components by their metachromatic properties.

Mast cell stain.

(Metachromasia is a constant feature of mast cell granules, presumably due to their heparin content.)

FIXATION. 10% buffered neutral formalin or 10% alcoholic formalin recommended. Avoid fixatives that contain strong oxidants, especially chromic acid.

TECHNIQUE. Paraffin or frozen sections. Process with control section if one is available.

DISCUSSION. Staining is more intense at pH values of 2.5 to 3.0.

Some metachromasia is "alcohol labile," i.e., it will be leached out by alcoholic dehydration, whereas other strongly metachromatic reactions will remain fast.

Occasionally the mounting media will reverse metachromasia; this can be avoided if the section is water mounted immediately after staining and promptly examined.

Loss of metachromasia is reduced if sections are blotted dry with filter paper, air-dried, and then mounted in a permanent media.

For all of the reasons given, a variety of methods of preserving the metachromasia follows.

Staining Solution

TOLUIDINE BLUE 0.5%

Toluidine blue	0.5 gm.
20% ethyl alcohol	100.0 ml.

Combine. When dye is completely dissolved, filter. Stain improves when aged.

Staining Procedures

Follow steps 1 through 3 and then complete staining technique with any one of the methods given below.

1. Deparaffinize sections and bring to water as usual.
2. Treat in toluidine blue for *5 to 20 minutes.*
3. Wash briefly in tap water.

METHOD I

4. Coverslip from the water and immediately examine the wet mount. This is impermanent.

METHOD II

4. Following step 3 above, dehydrate in two changes of 95% alcohol and two changes of absolute alcohol for *1 minute each.*
5. Clear in xylene, two changes, and mount in Permount.

METHOD III

4. Following water wash, blot dry (or dehydrate in acetone), clear in xylene, and mount in Permount.

METHOD IV (MOWRY)

4. Dehydrate in two changes of 95% alcohol and two changes of absolute alcohol, for *1 minute each.*
5. Air dry sections.
6. Clear in two or three changes of xylene, and mount in Permount.

RESULTS.   Mast cell granules of most species turn brilliant red to purple.
Acid mucopolysaccharides — red to pink
Nuclei — shades of blue
Erythrocytes — green to yellow

REFERENCE.   McManus, J. F. A., and Mowry, R. W. *Staining Methods, Histologic and Histochemical.* New York: Hoeber Med. Div., Harper & Row, 1960, pp. 132 and 261.

VERHOEFF'S ELASTIC-TISSUE STAIN
(Modified)

INDICATIONS. Staining elastic fibers in sections.

FIXATION. Helly's, Zenker's fluid or 10% formalin preferred.

TECHNIQUE. Paraffin

Staining Solutions

ELASTIC-TISSUE STAIN

Hematoxylin	1 gm.
Absolute alcohol	50 ml.

Combine in a small Erlenmeyer flask and dissolve hematoxylin with the aid of gentle heat. Filter and add in order given:

Ferric chloride, 10% aqueous solution	25 ml.
Lugol's iodine (page 29)	25 ml.

After deparaffinization, it is not necessary to treat Zenker-fixed or Helly-fixed sections with iodine before staining. Any mercurial precipitates which may be present will be removed by the staining solution. For best results the solution should be used within 24 hours.

10% FERRIC CHLORIDE

Ferric chloride lumps	10 gm.
Distilled water	100 ml.

Pulverize ferric chloride with mortar and pestle. Add water.

2% FERRIC CHLORIDE
(DIFFERENTIATING SOLUTION)

10% ferric chloride	20 ml.
Distilled water	80 ml.

VAN GIESON'S STAIN
(See page 270.)

Staining Procedure

1. Deparaffinize sections to water.
2. Immerse sections in elastic-tissue stain for *15 minutes to 1 hour*

or until perfectly black. Check after 15 minutes, which is usually ample time. Rinse off excess stain in distilled water.

3. Differentiate in 2% aqueous solution of ferric chloride. This requires only a few minutes. Sections may be rinsed quickly in water and checked with the microscope under low power magnification. As a guide for differentiation, look for the elastic tissue within arteries and large veins to determine if the elastic fibers have been sufficiently decolorized. Elastic tissue has the kinked appearance of a hairpin. Cytoplasm should be clear or only slightly colored. Elastic fibers should appear clear black. (If tissue has been overdifferentiated, the slide may be returned to the staining solution and restained.) When differentiation is complete, rinse with water.

4. Place sections in 95% alcohol to remove iodine (optional).

5. Rinse rapidly in distilled water.

6. Counterstain in van Gieson's stain for a few seconds or longer. Dip slide (use Coplin jar) until desired color is obtained. Control staining with microscope. Collagen should be bright red and the background yellow. Stain may be saved and reused.

7. Dehydrate rapidly in two changes of 95% alcohol, followed by three changes of absolute alcohol. Some of the yellow color (picric acid) will be lost here.

8. Clear in several changes of xylene and mount in Permount, or some neutral mounting medium.

RESULTS.   Elastic fibers — blue-black to black
Nuclei — blue to black
Collagen — red
Other tissue elements — yellow

REFERENCE.   Mallory, F. B. *Pathological Technique.* Philadelphia: Saunders, 1938, p. 170.

VAN GIESON'S STAIN

INDICATIONS.   Connective-tissue stain, generally used in combination with another stain. It is frequently used with Weigert's iron hematoxylin. The Weigert's is applied to the nuclei and the slides counterstained with van Gieson's stain. Picric acid solutions somewhat decolorize nuclei so that it is necessary to overstain nuclei slightly before placing in these solutions. As an alternative, the period of counterstaining may be shortened. Picric acid solutions combine with many dyes to form a compound that has an affinity for collagen.

Staining Solution

Saturated aqueous solution of picric acid (about 1.22%)	100 ml.
Acid fuchsin, 1% aqueous solution	5 to 15 ml.

Combine and store. This is a stable solution and may be reused indefinitely. In our experience a ratio of 10 ml. of 1% acid fuchsin to 100 ml. of the saturated picric acid has proved most satisfactory with our method of fixation. For your use, remember that the formula with the lesser strength of fuchsin will give a more intense yellow cytoplasm. When the concentration of fuchsin is too heavy, the yellow-stained elements of the tissue will be masked with the red dye.

Apply counterstain by dipping slides individually in a Coplin jar until the desired depth of coloration is acquired. Slides may be rinsed in distilled water and checked under the microscope. They are dehydrated and cleared in the routine manner.

RESULTS.   Connective tissue — red
Other tissue elements — yellow

WARTHIN-STARRY METHOD FOR STAINING SPIROCHETES

INDICATIONS.   For staining spirochetes.

FIXATION.   10% buffered neutral formalin

TECHNIQUE.   Paraffin

DISCUSSION.   All glassware must be chemically clean. Any impurities will cause precipitation of the silver. Use chemicals of reagent grade. When transferring slides in steps 2 and 3, handle sections with paraffin-coated forceps. Results are controlled by microscopic examination of stained sections. Process a "control" slide (known positive), if available, with test slide.

Before placing the slides in the 1% prewarmed silver nitrate, (step 2), measure the required amounts of 2% silver nitrate, gelatin, and hydroquinone into individual 50 ml. Erlenmeyer flasks, stopper, and place these in the hot water flotation bath at 43°C. The developer is a combination of these solutions, all of which must be prewarmed. By the time the impregnation has taken place, the components of the developer will be ready.

Staining Solutions

ACIDULATED WATER

One liter of triple-distilled water acidulated with a weak solution of citric acid (1% or less) to bring the solution to a pH of 3.8 to 4.4.

1% SILVER NITRATE SOLUTION
(For impregnation)

Silver nitrate, C.P. crystals	1 gm.
Acidulated water	100 ml.

2% SILVER NITRATE SOLUTION
(For developer)

Silver nitrate, C.P. crystals	2 gm.
Acidulated water	100 ml.

0.15% HYDROQUINONE SOLUTION

Hydroquinone crystals, photographic quality	0.15 gm.
Acidulated water	100.00 ml.

5% GELATIN SOLUTION

Sheet gelatin (high grade)	10 gm.
Acidulated water	200 ml.

Staining Procedure

1. Pass sections through xylene and alcohols to triple-distilled water. Rinse twice in distilled water. (For steps 2 and 3 handle sections with paraffin-coated forceps.)

2. Place in a preheated 1% solution of silver nitrate at 43°C. for *30 minutes.* (A water bath is a satisfactory method of warming.)

3. Cover sections with the developer which is mixed by combining the ingredients (warmed to 43°C. in a water bath) in the order given, rotating the container and mixing well after each addition. The developer must be used as soon as it is mixed. Do not wait more than a few seconds after the addition of the hydroquinone before putting the developer on the sections.

D E V E L O P E R

2% silver nitrate in acidulated water	1.50 ml.
5% gelatin in acidulated water	3.75 ml.
0.15% hydroquinone	2.00 ml.

Allow sections to develop until they are light brown or yellow. Check known control under the microscope. The spirochetes should be black and the background light brown or yellow. Time of development varies from *3 to 12 minutes.*

4. Rinse quickly and thoroughly in hot tap water (approximately 56°C.).

5. Rinse in distilled water, dehydrate through alcohols.

6. Cléar through two changes of xylene.

7. Mount in Permount.

RESULTS.   Spirochetes — black
Background — pale yellow to light brown

REFERENCES.   Kerr, D. A. *Amer. J. Clin. Path., Tech. Suppl.* 8:63, 1938.
Bridges, C. H., and Luna L. *Lab. Invest.* 6:357, 1957 (report on Armed Forces Institute of Pathology adaptation, 1957 edition of *Manual*).

WILDER'S METHOD FOR RETICULUM

FIXATION.   10% formalin

TECHNIQUE.   Paraffin sections cut at 6μ.
Use acid clean glassware throughout.

Staining Solutions

10% PHOSPHOMOLYBDIC ACID SOLUTION

Phosphomolybdic acid	10 gm.
Distilled water	100 ml.

1% URANIUM NITRATE SOLUTION

Uranium nitrate	1 gm.
Distilled water	100 ml.

AMMONIACAL SILVER SOLUTION

To 5 ml. of a 10% aqueous solution of silver nitrate, add 58% ammonium hydroxide, drop by drop, until the precipitate which forms is almost dissolved. Add 5 ml. of 3% sodium hydroxide and barely dissolve the resulting precipitate with a few drops of ammonium hydroxide. Make the solution up to 50 ml. with distilled water. Prepare *just* before use.

REDUCING SOLUTION

Distilled water	50.0 ml.
Neutral formalin,* full strength	0.5 ml.
Uranium nitrate, 1% aqueous solution	1.5 ml.

Make fresh, just before use.

0.2% GOLD CHLORIDE
(See page 28.)

5% SODIUM THIOSULFATE
(See page 30.)

NUCLEAR FAST RED STAIN
(See page 378.)

* See page 36.

Staining Procedure

1. Deparaffinize and hydrate to distilled water.
2. Oxidize in phosphomolybdic acid solution for *1 minute.*
3. Rinse well in running water or cells will hold yellow color.
4. Sensitize in uranium nitrate solution for *1 minute.*
5. Rinse in distilled water for *10 to 20 seconds.*
6. Immerse in ammoniacal silver solution for *1 minute* (change solution frequently).
7. Dip very quickly in 95% alcohol and go immediately into:
8. Reducing solution for *1 minute* (change solution frequently).
9. Rinse well in distilled water.
10. Tone in gold chloride solution for *1 minute* or until sections lose their yellow color and turn lavender. Too much toning will make sections red. Check individually under microscope.
11. Rinse in distilled water.
12. Place in sodium thiosulfate solution for *1 minute.*
13. Wash well in tap water.
14. Counterstain, if desired, with nuclear fast red solution. Rinse well in distilled water.
15. Dehydrate in 95% alcohol, absolute alcohol, and clear in xylene, two changes each.
16. Mount with Permount or Histoclad.

RESULTS. Reticulum fibers — black
Collagen — rose
Other tissue elements — red

REFERENCES. Wilder, H. C. *Amer. J. Path.* 11:817–821, 1935.
Luna, L. (Ed.), *Manual of Histologic Staining Methods of the Armed Forces Institute of Pathology* (3d ed.). New York: McGraw-Hill, 1968, p. 92.

ZIEHL-NEELSEN'S ACID-FAST STAIN FOR SMEARS

INDICATIONS. Rapid method of identifying acid-fast bacilli in smears.

TECHNIQUE. Air-dry smears and fix by passing through a gentle flame.

Staining Solutions

ZIEHL-NEELSEN ACID-FAST STAIN

Basic fuchsin, saturated alcoholic solution (about 5.95%)	10 ml.
Carbolic acid water, 5%	90 ml.

(Carbolic acid water is made by shaking together 5 ml. of melted carbolic acid crystals with 95 ml. of distilled water.)

Combine and store at room temperature. Filter before use.

1% ACID ALCOHOL

Hydrochloric acid, concentrated	1 ml.
70% ethyl alcohol	99 ml.

Staining Procedure

1. With eyedropper, apply filtered Ziehl-Neelsen stain to smear. Steam gently for *3 to 5 minutes.* Keep smear covered with staining solution.

2. Wash in tap water.

3. Decolorize in acid alcohol for approximately *10 seconds.*

4. Finish decolorizing in 70% alcohol, until no more color comes off (usually about *20 seconds* longer).

5. Wash in water.

6. If desired, counterstain lightly in 0.5% aqueous methylene blue or in 0.5% aqueous light green for approximately *10 seconds.*

7. Wash in water.

8. Dry and examine with oil-immersion objective without mounting.

RESULTS. Acid-fast bacteria — bright red

Background — pale blue or pale green, depending on the counterstain used

REFERENCE. Mallory, F. B. *Pathological Technique.* Philadelphia: Saunders, 1938, p. 275.

15

"How To" Chapter

The histologic technician is faced daily with many small problems that are easily solved with a few helpful hints.

GENERAL INFORMATION

How to Test Unknown Strengths of Alcohol

If there is a question as to the percentage of an alcohol, float an alcoholometer in the solution. The alcoholometer, a device for determining the strength or percentage of alcohol, is a kind of hydrometer with a scale marked to indicate the different percentages of alcohol. The number on the scale just at the surface of the liquid indicates its strength.

How to Deformalinize Tissue Sections

Occasionally it is desirable to refix formalin-fixed sections in some other fixative (e.g., Zenker's, Helly's, or Bouin's fluid) in order to produce a more brilliant stain, or because a specific fixative is required as a mordant for a particular stain.

1. Deparaffinize and place sections for 1 hour in ammonia water (to 100 ml. of water add 30 drops of 58% ammonium hydroxide).
2. Wash for 1 hour in running water.

POSTMORDANTING. *For Zenker Mordanting.* Refix sections on the slide for 30 to 60 minutes in Zenker's or Helly's fluid. Wash for 15 minutes in running water. Remove mercuric chloride crystals by treating the slides with alcoholic iodine, followed by hypo as usual. Wash thoroughly. Slide is ready to be stained.

For Bouin's Mordanting. Refix sections on the slide in Bouin's fluid or in saturated picric acid for 1 hour. Remove excess fixative in 50% and 70% alcohols, several changes, 30 to 60 minutes, or wash sections in running water for 30 minutes. Rinse with distilled water. Slide is ready to be stained.

How to Remove Mercuric Chloride Crystals

Fixatives containing mercuric chlorides leave a deposit of crystals on the tissue. These must be removed, as they interfere with the staining and reading of the slides.

1. Deparaffinize slides through xylene, absolute, and 95% alcohols.
2. Place in an alcoholic iodine solution (0.5% iodine in 80% alcohol) to remove the deposit (page 28). Leave in this solution for 5 to 10 minutes.
3. Wash in water or rinse in 80% alcohol.
4. Place in a 5% solution of sodium thiosulfate (hypo) for 2 to 5 minutes to bleach out the iodine.
5. Wash thoroughly in running tap water to remove the hypo. Proceed with staining technique.

How to Remove Formalin Pigment Deposits

Formalin sometimes produces a fine dark-brown or black crystalline precipitate, said to be the product of laked hemoglobin. To remove this precipitate, deparaffinize the sections to water and place in any of the following solutions.

Solution i

Ammonium hydroxide, 58%	2 ml.
Alcohol, 70%	100 ml.

Place in the solution for 30 to 60 minutes. Wash thoroughly in tap water to remove excess ammonia and stain as desired.

SOLUTION II

Hydrogen peroxide, 3% aqueous	50 ml.
Acetone	50 ml.
Ammonium hydroxide, 58%	1 ml.

Place in the solution for 5 to 10 minutes. Wash thoroughly in running water to remove excess ammonia and stain as desired.

SOLUTION III

Place sections in a saturated alcoholic picric acid solution for 2 to 3 hours. Wash well in running tap water.

How to Remove Melanin Pigment

In order to stain slides without the interference of the pigment, or to ascertain whether the pigment in question is melanin (since melanin will be bleached by this method):

1. Deparaffinize sections through to water.
2. Treat with 0.25% aqueous potassium permanganate solution for 1 to 4 hours.
3. Wash well in running tap water.
4. Bleach in 5% aqueous oxalic acid solution for 5 to 10 minutes.
5. Wash in running tap water for 10 minutes and rinse with distilled water. Slide is ready to be stained.

How to Remedy Improperly Dehydrated Tissue Blocks

When tissue sections are not completely dehydrated, the paraffin cannot infiltrate properly and the block is impossible to cut. The only way to secure a satisfactory section when this occurs is to remove the paraffin and redehydrate the tissue. Trim all residual paraffin from around the tissue. Melt remaining paraffin by placing tissue in the paraffin oven or on the embedding table. Place tissue in several changes of xylene to clear. Placing the xylene jar within the paraffin oven will accelerate dissolution of the paraffin. When the paraffin is completely dissolved, pass tissue slowly through several changes of absolute and 95% alcohols. The use of a mechanical mixer to speed up the rate of diffusion will shorten considerably the time required and 30 minutes in each solution will be adequate. Then start the slow dehydration process again. Dehydrate tissue thoroughly in 95% alcohol and absolute alcohol, clear in xylene, and reinfiltrate tissue with paraffin. Embed (cast) and section.

How to Remedy Improperly Fixed Tissue Blocks

Without adequate fixation, satisfactory cutting and staining is improbable. If tissue has been infiltrated and blocked, but it is impossible to cut an acceptable section, the following procedure will be necessary.

Remove paraffin (see p. 278) and run block through xylene, absolute, 95%, and 80% alcohols down to water. Refix tissue. The time required will depend on the nature and size of the tissue. After complete fixation the tissue is reprocessed through the dehydrants, reinfiltrated, and blocked.

How to Reclaim Tissues Ending Series in Wrong Solution

All of us have at one time or another arrived to find the basket of tissues (completely impregnated with paraffin) moved a step beyond into formalin, water, or whatever the initial solution was on the processing series. Don't panic. The paraffin impregnation prevents penetration of fixatives, water, or alcohols. (1) Rinse basket of tissues briefly under cold tap water and shake free of excess water. (2) Empty capsules onto cloth toweling and blot excess moisture from capsules. (3) Put capsules back into a dry basket carrier and place in paraffin oven (on a tray) for approximately 10 minutes. (4) Return basket of tissues to Autotechnicon paraffin bath for an additional 15 to 30 minutes of infiltration. (5) Embed (cast) and cut. Decant paraffin in the bath that was used for the reinfiltration and replace with new supply.

CUTTING PROBLEMS

How to Soften Tissue

Thyroid blocks, uterine fibroids, keratinized epithelium, and very scirrhous tissue, are sometimes very difficult or impossible to cut. The technician usually becomes aware of this when cutting the tissue block on the microtome. In order to secure a better section or any section at all, it becomes necessary to treat the tissue. The possibility that a dull knife is the problem can be ruled out by changing knives or by having a colleague try the block on her knife.

A rapid and simple method of softening the block is to soak it in a small dish or bowl containing water to which has been added a small amount of any detergent. (Ratio: approximately ½ teaspoonful of dry detergent to 100 ml. of tap water.) Shave into the block until the tissue is exposed. Place block in this solution and leave for ½ hour to 3 hours. Blot solution from block and recut on microtome. Do not leave tissue in this solution longer than necessary. If block is still difficult to section after 3 hours' immersion, leave in tap water overnight.

How to Cut Blood-Containing Tissues

It is very discouraging to try to cut a section of bloody tissue that has become so brittle in processing that it shatters like sawdust across the knife edge. (1) Try soaking the block (after shaving it on microtome to expose tissue) in tap water for a few hours. If tissue will not cut within a few hours, leave block in tap water overnight. (2) An alternate method is to soak blocks for 1 to 2 hours or overnight in a 10% solution of glycerin in 60% alcohol. (3) With a camel's hair brush, paint the surface of the block with 58% ammonium hydroxide. Cut a few sections and discard. The third or fourth section should be acceptable.

How to Remove Folds from Pleated Paraffin Sections

To remove stubborn folds from a paraffin ribbon, run 50% alcohol over an extra glass slide with an eyedropper. Place cut section directly on the alcohol-moistened slide. Transfer tissue ribbon on the slide to the hot water bath. Tissue will spin and spread out. Pick up tissue from water bath on properly identified slide. Drain and dry as usual.

How to Remedy Tissue Sections Hung-up on Tissue Processor (*Becoming Air-dried, Brittle, and Glass-like*) *

This problem is a very serious one and complete restoration of the texture, cutting, and staining qualities of the tissue block is not likely if the basket has become hung-up following dehydration.

If the tissue is still hanging midair on your arrival at the laboratory and has been through the dehydrants or clearing agent, place tissue in 95% absolute alcohol and 80% alcohol (reversing the dehydration series) for approximately 30 minutes each. If a mechanical stirrer is available, use it. Alternatively, you can reverse solutions on the tissue processor, attach the basket, and manually activate the cycle at 30-minute intervals for this hydration phase. Once the tissues have been hydrated in 80% alcohol, allow them to soak in normal saline for 1 to 3 hours or until they appear plumped out. Then redehydrate, clear, and infiltrate in the usual processing sequence. If the tissues have gone through paraffin infiltration and the brittle condition is not discovered until sectioning, first remove the paraffin with xylene and then follow the steps above.

Using control material, in our laboratory we deliberately allowed blocks of old autopsy tissue to "hang" following dehydration and following clearing. These we processed under controlled conditions in several different ways. From our study we concluded that if tissues had hung in the air for as long as 2 hours following the *clearing agent* (xylene), they suffered only in a minor way, and rehydration with subsequent normal saline treatment did not produce slides superior to those blocks which were transferred directly into the paraffin baths. However, if the tissues hung in the air following *dehydration,* treatment as here recommended helped cutting considerably. *Note:* Whoever detaches the basket from the tissue processor should check the clock *daily* and see if it coincides with the correct time. A deviation will alert the technician that a problem with the machine or personnel may have altered the embedding process.

* Suggestion courtesy of Mona Ayers, St. Joseph's Hospital, Burbank, California.

STAINING

How to Restain Slides

From time to time it is necessary to restain a section because it has faded, or perhaps a different stain is required on a slide that has already been stained routinely. First, soak off the coverglass by immersing the slide in xylene. This may take several hours to several days, depending on how long the slide has been coverslipped. The process may be expedited by placing the slides in the xylene in the paraffin oven. Leave no longer than is necessary.

Remove the slides as soon as the coverglasses have loosened. When the coverslip has become detached, rinse the slide in another change or two of xylene to ensure removal of the mounting reagent. Then pass the section through a few changes of absolute alcohol and 95% alcohol, down to water. Decolorize the stain in acid alcohol (page 26) until the section is free of all or most of the color. Wash thoroughly in running water. Section is ready to be restained.

How to Restore Faded Microslides

1. Gently warm slide to loosen coverglass or soak coverglass off in xylene.

2. Wash slides in xylene thoroughly to remove all traces of mounting reagent.

3. Hydrate sections through graded alcohols — absolute, 95%, 80% and water.

4. Place in a 0.5% solution of potassium permanganate for 5 minutes.

5. Rinse with tap water.

6. Bleach in a 0.5% solution of oxalic acid for approximately 1 to 2 minutes. If old stain has not been removed, repeat permanganate bath and oxalic bleach treatments.

7. Wash in running tap water to free tissue of excess acid.

8. Restain as desired.

Note: After treatment with the potassium permanganate and oxalic acid it will usually be necessary to dilute stains or shorten staining time.

REFERENCE. McCormick, J. B. *Techn. Bull. Regist. Med. Techn.* 20:13, 1959.

How to Revitalize Staining of Old Formalin-fixed Tissue

Formalin-fixed tissue which has been in wet storage over a period of time often stains poorly. The following procedure has been recommended by Dr. C. Culbertson (P.O. Box 618, Indianapolis, Indiana). (1) Place cut tissue sections on the slide into a 25% sodium bisulfite solution for 5 minutes. (2) Wash slides in buffered saline (pH 7.2) containing 3% TWEEN 80. (3) Stain as desired.

How to Restore Hematoxylin Staining of Overzenkerized Tissue Sections (AFIP Recommendation)

(1) Deparaffinize slides, treat with iodine and hypo, and wash in water. (2) Transfer slides and leave in a 10% aqueous solution of sodium bicarbonate for 6 to 8 hours. (3) Wash in running tap water for 10 minutes and restain.

How to Decolorize Sections (for Hematoxylin Series)

Acid alcohol (page 26) is perhaps the most used solution for the extraction of excess color in sections. The procedure is as follows:

Dip sections quickly in a dish containing 0.5% or 1% acid alcohol. Wash immediately and thoroughly in running tap water to stop acid action. Place sections in any of the following: (1) A dish of tap water which has been slightly alkalinized with a few drops of ammonium hydroxide. (2) A saturated solution of lithium carbonate for 15 to 30 seconds. (3) Running tap water for 5 to 15 minutes. The lithium carbonate, ammonia water, or running tap water neutralizes the acid and restores the purple-blue color to the sections.

After blueing in ammonia water or lithium carbonate, wash slides in running tap water to remove the alkaline solution or else the counterstain (usually eosin) will not be taken up properly by the tissue. It is convenient to have two dishes set up on the side of the sink, one containing acid alcohol and the other containing saturated lithium carbonate. The acid alcohol and the lithium carbonate should be changed when they turn color.

The writer prefers lithium carbonate for neutralizing; it is very rapid, taking much less time than blueing in running water. Ammonia dissolves albumen, and sections may loosen from the slide if left for long in this solution.

How to Keep Sections from Floating off Slide (Collodionization)

If a paraffin ribbon contains air bubbles, or the section is torn or inadequately infiltrated, it is likely to float from the slide when it is placed in a deparaffinizing or staining solution. The sections may be more firmly attached by coating the slide with a very dilute celloidin solution (page 27).

After deparaffinizing in xylene, dehydrate through absolute alcohol. Directly from the absolute alcohol, dip slides individually in a Coplin jar containing the very dilute ether-alcohol solution of celloidin. Stand slide on end to drain for ½ to 1 minute or until the section begins to whiten around the edges. Wipe off the back of the slide, and place in 80% alcohol for 3 to 5 minutes to harden the celloidin coating. Proceed with the steps of the regular staining technique. All or most of the celloidin will be removed in the final dehydration in absolute alcohol prior to clearing and mounting. If the coating of celloidin is heavy and not removed in the final absolute alcohol, place briefly in a dish containing equal parts of absolute alcohol and ether, or in absolute acetone. Clear in two or three changes of xylene and mount.

This treatment (collodionization) is also recommended for sections which are to be subjected to strong alkaline or acid solutions, for bone sections, and for tissues which are to be stained for the purpose of demonstrating glycogen. *Note:* Staining may take slightly longer with tissues that have been coated with celloidin. It is recommended that a duplicate section be processed without the collodionization.

How to Remove Cloudy, Opaque Areas from Coverslipped Sections

If this condition is noted after sections have been stained and coverslipped, it usually indicates insufficient dehydration or clearing. Such sections will fade rapidly if the condition is not corrected. Simply remove coverslip by soaking in xylene. Wash off mounting reagent thoroughly in xylene, and return slide to absolute alcohol for complete dehydration (if absolute alcohol is the dehydrant used). Clear slide once more in three changes of xylene and reapply the coverslip. Sections that are very resistant to routine procedures may be cleared in carbol-xylene (page 26), followed by rinsing in three changes of pure xylene.

How to Remedy a Coverslipped Section Showing Highly Refractive Lines Outlining Cells and Tissues

This occurs when the clearing agent is allowed to evaporate from the surface of the tissue section before the mounting reagent is applied. Remove coverslip, return slide to clearing agent for a few minutes, and remount.

HANDLING SLIDES

How to Salvage Broken Slides

If the slide is broken only on an end away from the tissue, reaffix the broken fragment with cellophane tape. Slides sent through the mail are sometimes received in several pieces.

METHOD I. If enough of the pieces are present, the stained slide may be reconstituted on a blank slide, using mounting medium as the adhesive. If the coverslip has also been fractured, it will be necessary to loosen the broken pieces with xylene and apply a new coverslip. When the broken slide has been reconstituted on the second slide, wipe gingerly with xylene. Dry slide flat on a hot plate or in a 37°C. oven for several hours or overnight.

METHOD II. This technique consists of transferring the sections of tissue from the broken slide to a transparent plastic film and remounting the film on a slide.

1. Reassemble all pieces of the broken slide on top of another clean slide.

2. Align two sections of an applicator stick in a large Petri dish and mount slide on this support.

3. Cover slide with xylene until coverslip pieces can be removed.

4. Pick off coverslip fragments, and while the section is still soaking wet with xylene, pour plastic * on center of slide (enough to spread evenly to cover whole slide). A thin coating is best.

5. Allow to dry for 2 to 24 hours.

6. With a sharp scalpel cut film along edges of slide. Place slide in cold water (approximately 2 or more hours) until film which encloses section can be easily peeled from the glass slide.

7. Dry film with smooth filter paper.

8. Trim off excess plastic and remount the film (containing the tissue section) on a clean slide. Place a drop of Permount on the slide. Place a second drop on the film and coverslip immediately.

How to Prepare Slides for Mailing

Place slides in a cardboard slide mailer. Wrap elastic band around mailer. Insert mailer in mailing tube, taking care to stuff the free area below, above, and around the slides with cotton batting or some similar protective cushioning.

If a large number of slides is to be mailed, place slides in a slotted wooden or reinforced cardboard box. Lay a strip of cushioning across the top of the slides to prevent displacement of slides, and replace box cover. Secure lid with rubber band or adhesive tape. Wrap slide box with a slightly oversized strip of corrugated cardboard. Place in a tight-fitting manila envelope, or pack area around all sides of the box firmly with crumpled paper, cotton batting, or some other protection, cushioning it within a larger box. Styrofoam slotted boxes which provide built-in cushioning are available for mailing slides, and these provide maximum protection against breakage.

Be sure slides are well identified. Wrap and tie package securely. Write FRAGILE on wrapping.

How to Disengage Slides That Are Stuck Together

Slides that have been placed together before a proper drying interval has elapsed will stick to one another. If they cannot be gently

* Diatex is available from Scientific Products Inc., Evanston, Ill. 60201.

pried apart, soak slides in a dish of xylene to dissolve the sticky mounting medium. When the slides have separated, clean and recoverslip as necessary.

TIME SAVERS

How to Dry Slides Very Rapidly

Where speed is of paramount importance, an ordinary hair dryer may be used. Cut and mount sections and stand slide on edge. Allow to drain for a few minutes. When placed directly under the heat of the dryer, the sections will be dry enough to stain after 1 to 5 minutes. Allow slides to cool before processing.

How to Use Gelatin as an Adhesive on Slides

This time-saving technique eliminates the necessity of coating slides with the traditional albumen-glycerin fixative. Drop approximately ¼ teaspoonful of U.S.P. gelatin into the hot water bath (43°C.). The gelatin will dissolve in the water within a few minutes. Float sections on the water. Pick up ribbons on clean glass slides. Drain and dry as usual.

There are some cautions to be observed, however: (1) If an excess of gelatin is used, the gelatin (which is a protein) will pick up the dyes, resulting in an unattractive finished slide. (2) With some special stains the gelatin may produce artefactual staining results. (3) Whenever gelatin is used, the water flotation bath must be kept scrupulously clean to avoid growth of bacteria (page 22). This bacteria may appear on tissue sections and give a false picture.

16

Efficiency in the Laboratory

GENERAL RULES

1. Keep all equipment and utensils in order. Avoid a cluttered environment. Before leaving the laboratory, return all equipment and utensils to their proper place.

2. Keep a memorandum of the daily work schedule. Go over this carefully each day upon arrival at the laboratory.

3. Develop regular work habits and maintain regular work hours with scheduled rest periods.

4. Schedule coffee and lunch breaks so that one technician is always on duty in the laboratory.

5. If you use up reagents when completing a staining technique, prepare new solutions immediately thereafter. Do not wait until the next request comes through for the stain.

6. All data concerning the handling of tissue should be carefully recorded in a daily log (see illustration on page 291).

7. Use only clean glassware in preparing reagents. Rinse all used glassware while it is still moist.

8. Solutions which are used frequently should be prepared in gallon-sized bottles, e.g., dilutions of alcohol, hypo, alcoholic iodine, decalcifying solutions, acid alcohol, and Papanicolaou fixative.

9. *Do not throw solid waste material into the sink!* This applies especially to embedding media.

Paraffin. Pour melted paraffin into cardboard boxes or lids. Or pour paraffin into a newspaper-lined basin. Allow to solidify. Discard solid mass with other trash.

Celloidin. For large quantities, pour liquid celloidin into waste jars and allow to solidify. Discard with the trash. For small quantities, pour the fluid on top of a large pan of cold tap water. As soon as solution solidifies, allow to air-dry and discard.

10. Discourage the presence of visitors, children, and animals during working hours, as they promote inefficiency and increase the chance for errors.

11. Segregate eating, drinking, and smoking from slide preparation in space and time. Do not keep food in a laboratory icebox that contains specimens, stains, and reagents.

12. Encourage younger persons to take an interest in laboratory work and to assist part time, whenever possible, since in this way you may develop their talents in scientific pursuits.

TIME SAVERS

Equipment

Each technician should have a minimum of four knives in addition to a "bone knife." Mechanical knife sharpeners are a must. Mechanical stirrers save technician time.

Aides

If the laboratory is fortunate enough to have a laboratory aide, he or she can be of great help in freeing technician time. The aide can take over the duty of helping the pathologist with the grossing in addition to maintaining logs; ordering and maintaining supplies; filing blocks, slides, and wet tissue; filtering stains; setting up staining series; cleaning capsules, benches, and glassware; and providing messenger service.

Boxes of slides for autopsies may be prepared in advance, utilizing brief intervals of free time. For instance, if 25 slides on a case is the minimum number, then 25 slides are cleaned, etched, and labeled (frosted-end slides) in advance. No albumen is placed on these slides. They are stored in covered slotted wooden or plastic boxes which are identified on the outside as to number.

TIME MANAGEMENT

Special Stains

Unless the time intervals are very close, there is no necessity to devote your entire attention to *one special* stain. Other duties can be easily accomplished during waiting periods.

If you have more than one special stain to be done they can be processed during the same time interval. Start the special stain requiring the longest time first. We find the following method helpful:

1. Place on the bench a strip of butcher paper * long enough to accommodate the series of staining jars.

2. Set up Coplin jars with required solutions on the paper.

3. Directly in front of the Coplin jar write down the name of the solution it contains and the time interval necessary for staining or other treatment.

4. For each special stain, place an individual interval timer (clock) with the series.

Daytime Autopsy Processing

If the automatic tissue processor cannot accommodate the volume of tissue during the evening run, autopsy tissues can be scheduled in the following manner:

1. After fixation, allow tissue to set overnight in 80% alcohol.

2. First thing in the morning, attach the basket of tissues to the Autotechnicon. With 1 hour in 95% alcohol, three changes of fresh acetone of 1 hour each, two changes of xylene, ½ hour each and two changes of paraffin of 1½ hours each, the tissue will be ready to embed within the working day. Even if the tissue is attached to the machine later in the day, as long as the tissues have been infiltrated with paraffin for as little as 1 hour, the basket can be removed (tissues

---

* *Note:* An 18″ wide, 1100 foot roll of butcher paper (coated on one side) costs less than $10.00 and lasts for 8 to 12 months. The waxed side is placed down to protect counter surface. The uncoated side accepts pencil or pen notations very well. In addition to expediting the performance of several special stains simultaneously, the paper keeps the bench clean.

left in their trays) and allowed to stand at room temperature. The next morning, or whenever convenient, the basket is returned to the paraffin bath to complete infiltration.

RECORDS

Suggested Log for Recording Daily Data

Use a ruled composition notebook (Fig. 16-1).

SURGICAL NO.	NO. OF BLOCKS	NO. OF SLIDES	LEVELS	RIBBONS	SPECIAL STAINS	MEMBR. FILTERS	PAPS	AUTOPSIES	
			march 5, 1972						
S-71-681	6	6						A-12	25
682	B=1 C=2	B=1 C=2					A=2	A-13	30
683	12	12			1 A.F. 1 A.A.S.			A-14	12
684	A=1 B=1	A=1 B=2	A=3					A-15	40
685	1	1		5				A-16	9
TOTALS								TOTALS	

Figure 16-1. Suggested log for recording daily data

Complete and carefully kept logs should be kept of all work done in the histology laboratory, not only for day-to-day general information but also for compiling statistical reports for the various accreditation inspectors. In addition, if you are falling behind in your workload, a review of your statistics (by number count or graphing) will either indicate that improvement is needed or justify a request for additional personnel.

The suggested log can be modified to conform to a particular workload reporting system, i.e. the gynecologic and special cytology methods are recorded separately, frozen sections and decalcification procedures added to surgical pathology information, and a separate log kept for autopsy slide preparation.

Tissue Request Sheet

This form is used to request the technician to make additional sections or special stains on a particular specimen. The pathologist or resident fills in the sheet. The sheet is easily prepared by mimeographing. A stencil may be typed with the tissue request repeated several times. Individual copies are cut after mimeographing. If a print shop is available in your hospital, the request sheets could be offset printed, cut, and padded for convenience.

A particularly efficient way of doing the offset printing is to have the form made on N.C.R.–CFB (no carbon required, coated front and back) paper. The pathologist retains a carbon copy of his request and attaches it to the protocol so that he is always aware of why the diagnosis is still pending. The sample request sheet (Fig. 16-2) can easily be modified to meet the requirements of a particular laboratory.

Caution Chits

The pathology secretary or clerk can type the word "caution" over and over in rows to fill a 5 x 8 index card. These are cut up and boxed, or left in strips (cut nearly to the far edge) to be torn free at time of use. Sutures, clips, and calcareous material can ruin a good knife edge. If the pathologist encounters something gritty at the time he is grossing the tissue, he can insert the "caution" chit in the capsule. Alerted by means of this signal, the technician can cut the section first on the bone knife, and if it presents no problem it can then be transferred and sectioned on her own knife. If no "bone knife" is kept, the tissue should be cut last, protecting the knife edge and prolonging its use.

SAMPLE DAILY SCHEDULE

In a routine laboratory a schedule is necessary in order to process the steady stream of work that requires prompt attention. Surgical material must of course take precedence over autopsy, central nervous system, and research material, and projects of an academic nature. Each laboratory must work out a schedule that will allow maximum efficiency in processing the specimens without compromising the quality of the work. The following illustrates a schedule that has proved effective in our laboratory. Material processed varies from two to four baskets, with three baskets representing a daily average. There

HISTOLOGY REQUISITION

FROM: Dr._____

ACCESSION #_____Block:_____

NUMBER OF LEVELS_____
    Spacing of levels: close intervals_____
                     wide intervals_____

COPIES_____

    Special instructions:_____

H & E
Acid fast   — Kinyoun
Acid mucopolysacc.   — Alcian blue or AB-PAS
Amyloid   — Congo red or crystal violet
Argentaffin   — Fontana-Masson
Bone marrow   — Giemsa or May-Grünwald-Giemsa or Fe
Connective tiss.   — Masson trichrome
Elastic tissue   — Verhoeff-van Gieson
Fibrils   — PTAH
Fibrin   — PTAH or Weigert's
Fungus   — Gridley or Grocott
Gram   — Brown & Brenn
Glycogen   — PAS
Iron   — Gomori
Mucin   — Mayer's mucicarmine or AB-PAS
Myelin   — Luxol fast blue
Nerve fibers   — Bodian
Reticulum   — Foot's or Wilder's

OTHER_____

WHEN NEEDED_____

Figure 16-2. Sample request sheet — larger than actual size ($4\frac{1}{4}''$ × $5\frac{3}{8}''$)

are three full-time technicians and one part-time aide. The first technician works from 6:30 A.M. to 3:00 P.M., the second works from 7:30 A.M. to 4:00 P.M., and the third works from 9:00 A.M. to 5:30 P.M. In this way the laboratory is covered for 11 hours daily.

The technicians work a 5-day week, with the laboratory operating a full 6-day week, necessitating a rotating schedule to provide such coverage. *Schedule A* includes 4 days in one week (Monday through Thursday) and 6 days the following week (Monday through Saturday) — not to exceed a total of 80 hours in a 2-week period. *Schedule B* is a straight 5-day week, Tuesday through Saturday, and *Schedule C* includes 6 days in one week (Monday through Saturday) and 4 days the following week (Monday through Thursday). The technicians are assigned so that they alternate on monthly schedules.

The daily schedule is rather inflexible in the morning, since all effort is directed to providing the pathologists with the surgical slides as soon as possible. Afternoon duties are more flexible.

Morning Duties

6:30 First technician arrives, fills water baths, switches on equipment (slide warmer, slide dryers, and so on), and embeds the first basket of surgical material. Embedded blocks are placed in refrigerator. Embedding of second basket is started.

7:30 Second technician arrives, and excess paraffin is rapidly scraped from the face of chilled blocks with a cartilage knife (shaving it off on the microtome dulls knife unnecessarily and takes more time). Second technician begins embedding the third basket. First technician takes a coffee break. On her return, the slides are etched, marked with permanent ink, albumenized, and boxed, in numerical order.

8:15 Blocks are divided into two groups for sectioning. Both technicians cut surgical material.

9:00 Third technician arrives. The empty capsules (already soaked free of paraffin) are put on to wash. Special cytologic material (received during the previous evening or early morning) is processed. Autopsy tissues (fourth basket) are embedded or autopsy slides from previous day may be stained at this time. While surgical slides are drying, autopsy slides and cytologic material are coverslipped.

9:30 or 10:00 One technician deparaffinizes and stains the morning's surgical specimens. Two technicians coverslip, match protocols with slides, enter data in logs, and deliver the slides to the pathologist between 10:30 and 11:30 A.M.

11:30   Lunch for two technicians. The third prepares slides, and cuts duplicate sections, levels, ribbons, and sections for special stains. All blocks from the morning are filed.

12:30 P.M.   Cutting areas are cleaned. One microtome is left ready for afternoon sectioning of autopsy tissue. While slides are drying the third technician goes to lunch.

Afternoon Duties

Special stains are done.

Autopsies are cut.

Tissues are prepared for pathologist to gross. One technician or the aide helps pathologist with the grossing.

GYN cytology is processed.

Knives are checked, sharpened and stropped, if necessary.

Solutions and paraffin ovens are checked (including Autotechnicon).

Staining bench series are cleaned and replenished for next day.

Decal solutions are checked before leaving for the day.

Laboratory is tidied up before personnel leaves for the day.

It has probably become obvious that this steadily flowing schedule does not make allowance for mechanical failures, holidays, vacations, absenteeism, and equipment breakdown. Fortunately such disruptions are sporadic and one must work around them. Insofar as possible one should have a daily schedule and keep to it as closely as possible. It is important that the duties of the laboratory are rotated so that each technician has an opportunity to become proficient in all phases of microtechnique.

APPENDIX I

Histochemistry

The following material is in essence a definition of the subject with no intent of in-depth coverage. For more complete information the student is referred to the texts of Lillie, McManus and Mowry, Pearse, and Barka.* The purpose of this section is to give the student a glimpse of how histochemistry differs from pure histopathology. In a routine diagnostic pathology laboratory most of the material presented to the pathologist is prepared with the purpose of providing him with a morphologic view of the tissue. Histochemistry is a specialized branch of histology, one that attempts localization of chemical substances in tissue by histochemical means. Its practicality is that certain chemical substances in tissue are characteristic of a particular disease. Histochemistry does not supplant pure histologic diagnosis, it augments it. Some examples of histochemistry that have become routine in the histology laboratory are the Feulgen and periodic acid-Schiff reactions, the Prussian blue reaction, and many of the staining techniques that are used to identify acid mucopolysaccharides.

Fixation is doubly important when preparing material for histochemical evaluation. Most fixatives alter chemical composition. One must be careful not to introduce a foreign chemical substance during the fixing process. For instance, a simple fixative like cold alcoholic formalin is recommended for the preservation of polysaccharides, and cold acetone for certain enzymes. In some methods, fixation may be avoided in its entirety by freeze-drying or cryostat techniques.

* Barka, T., and Anderson, P. *Histochemistry.* New York: Harper & Row, 1965. Lillie, R. D. *Histopathologic Technic and Practical Histochemistry.* New York: McGraw-Hill, 1965. McManus, J. F. A., and Mowry, R. W. *Staining Methods, Histologic and Histochemical.* New York: Hoeber Med. Div., Harper & Row, 1960. Pearse, A. G. E. *Histochemistry, Theoretical and Applied.* Boston: Little, Brown and Co., 1960.

FREEZE DRYING

Routine fixation and embedding methods present many disadvantages from the histochemical standpoint. There are fixation artefacts, changes in the physical properties of the cell constituents, chemical alterations, and loss of enzymes and lipids.

Freeze drying was developed to minimize some of these alterations. Very small pieces of fresh tissue are quick-frozen at −160° to −180°C. and dehydrated under vacuum until all unbound water is removed. The rapid freezing inhibits as much as possible the formation of disrupting ice crystals. The dehydration is carried out at low temperatures to avoid the damaging effects brought about by abrupt thawing of the frozen material. Once dried in vacuo below the freezing point, the tissues are allowed to reach room temperature, are vacuum-embedded in degassed paraffin or Carbowax, and sectioned on a rotary microtome.

For practical reasons freeze drying is not an established procedure. Its disadvantages are that (1) only small samples can be processed; (2) tissue must be processed immediately upon removal, a step which makes it more a research tool than a routine procedure; a delay of a few minutes would allow bacterial, autolytic, or other changes to occur; (3) an expensive special apparatus is required; (4) it is a cumbersome and finicky process, one which is not readily incorporated into a routine histology schedule.

The tissue is quick-frozen (quenched) in isopentane that has been prechilled with liquid nitrogen. Following quenching, the drying is slowly carried out under low vacuum to allow controlled vaporization of the water content of the frozen specimen. The freeze-dried tissue is either surrounded by degassed paraffin within the apparatus or transferred into a vacuum-embedding bath containing melted paraffin wax. Following casting and cutting on a rotary microtome, the sections are *not floated out on water* but are either dry-mounted directly on the slide or alternatively floated out on a special inert flotation mixture (such as 70% alcohol at 40° to 50°C., which will also act as a fixative). The preferred method appears to be the finger method of mounting in which sections are applied dry to the slide and flattened with the finger. Some chemical reactions are carried out without removing the paraffin.

While its original intent may have been to avoid fixation, it is frequently necessary to postfix freeze-dried sections so as to prevent their components from dissolving in the incubating medium or to preserve morphologic structure. In most instances brief alcohol or acetone postfixation is applied. The choice of fixative or the necessity to postfix depends on the nature of the components to be studied. A step-by-step procedure for freeze drying is given below:

FREEZE-DRYING TECHNIQUE
(After Pearse)

Freezing (Quenching)

PHASE I

1. Small pieces of fresh tissue 2 to 5 mm. thick are flattened on narrow strips of aluminum foil.

2. The foil with tissue attached is immersed in a tube containing isopentane cooled to about −160°C. with liquid nitrogen.

3. The snap-frozen tissue is removed from the foil with forceps.

PHASE II

Drying (Dehydration)

4. The tube containing the quenched tissue is attached to the vacuum apparatus where it is dried under vacuum for 8 to 12 or more hours, at a higher temperature than that of the quenching (−30° to −40°C.).

Embedding (Infiltration)

5. When drying is complete, the tube is removed and the dehydrated blocks are immediately transferred to a vacuum-embedding bath containing paraffin at 56° to 58°C., or they may be embedded in Carbowax. Alternatively, with some freeze dryers, the embedding takes place within the freeze-drying apparatus without vacuum being broken. Infiltration will take 10 to 30 minutes, depending on the thickness of the specimen.

Sectioning

6. Paraffin sections are cut at 6 to 8μ and transferred directly to cool slides, thinly coated with egg albumen, avoiding all contact with water. The sections are flattened to the slide with the finger.

7. The slides are warmed slightly to melt the wax and allowed to cool. The slides are stored in the desiccator at 4°C. until they are stained in accordance with the histochemical method chosen.

Application of the Technique

Sections of unfixed materials can be examined by phase contrast microscopy, polarized light, or microincineration; or sections may be examined after treatment with buffer extractions for histochemical and histological findings. Sections may also be used for autoradiographic techniques.

SECTION FREEZE SUBSTITUTION

Simpson (*Anat. Rec.* 80:173–189, 1940) modified the freeze-dry method by substituting polar solvents (with or without fixation) instead of desiccation under vacuo to dehydrate the quick frozen blocks. Chang et al. (*J. Histochem. Cytochem.* 9:292–300, 1961) further modified Simpson's freeze-substitution technique with a method he termed "Section Freeze Substitution." Chang maintains that his technique had the advantage of retaining oxidative and hydrolytic enzymes and other chemical substances which may be lost either in the freeze-dry or in the freeze-substitution techniques. Instead of using paraffin-embedded blocks following the quick freeze, Chang used open-top cryostat sections.

Chang's Section Freeze Substitution Method

1. Freshly excised tissue is quenched in liquid nitrogen or in isopentane prechilled by liquid nitrogen (same as for freeze drying).

2. Following quenching, frozen blocks are ready for immediate sectioning or they may be stored in airtight vials at dry ice temperature for weeks.

3. For sectioning, the frozen tissue is mounted by placing the block holder in a wide-mouth Dewar flask, partially filled with dry ice. A drop or two of water is applied to the holder, the block of tissue is mounted and frozen thereon, and the holder is immediately transferred to the cryostat.

4. Sections are cut in an open-top cryostat at −15° to −20°C. and flattened with the aid of a camel's-hair brush, and with the brush the free-frozen section is transferred directly to a wide-mouth, screw-cap vial containing absolute acetone prechilled to −70°C. by crushed dry ice in a Dewar flask. The author of the technique stresses the necessity of transferring the free sections within 1 minute to prevent morphological alteration due to partial dehydration or ice crystal formation.

5. The vial is capped, returned to the Dewar flask, and buried in the dry ice to complete the freeze-substitution process. Dehydration usually takes about 12 hours. These sections will keep well in acetone at dry ice temperatures for 1 month.

6. After dehydration in acetone, the sections may be mounted by floating them in chilled acetone over dry ice and picking up the section on a clean coverglass, rinsed in acetone. To promote greater adherence of the tissue to the coverglass, sections may be celloidin coated (1% celloidin at −70°C.), depending on the specific histochemical or staining method employed.

Summary of Technique

1. Tissue is quenched as with freeze-drying.

2. Tissue is sectioned on an open-top cryostat.

3. Free sections are frozen-substituted in absolute acetone at dry ice temperature overnight or for longer intervals.

4. Sections are mounted on coverglasses and stained or incubated.

ENZYME LOCALIZATION

Preservation of enzymes is difficult. For precise localization cryostat, freeze-dry, or freeze-substitution techniques may be used to avoid fixation which may alter or destroy the enzyme. Most enzymes are destroyed at temperatures above 53°C., and for this reason paraffin-embedding is not suitable. The identification of enzymes is sometimes masked or obscured by their association or combination with other substances. For instance, lipids must be removed before adequate localization of some proteolytic enzymes may be achieved.

An additional problem is that the enzyme may diffuse out of its precise localization into surrounding tissue or into the incubating medium, and consequently a short period of fixation (usually in acetone) is allowed or recommended. With some enzymes that are particularly stable, neutral buffered formalin can be used to stop diffusion and yet not interfere with techniques for their identification.

ENZYME DIGESTION

Enzyme digestion is a histochemical procedure particularly valuable in polysaccharide histochemistry. In this area an enzyme is used to remove a particular component (carbohydrate) in order to provide positive identification of the substance. For example, glycogen stains positively with the PAS-technique. To verify that the material is truly glycogen (since mucin is also strongly PAS-positive), a control slide of the same material is pretreated with malt diastase and stained together with the test slide. What was stained positively as glycogen with the Schiff reagent will be selectively eliminated in the control section.

Other commonly employed enzymes which are used as *controls* are hyaluronidase (bovine testicular type) for digestion of hyaluronic acid and chondroitin sulfate, sialidase for removing sialomucins, desoxyribonuclease for DNA (Feulgen), and ribonuclease for digestion of ribonucleic acid. Pectinase will remove elastica, mucin, basement membranes, and many hyaline substances but *will not* digest out amyloid, which is resistant to pepsin digestion. The enzymes, commercially available, are generally made in buffered solutions, and the control sections are immersed in them for a prescribed length of time at 37°C. or at room temperature.

HISTOCHEMICAL BLOCKADE METHODS

In this technique components are deliberately altered chemically so that they will predictably fail to react. The interference with the normal reaction and the failure to react following a specific procedure is considered to be proof of the presence of special chemical groupings. This introduction of specific chemical groups into tissue sections can contribute as much to histochemistry in this "negative" blockade method as in a positive or additive fashion in which a chemical reaction may be used to identify or unmask a chemical group. The blockade reactions may be permanent or temporary. With the use of special procedures, the temporary blocks can be reversed and chemical reactivity restored. Irreversible methods totally destroy the reactive groups.

Examples: Aldehyde groups, for example, can be produced in carbohydrates by oxidation (i.e. use of periodic acid in the PAS technique), and can be blocked by different aldehyde reagents, such as dimedone. Blockade methods include aldehyde blockades, methylation, saponification, sulfation, acetylation and so on. Sulfation will bring about strong basophilia and often metachromasia. Methylation on the other hand will eliminate metachromasia and basophilia in certain acidic polysaccharides. Sulfation can often be reversed by methylation. To bring about these chemical couplings, the tissue sections are treated in a solution of the chemical. For example: *methylation* — sections are treated with methanol-hydrochloric acid solution to produce methyl esters; *sulfation* — sections are treated with sulfuric acid solution to produce sulfates; *nitrosation* — sections are treated with sodium nitrite in acetic acid.

OXIDATION AND REDUCTION

To bring about a required reaction, both oxidizing and reducing chemicals are used to alter chemical reactivity. In the routine histology laboratory the staining techniques frequently employ oxidizers such as potassium permanganate, chromic acid, periodic acid, and sodium iodate, and reduce by using formalin solutions or the classic ferric chloride-potassium ferricyanide solution of Schmorl.

MICROINCINERATION

Microincineration is a histochemical method of tissue preparation for the study of inorganic constituents, pigments, and foreign materials like uranium. Cut sections of paraffin-embedded material mounted on the slides are reduced to an ash with heat until everything organic is destroyed and only inorganic components remain. The slide is allowed to cool and the ash is examined microscopically, usually by means of dark-field microscopy. Another name for the ashed section is a *spodogram.*

Technique

1. Tissues to be microincinerated are generally fixed in 10% buffered neutral formalin or in 10% alcoholic formalin. Avoid metal-containing fixatives.

2. Slides are placed on quartz plate in an electric furnace or on a Corning hot plate. The temperature is increased in increments, slowly at first and then more rapidly, so that a maximum temperature of 600° to 650°C. is reached in approximately 30 to 40 minutes.

3. The section will turn brown, then white, and finally it will be charred to a fine almost invisible ash (approximately 50 to 60 minutes).

4. The oven is shut off and the slides are carefully removed with heated forceps, placed on asbestos, covered with an inverted pie tin, and allowed to cool gradually so as not to crack the glass slide. This step may take 12 to 24 hours.

5. The preparation may be coverslipped with glycerol and examined with dark-field illumination. If the section is to be preserved, the coverglass is ringed with melted paraffin.

6. INTERPRETATION. Carbon will appear black or brown, iron oxide will appear light yellow-orange to dark red in color, calcium oxalate will show no bubbles, and calcium carbonate will show bubbles. Cal-

cium and magnesium look alike and have a white amorphous appearance. Silica may be recognized by its birefringent crystals.

There are some iron-staining materials that cannot be stained directly but will stain after microincineration. Following the routine staining method, if confirmation of the interpretation is indicated, a duplicate section (microincinerated) can be stained with the Prussian blue reaction for the histochemical demonstration of iron.

POLYSACCHARIDE HISTOCHEMISTRY

Many pathogenic organisms (bacteria, fungi, and parasites) are able to be stained and identified because of their carbohydrate content. Although a normal constituent of tissue protoplasm, an excessive amount or special types of carbohydrates such as glycogen, amyloid, fibrin, and other polysaccharide and carbohydrate-containing complexes are criteria for disease diagnosis. Chemically classified as glycol compounds, carbohydrates fall into two main categories including *simple* sugars (sucrose and glucose) and *complex* carbohydrates. The simple sugars are water-soluble and in processing are not preserved for histologic examination. Complex carbohydrates are a combination of simple sugars bound to other tissue components. Enzymes may be used as histochemical controls in the identification of carbohydrates (page 304), for their use will selectively eliminate the carbohydrate from the tissue section.

Polysaccharides are units joined together in groups of at least five. Of these the acid mucopolysaccharides have the widest staining range and will stain with iodine solutions, metachromatic dyes, alcian blue, and the colloidal iron-binding technique of Hale. Because of the affinity of acid groups for the basic dyes which are used, pH is very important in staining acid mucopolysaccharides. Using the dye solution of alcian blue as an example, at pH 2.5 both types of acidic mucopolysaccharides stain, whereas at pH 1.0 alcian blue selectively stains acidic sulfomucins. A 2.5 to 3.0 pH is routinely used for the demonstration of mucopolysaccharides or nucleoprotein. Both nucleic acid and acid mucopolysaccharides react with the dye at this pH. The strongest acidic components are the sulfated mucopolysaccharides and these stain below a pH of 2.0.

Fixation

1. Performed optimally at refrigerator temperature.
2. Avoid chromate-containing fixatives (Zenker's and Helly's).
3. Ice-cold buffered neutral formalin is the most widely recommended fixative. Bouin's fluid may be used for glycogen fixation. Also ice-cold 95% alcohol may be used, however it makes tissue brittle and difficult to section.

Polysaccharide Histochemical Staining

METACHROMASIA. Metachromasia, because it indicates chemical composition of the tissue components, is important. The primary group of substances which shows metachromasia are acid mucopolysaccharides found in the ground substance of collagen, in cartilage, and in connective tissue mucin. The strongest metachromatic reaction occurs with the sulfated acid mucopolysaccharides. Mast cells also are metachromatic, presumably owing to the heparin in the granules. Negative periodic surface charges bring about these metachromatic changes. Some metachromasia, e.g., "alcohol labile" metachromasia, will be leached out by alcoholic dehydration, whereas other strongly metachromatic reactions will remain fast.

PH FACTOR. The pH of reagents and dye solutions is critical in several staining procedures and particularly in those involving acid mucopolysaccharides. Alcian blue staining at a higher pH will give a more intense reaction. A constant pH is maintained by prerinses and postrinses in a solution buffered at the same pH as the stain. The use of solutions at various pH values increases specificity and helps to distinguish between sulfated and nonsulfated acid mucopolysaccharides. At a pH of 2.5 to 3.0 most acid mucopolysaccharides stain deep blue. At low pH values (0.4), only strongly acid substances like sulfated acid mucopolysaccharides will be positive. Aldehyde fuchsin and toluidine blue are also pH-dependent stains like alcian blue. If the pH is reduced, there is less affinity. At low pH in solutions, sulfated groups seem to be the only entities that stain.

PAS-REACTION. The periodic acid-Schiff reaction deserves special consideration. Schiff originated the formula in 1866, and since that time many variations of its formula and preparation have been introduced. A carefully calculated combination of sulfurous acid with the red dye basic fuchsin results in a bleaching of the dye solution into a colorless or near-colorless reagent (leucofuchsin). When this solution is applied to a section containing aldehydes, a colored product is formed at the site of the aldehydes. Mild oxidation with periodic acid oxidizes 1,2 glycol groups to liberate the aldehydes, which are subsequently colored red to magenta by the Schiff reagent.

Both chromic acid (Bauer) and potassium permanganate (Casella) have been used for oxidation, but their use is limited because the oxidation process is prolonged beyond liberation of the aldehydes; in fact they can overoxidize and destroy the aldehyde-Schiff reaction. Oxidation with periodic acid has become the method of choice. Because this reaction is for the most part observed in materials that consist of or contain carbohydrates, the PAS-reaction is fundamental to carbohydrate histochemistry.

STEPS OF THE PAS-REACTION. These include:

1. Oxidation in aqueous periodic acid followed by a water wash.
2. Treatment in Schiff reagent for 10 minutes.
3. Direct transfer to two or three successive baths of sulfurous acid solution.
4. Water wash to develop magenta coloration.

PAS USES AND STAINING REACTION. Although the Schiff reagent is employed following hydrolysis for the demonstration of DNA, it is used primarily after mild oxidation for the demonstration of polysaccharides. Materials colored with the PAS-reaction are said to be "PAS-positive." Those that do not color are said to be "PAS-negative." Tissues that have a high polysaccharide content and stain red are the reticulum of glandular tissue and blood vessels, basement membranes, mucins, colloids, and glycogen. Mucoproteins and certain complex lipids also stain positively, probably because of carbohydrate complexes joined with the protein.

Originally believed to be highly specific, the scope of the periodic acid-Schiff staining reaction is so extensive that it is frequently necessary to use controls (i.e., diastase digestion) or blockade techniques (acetylation) when explicit results are critical. It is a very versatile method in that it can be combined successfully with multiple other stains. Commonly used combinations are alcian blue-PAS, Luxol fast blue-PAS, PAS-oil red O, colloidal iron-PAS, PAS-orange G, and PAS-trichrome.

SCHIFF SOLUTIONS. Solutions are made up in strengths varying from 0.25 to 2.0%, but the 0.5 to 1.0% concentration is most generally used. In most cases the different variations of Schiff solution can be interchanged, allowing for additional staining time if the weaker concentrations are used. Lillie prefers a 1.0% strength solution and a shortening of the time interval to 10 minutes, in my experience a combination that is optimal.

The traditional method of preparing the reagent calls for boiling water, adding the dye, and filtering the solution while hot, followed by bleaching with sulfurous acid. Lillie's cold Schiff's reagent combines all the constituents, which are agitated manually or mechanically until the dye is bleached. In either case the final solution will be a clear light-yellow or water-white. Activated charcoal is used to remove residual color from the bleached dye solution. With refrigerator storage the reagent remains stable for as long as 4 months. On storage a white precipitate or pink color may occur. The reagent should be discarded if either of these features is evident. On storage and use the reagent gradually loses its potency and should be replaced. To test the efficiency of the reagent, Mowry recommends that a section of duodenum be used as a control, and Lillie recommends that a section of tunica muscularis of the human appendix be used.

The classic technique calls for removal of the excess reagent with three baths of dilute sulfurous acid following exposure to the Schiff reagent. The AFIP Manual and Pearse have abandoned this step and simply wash in water, but Lillie, McManus-Mowry, Davenport, and most other authorities in the field still use three rinses in the sulfurous acid. In my own experience two 2-minute rinses are optimal for this step, since they appear to eliminate some of the objectionable background staining and permit a clearer counterstain.

REFERENCES

Barka, T., and Anderson, P. *Histochemistry*. New York: Hoeber Med. Div., Harper & Row, 1965.

Chang, J. P., and Hori, S. H. A frozen section freeze-substitution technique and an improved cryostat. *J. Histochem. Cytochem.* 8:310, 1960.

Chang, J. P., and Hori, S. H. The section freeze-substitution technique: I. Method. *J. Histochem. Cytochem.* 9:292–300, 1961.

Chang, J. P., and Hori, S. H. The section freeze-substitution technique: II. Application to localization of enzymes and other chemicals. *Ann. Histochim.* 6:419–431, 1962.

Chang, J. P., and Hori, S. H. Survival of enzymes in section frozen-substituted tissue. *J. Histochem. Cytochem.* 10:592–595, 1962.

Johnson, W. C., Johnson, F., and Helwig, E. B. Effect of varying pH on reactions for acid mucopolysaccharides. *J. Histochem. Cytochem.* 10:684, 1962.

Lillie, R. D. *Histopathologic Technic and Practical Histochemistry*. New York: McGraw-Hill, 1965.

McManus, J. F. A., and Mowry, R. W. *Staining Methods, Histologic and Histochemical*. New York: Hoeber Med. Div., Harper & Row, 1960.

Pearse, A. G. E. *Histochemistry, Theoretical and Applied*. Boston: Little, Brown, 1960.

Simpson, W. L. An experimental analysis of the Altman technique of freeze drying. *Anat. Rec.* 80:173–189, 1941.

Staining Techniques: Advanced and Nonroutine

The stains in this appendix have been included in the interest of an up-to-date text, and because some of them have proved exceptionally valuable in helping to meet special challenges in laboratory work.

ALCIAN BLUE METHOD FOR ACID MUCOPOLYSACCHARIDES

INDICATIONS.   For staining acidic carbohydrates (see page 307).

FIXATION.   Ice-cold buffered neutral formalin is the most widely recommended fixative. Alcoholic fixation. Can be used following Helly's or Zenker fixation although the general rule is to avoid chromate-containing fixatives.

TECHNIQUE.   Paraffin

DISCUSSION.   Alcian blue has the property of coloring most epithelial and connective tissue mucins and mast cell granules. It is apparently the acid mucopolysaccharides that are particularly well colored by the alcian blue stain.

The length of time for staining is best kept to a minimum so that only acid mucopolysaccharides are colored. Nonspecific staining will result if sections are left in the alcian blue staining solution longer than necessary. Type of fixation will influence time factors. Counterstaining with nuclear fast red or collagen stains may mask the alcian blue stain.

Mowry states that currently supplied alcian blue (8GX) is more constant, more stable, more soluble, and less fast. With this dye he obtained satisfactory staining with a 1% dye solution in 3% acetic acid for 2 hours. (In our laboratory we found 5 minutes to be the optimum staining time.)

Prior to counterstains involving acid reagents (e.g., Feulgen), Mowry suggests that sections stained with alcian blue 8GX should be rinsed briefly, treated in alkali (e.g., 30 minutes in 0.3% sodium carbonate), and washed before proceeding with acidic counterstains. The alkali treatment changes alcian blue to an insoluble form.

Solutions

3% AQUEOUS ACETIC ACID

Glacial acetic acid	3 ml.
Distilled water	97 ml.

ALCIAN BLUE SOLUTION

Distilled water	97 ml.
Glacial acetic acid	3 ml.
Alcian blue	1 gm.

Combine and filter. Add crystal of thymol to prevent mold. The pH should be about 2.6. Solution remains stable for 2 to 4 weeks. Refilter as necessary.

HARRIS'S HEMATOXYLIN (page 227)

Staining Procedure

1. Deparaffinize as usual. Treat with iodine and hypo if necessary. Wash thoroughly.

2. Place in 3% acetic acid for *2 minutes.*

3. Place in 1% alcian blue solution and leave for *5 to 30 minutes.*

4. Wash in running tap water; counterstains — e.g., the Feulgen (page 325) or Harris's hematoxylin (page 227) — can be applied as desired.

5. Dehydrate in two changes of 95% alcohol, followed by two to three changes of absolute alcohol.

6. Clear in two to three changes of xylene, and mount in Permount.

RESULTS. Mucinous substances of connective tissues and goblet cells, mast cell granules, and certain microbial capsules — bright turquoise-blue.

Cytoplasm of cells lacking acidic carbohydrates is uncolored except by counterstains that may be used.

ALCIAN BLUE-PERIODIC ACID-SCHIFF STAIN

Solutions

ALCIAN BLUE STAIN (page 313)

0.5% PERIODIC ACID (page 262)

SCHIFF'S REAGENT (page 262)

SULFUROUS ACID RINSE (page 263)

Staining Procedure

1. Deparaffinize as usual.
2. Stain in alcian blue stain for *5 to 30 minutes* (page 312).
3. Wash in running tap water *2 minutes* and then rinse in distilled water.
4. Place in 0.5% periodic acid for *10 minutes.*
5. Wash in running tap water *5 minutes* and then rinse in distilled water.
6. Place in Schiff's reagent for *10 minutes.*
7. Place in two changes of sulfurous acid rinse, *each of 2 minutes* duration.
8. Wash in running tap water for *5 minutes.*
9. Dehydrate in two to three changes of 95% alcohol and two to three changes of absolute alcohol.
10. Clear in xylene, and mount in Permount.

RESULTS. Exclusively acid substances (e.g., various connective-tissue mucins) — blue.

Neutral polysaccharides (e.g., glycogen) — magenta.

Certain substances (e.g., most epithelial mucins and cartilage ground substance) are colored by both alcian blue and PAS, yielding varying shades of purple to a very deep blue.

Cell bodies of fungi are red to purple, whereas mucoid capsules are blue.

Other features appear about the same as with the ordinary PAS stain.

REFERENCE. McManus, J. F. A., and Mowry, R. W. *Staining Methods.* New York: Hoeber Med. Div., Harper & Row, 1960, pp. 63 and 137.

STAINING REACTION FOR BILIRUBIN IN SECTIONS OF TISSUE

PRINCIPLE OF METHOD. When oxidized in acid mediums, bilirubin develops a specific and easily identifiable green color caused chiefly by biliverdin. The oxidation is rapidly completed by ferric chloride in trichloracetic acid mediums.

INDICATION. Demonstration of bile pigment.

FIXATION. 10% formalin, Müller's fluid, Orth's fluid are recommended.

Bouin's or Carnoy's solution can be used.

Zenker's solution is unsatisfactory.

TECHNIQUE. Paraffin sections

Solutions

FOUCHET'S REAGENT

Trichloracetic acid	25 gm.
Distilled water	100 ml.
10% ferric chloride	10 ml.

VAN GIESON'S STAIN

Acid fuchsin, 1% aqueous solution	5 ml.
Picric acid, saturated solution (about 1.22%)	100 ml.

Staining Procedure

1. Deparaffinize and hydrate sections of tissue in the usual way.
2. Wash in distilled water.
3. Stain for *5 minutes* in freshly filtered Fouchet's reagent.
4. Wash in tap water, then distilled water.
5. Stain in van Gieson's stain for *5 minutes.*
6. Place directly into 95% alcohol.
7. Dehydrate in two changes of absolute alcohol.
8. Clear in two to three changes of xylene.
9. Mount in Permount.

RESULTS.   Bilirubin oxidized to biliverdin will be olive-drab green to emerald green, depending upon the concentration of bilirubin in the tissue.

REFERENCE.   Hall, M. J.   *Amer. J. Clin. Path.* 34:313, 1960.

BODIAN METHOD FOR NERVE FIBERS AND ENDINGS

All glassware must be chemically clean. Use no metallic instruments.

FIXATION.   10% formalin, alcohol-formalin, or Bouin's solution.

TECHNIQUE.   Paraffin sections 8 to 10μ thick

Solutions

1% PROTARGOL SOLUTION

Protargol S* (silver albumose)   1 gm.
Distilled water   100 ml.

Pour distilled water in dish or wide-mouth beaker and set on hot plate regulated at 37°C. Slowly sprinkle protargol on the surface of the water and allow it to remain undisturbed until it has dissolved.

* Protargol S is available from Allied Chemical Corporation, P.O. Box 431, Morristown, N.J. 07960.

AQUA REGIA

(By volume)

| Nitric acid | 1 part |
| Hydrochloric acid | 3 parts |

REDUCING SOLUTION

Hydroquinone	1 gm.
Sodium sulfite	5 gm.
Distilled water	100 ml.

1% GOLD CHLORIDE SOLUTION

Gold chloride	1 gm.
Distilled water	100 ml.
Glacial acetic acid	3 drops

2% OXALIC ACID

| Oxalic acid | 2 gm. |
| Distilled water | 100 ml. |

Staining Procedure

1. Deparaffinize sections to distilled water.

2. Transfer slides to a staining dish containing the 1% protargol solution. Add 5 gm. of clean bright copper shot per 100 ml. of solution just before placing slides in dish. Copper should *not* be in contact with tissue sections. Place dish in oven at 37°C. for *12 to 48 hours.* (Clean copper with aqua regia.)

3. Wash in distilled water, three changes.

4. Place in reducing solution for *10 minutes.*

5. Rinse thoroughly in distilled water, several changes.

6. Tone in 1% gold chloride solution *5 to 10 minutes.*

7. Wash in distilled water, several changes.

8. Develop in 2% oxalic acid until entire section has a faint purple or blue tinge. Check with microscope. Slide is ready when background is gray and nerve fibers appear clearly. Usually requires *2 to 5 minutes.*

9. Rinse in distilled water, several changes.

10. Place in 5% sodium thiosulfate (page 30) to removal residual silver salts for **5 minutes.**

11. Wash in distilled water thoroughly.

12. If desired, counterstain at this point. A background coloration may be applied by dipping sections a few times in light green or in van Gieson's stain.

13. Dehydrate in 95% alcohol, followed by several changes of absolute alcohol.

14. Clear in several changes of xylene, and mount in Permount.

RESULTS.   Myelinated fibers, nonmyelinated fibers of the central and peripheral nervous system, and neurofibrils will stain black.

REFERENCE.   Jones, R. McClung. *Handbook of Microscopical Technique* (3d ed.) New York: Paul B. Hoeber, Inc., 1950, p. 373.

BOWIE STAIN FOR THE JG APPARATUS

Careful and proper preparation of the staining solution is a critical factor. The clove oil used for differentiation must be of high grade. Use of lesser grades of clove oil, when combined with xylene, will produce a milky solution unfit for differentiation.

INDICATIONS.   For staining the juxtaglomerular apparatus (JG cells) of the kidney.

FIXATION.   Helly's solution (Zenker-formol) preferred. Others may be used.

TECHNIQUE.   Paraffin sections 4μ thick

Staining Procedure

2.5% POTASSIUM BICHROMATE

Potassium bichromate	2.5 gm.
Distilled water	100 ml.

For best results make this solution just before use.

Bowie Stain (Stock Solution)

PREPARATION. Dissolve 1 gm. of Biebrich scarlet in 250 ml. of distilled water and filter through a rapid filter paper into a beaker. Dissolve 2 gm. of ethyl violet in 500 ml. of distilled water and filter a small amount at a time into the same beaker with frequent stirring. The ethyl violet solution is cautiously added just until the end-point of neutralization is reached.

The end-point of neutralization is indicated when a small amount of the mixture placed on a filter paper does not show any color other than that of the precipitate itself. A colorless halo with slight peripheral coloration by the precipitate will be noted. Test the dye solution often while filtering. The end-point is a critical factor in obtaining a satisfactory dye solution.

The mixture is then filtered, and the precipitate remaining on the filter paper is dried in a desiccator or in a 37°C. oven.

The stock solution is made up by dissolving *0.2 gm. of the dried precipitate in 20 ml. of 95% ethyl alcohol.* Up to 100 ml. of stock solution can be obtained from one batch if the end-point is carefully determined.

Note: Unless using the stain in large quantities, make up only 20 ml. of the staining solution for stock purposes and store the remainder of the dried precipitate in a well-stoppered bottle.

Bowie Stain (Working Solution)

Bowie stock solution	10 to 15 drops
20% ethyl alcohol	100 ml.

Staining Procedure

1. Take sections rapidly through xylene and alcohols to alcoholic iodine (if Zenker-formol-fixed). Leave there for *no more than 3 minutes* and *no more than 3 minutes* in hypo. Wash in running tap water for *5 minutes.*

2. Mordant in 2.5% potassium bichromate at approximately 37°C. *overnight.*

3. Rinse with distilled water and immerse sections *overnight* in working solution of Bowie stain.

4. Blot sections thoroughly with bibulous paper. Dip quickly 2 to 3 times in two changes of acetone to remove excess stain.

5. Differentiate in equal parts of xylene and clove oil until sections appear red (or magenta) or red-purple grossly. Differentiation may be checked with the microscope; elastic tissue in arteries should appear deep blue-purple.

6. Rinse sections in three changes of xylene and mount in Permount.

RESULTS. Renal parenchyma — red (or magenta) in contrast to elastic tissue of vessels which should be blue-purple.

Granulated juxtaglomerular cells — when present will be same color as elastic tissue.

Red blood cells — amber due to previous chromation.

REFERENCE. Pitcock, J. A., and Hartroft, P. M. *Amer. J. Path.* 34:863–864, 1958.

BROWN AND BRENN STAIN FOR BACTERIA IN TISSUE

INDICATIONS. To demonstrate bacteria in tissue.

FIXATION. 10% buffered formalin preferred.

TECHNIQUE. Paraffin

Solutions

1% CRYSTAL VIOLET SOLUTION

Crystal violet	1 gm.
Distilled water	100 ml.

5% SODIUM BICARBONATE SOLUTION

Sodium bicarbonate	5 gm.
Distilled water	100 ml.

GRAM'S IODINE SOLUTION

Iodine	1 gm.
Potassium iodide	2 gm.
Distilled water	300 ml.

Ethyl Ether-Acetone Solution

Ethyl ether	50 ml.
Acetone	50 ml.

Saturated Basic Fuchsin Solution

Basic fuchsin	approx.	0.25 gm.
Distilled water		100.00 ml.

Working 0.1% Basic Fuchsin Solution

Basic fuchsin, saturated solution	25 ml.
Distilled water	25 ml.

0.1% Picric Acid-Acetone Solution

Picric acid	0.1 gm.
Acetone	100.0 ml.

Staining Procedure

1. Deparaffinize through two changes of xylene, two changes of absolute alcohol and 95% alcohol to distilled water. If Zenker-fixed, treat with iodine and hypo solutions as usual.

2. Place slides on staining rack. Pour on approximately 1 ml. (20 drops) of 1% crystal violet solution, and add 5 drops of 5% sodium bicarbonate solution for *1 minute.* Agitate gently. If preferred, the two solutions may be mixed just before use.

3. Wash in water.

4. Flood slides with Gram's iodine solution for *1 minute.*

5. Rinse in water and blot with filter paper.

6. Decolorize in a Coplin jar with a mixture of equal parts of ether and acetone until no more blue color runs off, *5 to 15 seconds.*

7. Stain with working 0.1% basic fuchsin solution for *1 minute.*

8. Wash in water; blot gently, but not completely dry.

9. Dip quickly in acetone to start reaction.

10. Differentiate immediately with 0.1% picric acid-acetone solution until sections are yellow-pink. This is the most critical stage of the process. Most of the basic fuchsin should be decolorized from the tissue.

11. Rinse quickly in acetone and in a mixture of equal parts of acetone and xylene.

12. Clear in several changes of xylene and mount in Permount.

RESULTS.　Gram-positive bacteria — blue
Gram-negative bacteria — red
Nuclei — red
Filaments of Nocardia and actinomyces — blue
Other tissue elements — yellow

REFERENCE.　Brown, J. H., and Brenn, L. *Bull. Hopkins Hosp.* 48:69, 1931 (Armed Forces Institute of Pathology adaptation).

CAJAL'S GOLD SUBLIMATE METHOD FOR ASTROCYTES

FIXATION.　Fix thin blocks of tissue in formalin-ammonium bromide (FAB) solution for *1 day* in the incubator at 37°C.

TECHNIQUE.　Cut frozen sections at 15 to 30μ and place them in a solution of 1% formalin in distilled water.

Solutions

FORMALIN-AMMONIUM BROMIDE SOLUTION

Formalin, full-strength Merck's blue label	15 ml.
Ammonium bromide	2 gm.
Distilled water	85 ml.

CAJAL'S GOLD CHLORIDE SUBLIMATE SOLUTION

Mercuric bichloride crystals	0.5 gm.
Gold chloride (*Merck's brown*), 1% aqueous solution	6.0 ml.
Distilled water	35.0 ml.

Prepare the solution fresh each time, using chemically clean glassware. Pulverize the mercuric bichloride crystals and add them to the distilled water. Heat gently to dissolve the crystals; do not overheat. When dissolved, add the gold chloride to the hot solution and filter. Allow to come to room temperature for use.

5% Sodium Thiosulfate Solution (Hypo)

Sodium thiosulfate   5 gm.
Distilled water   100 ml.

Hortega's Carbol-Xylene-Creosote Mixture (Optional)

Creosote   10 ml.
Phenol crystals, melted   10 ml.
Xylene   80 ml.

Staining Procedure

Use acid-clean glassware throughout. Handle free-floating frozen sections with a glass rod.

1. Wash sections quickly in two changes of distilled water.
2. Place sections flat (avoid overlapping of sections) in the freshly prepared gold chloride sublimate solution for *4 to 6 hours* in the dark at room temperature. When the tissue turns an intense purple, remove from the solution and check wet sections under the microscope. At this time the astrocytes should be stained darkly with a light background.
3. Wash in distilled water for *5 to 10 minutes.*
4. Fix for *5 to 10 minutes* in 5% sodium thiosulfate solution.
5. Wash well in several changes of distilled water.
6. Float sections onto slide and dehydrate in 95% alcohol.
7. Clear in Hortega's carbol-xylene-creosote mixture. As soon as the sections are clear, blot them with fine grained filter paper and mount in Permount.

Note: For steps 6 and 7 the McManus-Mowry method is as follows:

6. Float sections onto slide, blot with bibulous paper, and dehydrate in 95% and absolute alcohol. This prevents sections from curling and shrinking in alcohol.
7. Clear in xylene and mount.

RESULTS.   Astrocytes and their processes — black
                  Background — unstained or light brown-purple

Nerve cells — pale red
Nerve fibers — unstained

REFERENCE. Mallory, F. B. *Pathological Technique.* Philadelphia: Saunders, 1938, p. 248.

DAHL'S METHOD FOR CALCIUM
(AFIP Modification)

FIXATION. 95% ethyl alcohol or 10% buffered neutral formalin.

TECHNIQUE. Cut paraffin sections at 6μ.

Solutions

1% ALIZARIN RED S SOLUTION

Alizarin red S	1 gm.
Distilled water	100 ml.

Stir dye into the distilled water so that only a few small grains of dye remain undissolved. *Add 10 ml. of 0.1% ammonium hydroxide* slowly with constant stirring. Resulting pH should be 6.36 to 6.40. Solution is stable for one month.

0.1% AMMONIUM HYDROXIDE SOLUTION

Ammonium hydroxide, C. P. 58%	0.1 ml.
Distilled water	100 ml.

1% LIGHT GREEN SOLUTION

Light green, SF yellow	1 gm.
Distilled water	100 ml.
Glacial acetic acid	1 ml.

Staining Procedure

1. Deparaffinize and hydrate to 95% alcohol (drain off excess 95% alcohol).

2. Immerse in alizarin red S solution for *2 minutes.*

3. Remove excess stain with distilled water, five or six rinses.

4. Counterstain in light green solution for *1 minute.*

5. Rinse in distilled water for *5 to 10 seconds.*

6. Dehydrate in 95% alcohol, absolute alcohol, and clear in xylene, two changes each.

7. Mount with Permount or Histoclad.

RESULTS. Calcium salts — intense red-orange
Background — pale green

REFERENCES. Dahl, L. K. *J. Exp. Med.* 95:474–479, 1952. Permission by The Rockefeller University Press.
Modified by and published in *Manual of Histologic Staining Methods of the Armed Forces Institute of Pathology* (3d ed.). New York: McGraw-Hill, 1968, p. 175.

FEULGEN STAIN

This is a specific chemical test for desoxyribonucleic acid (DNA). Its reaction depends on the treatment of fixed tissue by mild acid hydrolysis, which releases aldehyde groups from the desoxypentose sugar of ribonucleic acid. Following hydrolysis the tissues are washed and transferred to a solution of Schiff's reagent, which reacts with the exposed aldehyde groups to produce a purple dye in the nuclear chromatin alone. Any one of the Schiff variants may be used.

INDICATIONS. Specific test for desoxyribonucleic acid (DNA). A section of lymph node may be used as a control.

FIXATION. Practically all fixatives with the exception of Bouin's may be used. The duration of hydrolysis varies somewhat with the fixative employed, but most workers find that hydrolysis for 10 to 15 minutes is adequate for the most commonly used fixatives.

TECHNIQUE. Paraffin

Solutions

NORMAL HYDROCHLORIC ACID

Hydrochloric acid, concentrated, s.g. 1.19	83.5 ml.
Distilled water	916.5 ml.

LEUKOFUCHSIN SOLUTION (COLEMAN'S) *

Dissolve 1 gm. of basic fuchsin in 200 ml. of boiling distilled water. Cool to 50°C. Filter and add *10 ml. of normal hydrochloric acid.* Add *2 gm. of potassium metabisulfite.* Stopper and allow to bleach in the dark at room temperature overnight or for 24 hours. Then add 0.5 gm. of neutral activated charcoal; shake for 1 minute and filter through coarse filter paper. The solution should be almost water-white. Repeat filtration until solution is colorless. Bottle and store in refrigerator.

SULFUROUS ACID RINSE

10% aqueous potassium metabisulfite or sodium bisulfite	6 ml.
Normal hydrochloric acid	6 ml.
Distilled water	120 ml.

Staining Procedure

1. Deparaffinize sections through xylene and the alcohols to water as usual. Remove mercuric chlorides, if necessary, in iodine followed by hypo. Wash well in tap water.

2. Place sections in preheated normal hydrochloric acid at 60°C. for *10 to 15 minutes.*

3. Immerse for *10 to 20 minutes* in leukofuchsin solution at room temperature.

4. Drain and treat sections with two successive changes of freshly prepared sulfurous acid rinse in covered Coplin jars for *2 minutes* each. Discard solutions.

5. Wash in running tap water for *5 minutes.* Rinse with distilled water.

6. If desired, counterstain lightly by dipping sections in 0.25% light green or in 0.25% alcoholic fast green. Rinse and check counterstain with microscope.

---

* Schiff's reagents are interchangeable. If dye strengths vary, modify time intervals.

7. Rinse slides in distilled water.

8. Dehydrate in two changes of 95% alcohol, followed by two to three changes of absolute alcohol.

9. Clear in two to three changes of xylene, and mount in Permount.

RESULTS. Desoxyribonucleic acid (DNA) — shades of purple-red
Background — pale green if counterstain is used

REFERENCE. Lillie, R. D. *Histopathologic Technic and Practical Histochemistry* (2d ed.). New York: McGraw-Hill, 1954, p. 132.

FONTANA-MASSON METHOD FOR ARGENTAFFIN GRANULES

INDICATIONS. This is a stain used to aid in the diagnosis of carcinoid tumors, pheochromocytomas, and melanomas. Argentaffin cells exhibit the property (capacity of the tissue component itself) of reducing ammoniacal silver solutions to metallic silver. Argentaffin cells are found in the digestive tract (enterochromaffin) and in the adrenals. The tumor termed "carcinoid" appears to arise from argentaffin cells. The pigment melanin is also argentaffin.

FIXATION. Bouin's fluid or 10% formalin.

TECHNIQUE. Paraffin.
Chemically clean glassware should be used throughout.

Solutions

STOCK 10% SILVER NITRATE SOLUTION

Silver nitrate	10 gm.
Distilled water	100 ml.

Combine and place in a dark bottle. Store away from light.

FONTANA-MASSON SILVER NITRATE SOLUTION

To *50 ml. of 10% silver nitrate solution, add ammonium hydroxide* (58%) by degrees. The first drop or two will cause a dark-brown precipitate. Continue to add the ammonia water drop by drop just until the solution becomes clear. From the stock 10% solution add a little more silver nitrate drop by drop, shaking vigorously to dissolve the brown clouds of silver oxide. Continue to add the silver nitrate drop by drop until a faint permanent turbidity is attained. Let stand overnight to settle. Before using, decant silver solution, filter, and dilute with an equal amount of *distilled water*. Prepare a small quantity fresh each time.

1% GOLD CHLORIDE SOLUTION

Gold chloride	1 gm.
Distilled water	100 ml.

Break glass vial of 15 grains (15 grains = 1 gram) into the distilled water.

0.2% WORKING GOLD CHLORIDE SOLUTION

Gold chloride, 1% aqueous	10 ml.
Distilled water	40 ml.

5% SODIUM THIOSULFATE SOLUTION (HYPO)

Sodium thiosulfate	5 gm.
Distilled water	100 ml.

Staining Procedure

1. Deparaffinize sections down to distilled water.

2. Immerse slides in Fontana-Masson silver nitrate solution in paraffin oven at 56° to 58°C. for *1 hour,* or in the dark at room temperature in a covered dish for *12 to 48 hours.* Sections will appear light brown.

3. Rinse in distilled water.

4. Tone in working solution of gold chloride for *5 minutes.*

5. Rinse in distilled water.

6. Place in 5% sodium thiosulfate solution for *2 minutes.*

7. Wash thoroughly in running tap water followed by a rinse with distilled water.

8. For contrast, counterstain if desired in 0.1% aqueous safranin, eosin, or nuclear fast red (page 378). Rinse in distilled water.

9. Dehydrate in two changes of 95% alcohol, two to three changes of absolute alcohol.

10. Clear in two to three changes of xylene and mount.

RESULTS. Argentaffin granules — black (carcinoid granules appear brown).

Other tissue elements stained according to counterstain used.

REFERENCE. Lillie, R. D. *Histopathologic Technic and Practical Histochemistry* (2d ed.). New York: McGraw-Hill, 1954, p. 164.

GALLOCYANIN STAIN FOR NISSL SUBSTANCE
(Einarson Method)

FIXATION. Any fixative that preserves chromophil substances — Zenker's fluid, Zenker-formalin, 10% formalin, or Carnoy's fluid.

TECHNIQUE. Paraffin

Solutions

GALLOCYANIN SOLUTION

Chrome alum (chromium potassium sulfate)	10.0 gm.
Distilled water	200.0 ml.
Gallocyanin	0.3 gm.

Dissolve the chrome alum in distilled water, add gallocyanin, and mix by shaking. Warm gradually, finally allowing solution to boil gently for *10 to 15 minutes.* Cool slowly to room temperature and filter. Solution keeps for only 1 week.

Staining Procedure

1. Deparaffinize in two changes of xylene, absolute alcohol, and 95% alcohol. If necessary treat with iodine followed by sodium thiosulfate. Wash thoroughly in tap water. Place sections in distilled water.

2. Place sections *overnight* in gallocyanin solution at room temperature or for *1 hour* in 58°C. oven.

3. Wash in distilled water.

4. Dehydrate in two changes of 95% alcohol, two to three changes of absolute alcohol.

5. Clear in several changes of xylene, and mount in Permount.

RESULTS. Nissl substance — blue

REFERENCE. Einarson, L. *Amer. J. Path.* 8:295, 1932. (Permission of *American Journal of Pathology.*)

GOMORI'S ALDEHYDE-FUCHSIN STAIN

INDICATIONS. For staining beta cells of the pancreas
For staining elastic fibers
For staining mucin

FIXATION. Formalin preferred. Other fixatives may be used. Dichromate fixation not recommended for polysaccharide staining.

TECHNIQUE. Paraffin. Do not use on celloidin blocks or celloidin-coated paraffin sections. This stain will not diffuse through celloidin.

Solutions

ALDEHYDE-FUCHSIN SOLUTION (pH 1.7)

Basic fuchsin	1 gm.
70% ethyl alcohol	200 ml.
Hydrochloric acid, concentrated	2 ml.
Paraldehyde, U.S.P.	2 ml.

Allow to stand at room temperature for *1 to 3 days* or until the solution is a deep purple color. As soon as this color change takes place, the dye is ready for use. The solution stains rapidly and strongly when new but weakens and deteriorates with age. It is stable for about 2 months. Store in refrigerator.

Staining Procedure

1. Deparaffinize sections through two changes of xylene and two changes of absolute and 95% alcohols as usual.

2. Remove mercuric precipitates if necessary in iodine (0.5% in 80% alcohol). Gomori recommends treatment (oxidation) in iodine, no matter what the fixative, for *10 minutes to 1 hour.* Wash in water.

3. Transfer to 5% sodium thiosulfate (hypo) for *2 to 3 minutes* to bleach iodine.

4. Wash well in running water.

5. Rinse with 70% alcohol.

6. Stain in aldehyde-fuchsin solution for *5 minutes to 2 hours,* depending on tissue component to be stained:

for elastic fibers — 5 to 10 minutes
for beta cells — 15 to 30 minutes
for pituitary cells — 30 minutes to 2 hours
for mast cell granules — 5 to 10 minutes

7. Rinse off excess stain in 70% alcohol.

8. Wash in water. Check staining with microscope. The stain can be rinsed and inspected under the microscope any number of times.

9. If desired, counterstain lightly with Masson's trichrome or van Gieson's stain (page 270).

10. Dehydrate in 95% alcohol followed by absolute alcohol.

11. Clear in two to three changes of xylene, and mount in Permount or balsam.

RESULTS. Elastic fibers and sulfated mucosubstances — deep blue to purple

Beta cells of pancreas — deep blue to purple

Other tissue elements stained according to counterstain used.

REFERENCE. Gomori, G. L. *Amer. J. Clin. Path.* 20:665, 1950. (Permission of Williams & Wilkins Co., Baltimore.)

GOMORI'S CHROMIUM-HEMATOXYLIN-PHLOXINE
STAIN (CHROME ALUM-HEMATOXYLIN STAIN)

INDICATIONS. Differential stain for islet cells of pancreas.

FIXATION. Bouin's solution, 10% formalin, or Zenker-formol. Bouin's solution is the preferred fixative.

TECHNIQUE.   Paraffin sections, 4 to 6μ thick

Solutions

BOUIN'S FLUID

Picric acid, saturated aqueous solution (approximately 1.22%)   75 ml.
Formalin, concentrated   25 ml.
Glacial acetic acid   5 ml.

POTASSIUM PERMANGANATE SOLUTION

Potassium permanganate	0.3 gm.
Distilled water	100.0 ml.
Sulfuric acid	0.3 ml.

SODIUM BISULFITE SOLUTION 5%

Sodium bisulfite	5 gm.
Distilled water	100 ml.

CHROMIUM HEMATOXYLIN SOLUTION

Hematoxylin, 1% aqueous solution	50 ml.
Chrome alum,* 3% aqueous solution	50 ml.

To *100 ml. of chromium hematoxylin add 2 ml. of a 5% potassium dichromate and 2 ml. of a 2N sulfuric acid* (about 2.5%). The mixture is ripe after 48 hours and can be used as long as a film with a metallic luster forms on its surface in a Coplin jar. Filter before use.

PHLOXINE B SOLUTION 0.5%

Phloxine B	0.5 gm.
Distilled water	100.0 ml.

PHOSPHOTUNGSTIC ACID SOLUTION 5%

Phosphotungstic acid	5 gm.
Distilled water	100 ml.

Staining Procedure

1. Deparaffinize sections down to water.
2. Refix in Bouin's fluid for *12 to 24 hours.*

* Chromium potassium sulfate.

3. Wash thoroughly in running tap water to remove picric acid.

4. Treat sections by oxidizing in potassium permanganate solution for about *1 minute.*

5. Decolorize with a 5% solution of sodium bisulfite until colorless.

6. Wash well in running tap water.

7. Stain in chromium hematoxylin solution for *10 to 15 minutes.* Stain until beta cells stand out deep blue. Check staining with microscope.

8. Differentiate in 1% hydrochloric acid alcohol for about *1 minute.*

9. Wash in tap water until the section is a clear blue.

10. Counterstain with phloxine B solution for *5 minutes.*

11. Rinse in distilled water.

12. Immerse in 5% phosphotungstic acid solution for *1 minute.*

13. Wash in running tap water for *5 minutes.* The section should regain its red color.

14. Differentiate in 95% ethyl alcohol. If the section is too red and the alpha cells do not stand out clearly enough, rinse the section for about *15 to 20 seconds* in 80% alcohol.

15. Transfer and complete dehydration in absolute alcohol.

16. Clear in several changes of xylene.

17. Mount in Permount.

RESULTS.   Pancreatic islets: Alpha cells — red

Beta cells — blue

D cells — from pink to red and indistinguishable from alpha cells

REFERENCE.   Gomori, G. *Amer. J. Path.* 17:398, 1941. (Permission of *American Journal of Pathology.*)

GOMORI'S METHENAMINE SILVER METHOD FOR URIC ACID

INDICATIONS.   For demonstration of urate crystals (See also page 199).

FIXATION.   Absolute alcohol, refrigerator temperature for 24 hours. Change alcohol at least once during this period.

TECHNIQUE.   From absolute alcohol, transfer sections to equal parts of xylene-paraffin for 1½ hours at 58°C. Transfer to paraffin for 1 hour. Cast, and cut sections at 8 to 10μ. Float sections onto slides with 95% alcohol. Dry slides (on warming table) at 43°C. for 2 hours.

Staining Solutions

3% METHENAMINE SOLUTION
(See page 342.)

5% SILVER NITRATE SOLUTION
(See page 342.)

BORATE BUFFER WORKING SOLUTION pH 8.2
(See page 343.)

GOMORI'S METHENAMINE SILVER SOLUTION

3% methenamine solution	100 ml.
5% silver nitrate solution	5 ml.
Borate buffer, pH 8.2	5 ml.

To the 100 ml. of 3% methenamine, add the silver nitrate. A precipitate forms and redissolves. Add the 5 ml. of borate buffer of approximately pH 8. Make up to 200 ml. with distilled water. Prepare this solution just before use.

5% SODIUM THIOSULFATE
(See page 30.)

Staining Procedure

1. Remove the paraffin with xylene, two changes, followed by absolute alcohol, two changes.

2. Transfer sections directly to methenamine-silver solution at 37°C. The slides should remain in this solution until uric acid deposits are black — *15 to 60 minutes.*

3. Treat in 5% sodium thiosulfate for *3 minutes.* Wash rapidly in tap water.

4. Counterstain with 1% alcoholic eosin for *1 minute.*

5. Dehydrate rapidly in 95% alcohol, followed by two changes of absolute alcohol.

6. Clear in xylene, two changes each.

7. Mount in Permount.

RESULTS.   Urate crystals — black
              Background — pink

REFERENCE.   Pearse, A. G. *Histochemistry.* Boston: Little, Brown, 1960, p. 949.

GROCOTT MODIFICATION OF GOMORI'S METHENAMINE-SILVER NITRATE STAIN

The use of Gomori's methenamine-silver nitrate method as a staining procedure for fungi in tissue sections and smears has the following advantages: (1) The method uses readily available reagents and stable solutions. (2) The technique produces highly photogenic black-and-white preparations of fungi in tissue. (3) The technique will stain old, nonviable fungi which could not be demonstrated by other fungi staining methods.

INDICATIONS.   Stain for fungi in tissue sections and smears.

FIXATION.   10% formalin

TECHNIQUE.   Paraffin sections or smears. Smears are prepared on albumen-treated slides and fixed in 95% alcohol.

Solutions

5% CHROMIC ACID

| Chromium trioxide | 5 gm. |
| Distilled water | 100 ml. |

5% BORAX SOLUTION

| Sodium borate, tetra | 5 gm. |
| Distilled water | 100 ml. |

Stock Methenamine-Silver Nitrate Solution

Silver nitrate, 5% aqueous solution	5 ml.
Methenamine,* 3% aqueous solution	100 ml.

Add the silver nitrate to the methenamine solution. A white precipitate forms but dissolves immediately on shaking. The clear solution remains usable for months at refrigerator temperature.

Working Methenamine-Silver Nitrate Solution

Prepare just before use.

Distilled water	25 ml.
Borax, 5% solution	2 ml.

Combine and add:

Stock methenamine-silver nitrate solution	25 ml.

1% Sodium Bisulfite Solution

Sodium bisulfite	1 gm.
Distilled water	100 ml.

0.1% Gold Chloride Solution

Gold chloride, 1% aqueous solution	10 ml.
Distilled water	90 ml.

2% Sodium Thiosulfate Solution (Hypo)

Sodium thiosulfate	2 gm.
Distilled water	100 ml.

Staining Procedure

If possible, process a control slide with the other sections.

1. Deparaffinize sections as usual. If previously stained with eosin and hematoxylin, remove coverglass, rinse with xylene, and run through alcohols to water. Subsequent chromic acid treatment will remove any remaining stain.

* Hexamethylenetetramine. Fisher Scientific Company.

2. Oxidize in 5% chromic acid for *1 hour.*

3. Wash in running tap water for *2 to 5 minutes.*

4. Treat with 1% sodium bisulfite for *1 minute* to remove any residual chromic acid.

5. Wash in tap water for *5 minutes.*

6. Rinse with three changes of distilled water.

7. Place in silver methenamine working solution in oven at 56° to 58°C. (or place in a covered Coplin jar in a hot water bath regulated at 43°C.). Fungi and mucin will begin to stain yellow-brown in *20 to 30 minutes,* and will be adequately stained at the end of *1 hour.* Check progress with microscope from time to time. Fungi should be dark brown with pale yellow background.

8. Rinse slides thoroughly in several changes of distilled water.

9. Tone in 0.1% gold chloride solution for *5 minutes.* This will also bleach the background.

10. Rinse in distilled water.

11. Remove unreduced silver by treating with 2% sodium thiosulfate solution for *2 minutes.*

12. Wash thoroughly in tap water.

13. Counterstain if desired. If a red nuclear stain is preferred, nuclear fast red or aqueous safranine may be used. A light hematoxylin and eosin combination may be used. If only contrast is desired, counterstain by dipping slides lightly in a very dilute solution of light green (page 250).

14. Dehydrate with two changes of 95% alcohol followed by two to three changes of absolute alcohol.

15. Clear in two to three changes of xylene, and mount in Permount.

RESULTS.   Fungi — sharply delineated in black
　　　　　　Inner parts of mycelia and hyphae — old rose (gray-red)
　　　　　　Mucin — taupe (brown-gray)
　　　　　　Background — dependent on counterstain used

REFERENCE.   Grocott, R. G.   *Amer. J. Clin. Path.* 25:975, 1955. (Permission of Williams & Wilkins Co., Baltimore.)

HEIDENHAIN'S IRON HEMATOXYLIN

INDICATIONS.   Stain for chromatin.
Stain for amebae.
Stain for secretory granules.

FIXATION.   Zenker's or Helly's preferred. Others may be used.

TECHNIQUE.   Paraffin sections cut 5μ thick.

Solutions

AMMONIO-FERRIC ALUM SOLUTION

Ammonio-ferric alum	2.5 gm.
Distilled water	100.0 ml.

ALCOHOLIC HEMATOXYLIN

Hematoxylin	0.5 gm.
Alcohol, 95%, ethyl	10.0 ml.
Distilled water	90.0 ml.

Dissolve the hematoxylin in the alcohol and add the water. Allow to ripen for *4 to 5 weeks.* For use, dilute the hematoxylin with equal parts of distilled water. This solution may be reused.

VAN GIESON'S STAIN

Acid fuchsin, 1% aqueous solution	5 to 10 ml.
Picric acid, saturated aqueous solution (about 1.22%)	100 ml.

Use the lesser strength of fuchsin if a more yellow cytoplasm is desired.

Staining Procedure

1. Deparaffinize in two changes of xylene, two changes of absolute alcohol, and two changes of 95% alcohol.

2. Place in alcoholic iodine for *5 minutes* to remove mercuric chlorides.

3. Rinse in 80% alcohol or wash in tap water.

4. Transfer to 5% sodium thiosulfate (hypo) for **2 minutes** to bleach iodine.

5. Wash well in running tap water.

6. Mordant sections in ammonio-ferric alum solution for **1 to 2 hours** (save solution to differentiate slides — step 10).

7. Wash quickly in distilled water.

8. Stain for **1 hour to 36 hours** in the alcoholic hematoxylin solution. The sections will be adequately stained when on being taken out of the hematoxylin they are a homogeneous jet black and microscopically show no cellular detail at all.

9. Wash in tap water.

10. Differentiate in the ammonio-ferric alum solution, controlling the results with a microscope. The section should be rinsed in tap water before each examination, which will immediately stop the decolorization.

11. Wash in running tap water **15 to 60 minutes.**

12. If desired, counterstain with van Gieson's stain or eosin.

13. Rinse with 50% alcohol.

14. Dehydrate in two changes of 95% alcohol and two changes of absolute alcohol.

15. Clear in two to three changes of xylene, and mount in Permount.

Note: Lillie modified this technique by using Weigert's iron hematoxylin, with the advantage that his method does not require a ripened hematoxylin.

Lillie's modification is as follows:

IRON HEMATOXYLIN STAINING SOLUTION. Mix 100 ml. of fresh 1% hematoxylin in 95% alcohol with 1 ml. of concentrated hydrochloric acid, 99 ml. distilled water, and 2.5 gm. ferric chloride (Fe $Cl_3 \cdot 6 H_2O$). Solution is stable for 2 to 3 weeks only. Follow steps 1 through 5 in the foregoing technique, and stain with Lillie's modified Weigert's hematoxylin for **5 minutes** followed by washing well in distilled water. Continue stain following steps 12 through 15.

RESULTS. Chromatin, nucleoli, mitochondria, centrioles, and certain parts of striated muscle fibers are stained black. Other tissue elements colored by the counterstain used.

Amebae — black

REFERENCE. Mallory, F. B. *Pathological Technique.* Philadelphia: Saunders, 1938, p. 74.

HOLZER'S METHOD FOR GLIAL FIBERS
(AFIP Modification)

FIXATION.   10% buffered neutral formalin or formol alcohol.

TECHNIQUE.   Cut paraffin sections at 6μ.

Solutions

PHOSPHOMOLYBDIC-ALCOHOL SOLUTION

Phosphomolybdic acid, 0.5%	50 ml.
Alcohol, 95%, ethyl	100 ml.

Make fresh.

ABSOLUTE ALCOHOL-CHLOROFORM SOLUTION

Alcohol, 100%	40 ml.
Chloroform	160 ml.

CRYSTAL VIOLET SOLUTION

Crystal violet	5 gm.
Alcohol, 100%	20 ml.
Chloroform	80 ml.

POTASSIUM BROMIDE SOLUTION

Potassium bromide	100 gm.
Distilled water	1000 ml.

DIFFERENTIATING SOLUTION

Aniline	120 ml.
Chloroform	180 ml.
Ammonium hydroxide, 58%	1 ml.

Staining Procedure

1. Deparaffinize and hydrate to distilled water. Carry slides through one at a time.

2. Immerse in phosphomolybdic-alcohol solution for *3 minutes.* Drain.

3. Immerse in absolute alcohol-chloroform solution until section becomes translucent.

4. Place slide on staining rack and flood section with crystal violet solution for *30 seconds.* Blot dry.

5. Flood section with potassium bromide solution for *1 minute.* Blot dry.

6. Place in differentiating solution for *30 seconds.* If overdifferentiated, restain.

7. Rinse in xylene, several changes. Check with microscope after first xylene.

8. Mount with Permount or Histoclad.

RESULTS.   Glial fibers — deep violet
Background — pale violet

Note: If a crystal violet precipitate forms on slide, it may be removed with straight aniline.

REFERENCES.   Holzer, W. Über eine neue Methode der Gliofaser-Farbung. *Z. ges. Neurol. Psychiat.* 69:354, 1921.
Luna, L. (Ed.), *Manual of Histologic Staining Methods of the Armed Forces Institute of Pathology* (3d ed.). New York: McGraw-Hill, 1968, p. 200.

JONES' PERIODIC ACID-SILVER METHENAMINE METHOD
(AFIP Modification)

INDICATIONS.   Valuable for study of glomular capillary basement membrane of kidney sections.

FIXATION.   10% buffered neutral formalin, Bouin's, or Helly's fluid

TECHNIQUE.   Paraffin sections cut 2μ thick

DISCUSSION.   Chemically clean glassware carefully rinsed in chloride-free distilled water is absolutely essential. Following the silvering, slides must be rinsed in chloride-free distilled water. Distilled water may be checked for free chloride by the addition of several drops of 5% silver nitrate. If a white cloud appears on the addition of the silver nitrate, discard the sample of water and replace.

Occasionally the methenamine-silver staining solution darkens before all the basement membranes are completely stained; it is advisable to transfer slides and continue staining in a fresh preheated solution. Keep several Coplin jars filled with distilled water in the incubator for rinsing slides when they are to be checked microscopically.

Best results are obtained if the periodic acid, methenamine, silver nitrate, and buffer solutions are made fresh or not used beyond 1 to 2 week's time.

Staining Solutions

0.5% PERIODIC ACID SOLUTION

Periodic acid	0.5 gm.
Distilled water	100.0 ml.

3% METHENAMINE* SOLUTION

Hexamethylenetetramine (methenamine)*	3 gm.
Distilled water	100 ml.

5% SILVER NITRATE SOLUTION

Silver nitrate	5 gm.
Distilled water	100 ml.

BORATE BUFFER SOLUTIONS (STOCK)
SOLUTION A: 0.2M BORIC ACID

Boric acid	12.36 gm.
Distilled water	1000.0 ml.

* Fisher Scientific Co.

SOLUTION B: 0.25 M SODIUM BORATE

Sodium borate	19.07 gm.
Distilled water	1000.0 ml.

BORATE BUFFER SOLUTION, pH 8.2 (WORKING)

Solution A	6.5 ml.
Solution B	3.5 ml.

1% GOLD CHLORIDE SOLUTION (STOCK)

(See page 28.)

GOLD CHLORIDE SOLUTION (WORKING)

Gold chloride stock solution	10 ml.
Distilled water	40 ml.

3% SODIUM THIOSULFATE (HYPO) SOLUTION

Sodium thiosulfate	3 gm.
Distilled water	100 ml.

METHENAMINE SILVER SOLUTION,
pH 8.2 (WORKING)

Methenamine, 3%	42.5 ml.
Silver nitrate, 5%	2.5 ml.
Borate buffer, pH 8.2	12.0 ml.

Prepare fresh just before use and filter. This solution is stable for approximately 60 to 75 minutes. After this time, there is a breaking down process, which produces a black precipitate and is picked up on the slides. (See paragraph two in DISCUSSION, p. 342.)

Staining Procedure

1. Deparaffinize and hydrate to distilled water.
2. Place in periodic acid solution for *11 minutes.*
3. Rinse in chloride-free distilled water.
4. Filter freshly prepared methenamine-silver solution into Coplin jar.

5. Place slides in methenamine-silver solution and then place Coplin jar in prewarmed 70°C water bath. Start timing at this point, *approximately 60 to 75 minutes.* Check under microscope when slides macroscopically show a medium brown color.

Note: Solution and slides should be allowed to come to 70°C together. While slides are in the silver solution they may be examined after they begin to show macroscopically a medium brown color reaction. Before checking under the microscope, they are first rinsed in hot 70°C chloride-free distilled water, checked, returned to hot water rinse, and then returned into hot staining solution. Slides should be checked every 10 minutes when they have reached the dark or medium brown stage. Slides should be checked as rapidly as possible because if the section cools there is an uneven staining of the section.

When the desired staining time has been reached, the slide should be checked as described above, every 1 to 2 minutes. Strict adherence to the timing is essential in order to obtain a uniform consistency in staining. A properly stained section at this point should have a dark brown-yellow background; the reticulum fibers will be intense black, as should the basement membranes. An overstained section will be too black. Differentiation will be very difficult, because the black will be so intense as to obscure many or all of the tissue elements. The section may be destained with an extremely dilute solution (0.1%) of potassium ferricyanide for one or two dips or until decolorized.

6. Rinse section well in distilled water.
7. Tone in working gold chloride solution for *1 minute.*

Note: If sections are overtoned, place in 3% sodium metabisulfite for *1 to 3 minutes,* checking periodically.

8. Rinse well in distilled water.
9. Reduce in sodium thiosulfate solution for *1 to 2 minutes.*
10. Wash in running tap water for *10 minutes.*
11. Rinse well in distilled water.
12. Counterstain with routine Harris's hematoxylin and eosin stain.
13. Dehydrate in 95% alcohol, absolute alcohol, and clear in xylene, three changes each.
14. Mount with Permount or Histoclad.

RESULTS.   Basement membrane — black
Reticulum fibers — black
Nuclei — blue
Cytoplasm, collagen, and connective tissue — pink to orange

REFERENCES.   Jones, D. B. *Amer. J. Path.* 27:991–1009, 1951. Modified by Avalone, F., G. U. Branch, Armed Forces Institute of Pathology.
Manual of Histologic Staining Methods of the Armed Forces Institute of Pathology (3d ed.). New York: McGraw-Hill, 1968, p. 97.

LEVADITI'S METHOD OF STAINING SPIROCHETES IN THE BLOCK

FIXATION.   Fix tissue blocks 1 mm. thick in 10% formalin for 24 hours.

TECHNIQUE.   Blocks of tissue are stained *prior* to processing with paraffin-embedding technique.

Solutions

SILVER NITRATE SOLUTION

Silver nitrate	1.5 to 3 gm.
Distilled water	100 ml.

For biopsy specimens the stronger solution of silver nitrate is preferable.

REDUCING SOLUTION

Pyrogallic acid	3 gm.
Formalin	5 ml.
Distilled water	100 ml.

Staining Procedure

1. Wash blocks of tissue thoroughly in tap water to remove excess fixative. It is important to remove the formalin.

2. Place blocks in 95% alcohol for **24 hours.**

3. Place in distilled water until the tissue sinks to the bottom of the container.

4. Place in the freshly prepared aqueous silver nitrate solution, and keep at 37°C. in the dark for **3 to 5 days,** changing the solution three times.

5. Wash in distilled water, several changes.

6. Place in the reducing solution at room temperature in the dark for **24 to 72 hours.**

7. Wash in several changes of distilled water.

8. Dehydrate in 80% and 95% alcohols followed by absolute alcohol. (This will take several hours.)

9. Clear in oil of cedarwood or toluene, and embed in paraffin in the usual manner.

10. Cut sections 5μ thick and mount on slides.

11. When dry, deparaffinize with xylene, and mount with Permount.

RESULTS.   Spirochetes — intense black
　　　　　　Background — yellow to brown

REFERENCE.   Mallory, F. B. *Pathological Technique.* Philadelphia: Saunders, 1938, p. 293.

LIEB CRYSTAL VIOLET STAIN FOR AMYLOID

DISCUSSION.   This is a reliable, specific stain for amyloid. However, the metachromatic reaction of crystal violet will be lost unless the sections are mounted in a water-soluble medium (Abopon recommended). See alternate mounting agents and conditions of their usage under subheading Abopon mounting medium, p. 347. Sections will fade if dehydrated in the usual manner with alcohols.

INDICATIONS.   To demonstrate amyloid in tissues.

FIXATION.   Formalin 10% or alcohol fixation.

TECHNIQUE.   Paraffin. Process with control slide if one is available.

Solutions

STOCK CRYSTAL VIOLET SOLUTION

Crystal violet, to saturate	approx. 14 gm.
Alcohol, 95% ethyl	100 ml.

Staining solution is stable.

WORKING CRYSTAL VIOLET SOLUTION

Crystal violet, stock solution	10 ml.
Distilled water	300 ml.
Hydrochloric acid, concentrated	1 ml.

ABOPON MOUNTING MEDIUM

Lieb's original staining method recommended a special mounting medium called Abopon which prevents the bleeding of crystal violet stains from amyloid. It is not available in solution but the crystals may be ordered from Valnor Corporation, Brooklyn, New York. The crystals are combined with an 0.2 M phosphate buffer at pH 7.

Any water-soluble mountant, e.g., gum syrup or glycerin, may be used in its place if sections are not to be stored. The stain should be examined immediately after mounting and should be photographed soon after preparation if a permanent record is desired.

Staining Procedure

Process a control slide with the sections.

1. Deparaffinize sections through two changes of xylene, absolute and 95% alcohols to distilled water as usual.
2. Stain in working solution of crystal violet for *1 to 5 minutes.* Check control with microscope after 1 minute. Amyloid should be purple-red. Excess background stain may be removed by differentiating in 1% acetic acid.
3. Rinse well in tap water.

4. Drain slide and mount in gum syrup or glycerin.

5. Edges of coverslip may be sealed with fingernail polish or Duco cement.

RESULTS. Amyloid — purple-red
Other tissue elements — blue

REFERENCE. Lieb, E. *Amer. J. Clin. Path.* 17:413, 1947. (Permission of Williams & Wilkins Co., Baltimore.)

LUXOL FAST BLUE-PERIODIC ACID-SCHIFF AND HEMATOXYLIN STAIN
(After Klüver and Barrera)

Luxol fast blue is a phthalocyanine dye specific for polysaccharides and with a marked affinity for myelin. It is the alcohol-soluble counterpart of alcian blue. The Luxol fast blue method may be incorporated into other staining techniques, e.g., Luxol fast blue and cresyl violet, Luxol fast blue and phosphotungstic acid hematoxylin, Luxol fast blue and oil red O. The most useful combination is perhaps the Luxol fast blue-periodic acid-Schiff method, which provides a correlative study of the cellular elements, the fiber pathways, and the vascular components of the nervous system.

INDICATIONS. Stain for myelin
Stain for nerve cells and fibers

FIXATION. Formalin 10%

TECHNIQUE. Paraffin

Solutions

0.1% LUXOL FAST BLUE SOLUTION

Luxol fast blue B	0.1 gm.
Alcohol, 95%	100.0 ml.

Dissolve the dye in the alcohol. Add *0.5 ml. of 10% acetic acid* to each 100 ml. Solution is stable.

0.05% Lithium Carbonate Solution

Lithium carbonate	0.05 gm.
Distilled water	100.00 ml.

Periodic Acid Solution 0.5%

Periodic acid	0.5 gm.
Distilled water	100.0 ml.

Schiff's Solution

(See page 262.)

Sulfurous Acid Rinse

10% sodium metabisulfite, aqueous	6 ml.
Hydrochloric acid, 1N aqueous solution	5 ml.
Distilled water	100 ml.

Papamiltiades's Hematoxylin

(Optional)

Hematoxylin	(1% aqueous solution)	100 ml.
Aluminum sulfate	(5% aqueous solution)	50 ml.
Zinc sulfate	(5% aqueous solution)	25 ml.
Potassium iodide	(4% aqueous solution)	25 ml.
Acetic acid, glacial		8 ml.
Glycerin		25 ml.

Note: Equally good results are obtained with Harris's hematoxylin.

This solution is ready for immediate use and keeps for approximately 2 months.

Staining Procedure

1. Deparaffinize in two changes of xylene, two changes of absolute and 95% alcohols.

2. Place in 0.1% Luxol fast blue solution in oven at 60°C. *overnight* or in the preheated stain in the paraffin oven (60°C.) for *1 to 3 hours.*

3. Rinse off excess stain in 95% alcohol.

4. Rinse in distilled water.

5. Place in 0.05% lithium carbonate for a *few seconds.*

6. Differentiate in 70% alcohol for *20 to 30 seconds.*

7. Rinse in distilled water.

8. Place in second solution of 0.05% lithium carbonate briefly (*10 to 25 seconds*).

9. Differentiate briefly in 70% alcohol.

10. Rinse in distilled water. Check with microscope. The white matter should be colored green-blue in contrast to colorless gray matter. If differentiation is incomplete, repeat steps 8 and 9.

11. Place in 0.5% periodic acid solution for *5 minutes.*

12. Rinse in two changes of distilled water.

13. Place in Schiff's reagent for *15 minutes.*

14. Place in sulfurous acid solution for two changes of *2 minutes each.*

15. Wash in tap water for *5 minutes.*

16. Stain in Papamiltiades's *or* Harris's hematoxylin for *1 minute.*

17. Wash in tap water for *5 minutes.* (If background is not clear after staining, dip once in acid alcohol and wash again.)

18. Dehydrate with two changes of 95% alcohol, two or three changes of absolute alcohol.

19. Clear with two or three changes of xylene and mount.

RESULTS.   Myelin — blue-green
Fungi and PAS-positive elements — rose to magenta
Nuclei — dark blue
Cytoplasmic nucleoproteins — blue-purple
Capillaries — red

REFERENCE.   Margolis, G., and Pickett, J. P.   *Lab. Invest.* 5:459, 1956.

MALLORY-HEIDENHAIN'S ANILINE BLUE STAIN
(AZAN STAIN)

INDICATIONS.   Stain for alpha cells of the pancreas
Stain for collagen

FIXATION.   Zenker's, Helly's, Bouin's, or Carnoy's

TECHNIQUE.   Paraffin

Solutions

AZOCARMINE G SOLUTION

Azocarmine G	1 to 1.5 gm.
Distilled water	200.0 ml.

Bring to boil. Filter through coarse filter paper in paraffin oven at 58°C. so that fine particles of dye (needle-like crystals) will also pass through. When cool, add 2 ml. of glacial acetic acid. Keep in refrigerator. Filter before use.

Note: Azocarmine B has been replaced with Azocarmine G because of the latter's greater solubility and staining power.

ANILINE-ALCOHOL SOLUTION

Aniline oil	1 ml.
Alcohol, 95%, ethyl	100 ml.

1% GLACIAL ACETIC ALCOHOL

Glacial acetic acid	1 ml.
Alcohol, 95%, ethyl	100 ml.

5% PHOSPHOTUNGSTIC ACID SOLUTION

Phosphotungstic acid	5 gm.
Distilled water	100 ml.

STOCK ANILINE BLUE SOLUTION

Aniline blue, water soluble	0.5 gm.
Orange G	2.0 gm.
Distilled water	100.0 ml.
Glacial acetic acid	8.0 ml.

WORKING ANILINE BLUE SOLUTION

Aniline blue stock solution	1 part
Distilled water	2 parts

Staining Procedure

1. Deparaffinize sections through xylene, absolute and 95% alcohols down to water. Remove mercuric chlorides with iodine, followed by hypo, if necessary.

2. Rinse in distilled water.

3. Stain in azocarmine G solution in a covered dish in the paraffin oven at 58°C. for *15 to 20 minutes.* Allow to cool for *5 minutes* at room temperature.

4. Rinse in distilled water.

5. Differentiate in the aniline-alcohol solution until cytoplasm and connective tissue are pale pink and nuclei stand out sharply. Control differentiation by rinsing slide in 1% glacial acetic alcohol and check with microscope. If section is too red, return to aniline-alcohol. Rinse with 1% glacial acetic alcohol.

6. Mordant in 5% phosphotungstic acid solution until the connective tissue is completely decolorized *15 minutes to 1 hour.* Check with microscope at 15-minute intervals.

7. Rinse quickly in distilled water.

8. Counterstain from *5 to 30 minutes* in the working aniline blue solution until the finest connective tissue fibers are sharply stained. Examine from time to time with microscope.

9. Rinse in distilled water.

10. Dehydrate quickly through 95% alcohol, two changes of absolute alcohol.

11. Clear with two or three changes of xlyene, and mount in Permount.

RESULTS.   Chromatin and neuroglia — red
Cytoplasm — pink to blue
Collagen and reticulum — blue
Muscle — red to orange
Alpha cells — red

REFERENCE.   Mallory, F. B. *Pathological Technique.* Philadelphia: Saunders, 1938, p. 154.

MASSON'S HEMATOXYLIN-PHLOXINE-SAFRAN (HPS) STAIN

INDICATIONS. Used in the same manner as hematoxylin and eosin staining for the study of morphology of tissue. It gives a wide range of coloration of different tissue components (see RESULTS).

FIXATION. Bouin's fluid or Brazil-Dubosco solution preferred. If initially fixed in other solutions, postmordant slides in saturated picric acid for 15 to 30 minutes.

TECHNIQUE. Paraffin

Solutions

BRAZIL-DUBOSCO SOLUTION

80% ethyl alcohol	150 ml.
Full-strength formalin (37–40%)	60 ml.
Acetic acid, glacial	15 ml.
Picric acid	1 gm.

SATURATED AQUEOUS PICRIC ACID
(See page 30.)

MAYER'S HEMATOXYLIN
(See page 228.)

1.0% AQUEOUS PHLOXINE B SOLUTION

Phloxine B	1 gm.
Distilled water	100 ml.

SAFRAN DU GATINAIS SOLUTION, 3.5%

Safran du Gatinais *	14 gm.
Absolute ethyl alcohol	400 ml.

* Safran du Gatinais, imported from Chroma-Gesellschaft, may be purchased from Roboz Surgical Instrument Co., 810 18th Street, N.W., Washington, D.C. 20006. Spice saffron may be purchased from Schoenfeld & Sons, 12 White St., New York, N.Y. 10013.

Keep solution in the incubator at 58°C. for 2 weeks, shaking bottle frequently. Filter before use. After use, filter solution back into stock bottle. Store in a dark bottle, tightly closed and away from light. Stock solution lasts indefinitely.

Note: Because Safran du Gatinais is relatively expensive, it is acceptable to use a spice saffron solution, adding it to the Safran du Gatinais in the staining dish to prolong its use. The dry spice saffron is ground in a mortar to a powder and made in the same manner and strength as the formula indicated.

Staining Procedure

1. Deparaffinize sections through to distilled water.

2. If sections are Zenker's, Helly's, or formalin-fixed, mordant slides for *5 to 15 minutes* in saturated picric acid, followed by washing in running tap water for *15 minutes.*

3. Stain nuclei in Mayer's hematoxylin for *5 to 10 minutes.*

4. Wash in warm running tap water (to blue nuclei) for *10 minutes.*

5. Stain in 1% phloxine B solution for *10 minutes* (see note below).

6. Wash in running tap water for *5 minutes.*

7. Drain and dehydrate rapidly in three changes of absolute alcohol. Keep slide in constant motion.

8. Stain in safran solution for *5 minutes.*

9. Rinse in two changes of absolute alcohol.

10. Clear in three or four changes of xylene for *2 minutes each.*

11. Mount in Permount.

RESULTS.   Nuclei — blue
Red cells — bright pink
Bone — yellow
Cartilage — yellow
Muscle — red
Collagen — yellow

REFERENCES.   Masson, P. Diagnostics de Laboratoire, pp. 684–686, part XXVII of *Traite de Pathologie Medicale et de Therapeutic.* Paris: A. Maloine et Fils, 1923.

Note: The method here described is a modification of Masson's technique. It was modified by the Surgical Pathology Laboratory at Columbia University Medical Center.

The AFIP modified the original technique by using (1) any fixative provided it is postmordanted in saturated aqueous picric acid for 5 minutes, (2) a 1.5% aqueous phloxine B for 2 minutes, and (3) a 2% Safran du Gatinais for 5 minutes.

MAY–GRÜNWALD GIEMSA STAIN FOR BONE-MARROW SECTIONS

The May-Grünwald and the Jenner stains are identical and may be interchanged. (See discussion of dyes on page 153.)

FIXATION. Zenker fixation preferred

TECHNIQUE. Paraffin

Solutions

STOCK MAY-GRÜNWALD SOLUTION

May-Grünwald dye	1 gm.
Methyl alcohol	400 ml.

WORKING MAY-GRÜNWALD SOLUTION

Stock May-Grünwald solution	25 ml.
Distilled water	25 ml.

STOCK GIESMA SOLUTION *

Giemsa powder	1 gm.
Glycerin	66 ml.

Mix glycerin and Giemsa powder. Place in 60°C. oven for 30 minutes to 2 hours. Finally add 66 ml. of *absolute methyl alcohol*.

WORKING GIEMSA SOLUTION

Stock Giemsa solution	3 ml.
Distilled water	50 ml.

Make solution fresh just before use. Do not reuse.

* If desired, stock Giemsa staining solution (ready-to-use from laboratory supply house) may be substituted for the formula above. Order Giemsa tissue stain, Wolbach's modification, Item #6203, Harleco Company.

1% ACETIC WATER

Glacial acetic acid	1 ml.
Distilled water	99 ml.

Staining Procedure

1. Deparaffinize sections through two changes of xylene, absolute alcohol and 95% alcohol.

2. Remove mercury precipitates with alcoholic iodine solution for *5 minutes*.

3. Wash in tap water or rinse in 80% alcohol.

4. Bleach out iodine in 5% sodium thiosulfate solution for *2 minutes*.

5. Wash in running tap water for *5 minutes*. Transfer to distilled water.

6. Place sections in absolute methyl alcohol for *3 minutes*.

7. Place in second change of methyl alcohol for *3 minutes*.

8. Stain in working May-Grünwald solution for *5 to 6 minutes*.

9. Transfer directly into working Giemsa solution for at least *45 minutes*.

10. Carrying forward one slide at a time, rinse quickly in distilled water and differentiate in 1% acetic water. Check slides individually with the microscope. Nuclei should be bright blue and clear, cytoplasm a soft pink.

11. Rinse in distilled water.

12. Dehydrate quickly in 95% alcohol followed by two or three changes of absolute alcohol.

13. Clear in two or three changes of xylene, and mount in Permount or some other neutral mounting medium.

RESULTS.   Nuclei — blue
Cytoplasm — pink to rose
Bacteria — blue

REFERENCES.   Strumia, M. M.   *J. Lab. Clin. Med.* 21:930, 1935–1936.
Armed Forces Institute of Pathology *Manual of Histologic and Special Staining Technics.* 1957, p. 113.

MAYER'S MUCICARMINE
(Modified by Southgate, 1927)

DISCUSSION. Mayer's original formula calls for 1.0 gm. carmine, 0.5 gm. anhydrous aluminum chloride and 2.0 ml. of distilled water. The constituents are combined and heated in a small test tube or in a small evaporating dish until the liquid becomes dark and syrupy. This is then diluted to 100 ml. with 50% alcohol. It is a fairly difficult solution to prepare and results are not always successful.

Southgate modified Mayer's method by using a greater volume of solvent in the original mixing and by adding aluminum hydroxide to neutralize the hydrochloric acid that is liberated when the aluminum chloride comes in contact with the solvent. The instructions for preparation of this dye solution call for a boiling water bath. If possible, this should be positioned under a hood with the fan running. *Cautions:* Wear rubber gloves when opening and weighing the aluminum chloride. It is anhydrous so do not use filter paper in measuring the dry weight. Use a small glass beaker. Take all precautions that you would when handling any acid or caustic material. *Use a larger flask than is necessary* for the volume amount of the solution. Add the aluminum chloride *slowly* to the previously mixed reagents.

INDICATIONS. For staining mucin in sections.
Will stain cryptococcus.

FIXATION. 10% formalin, Zenker's fluid, Helly's fluid, or Carnoy's fluid.

TECHNIQUE. Paraffin
Process with a control. A section of colon will serve as control material.

Solutions

MUCICARMINE STAIN (STOCK SOLUTION)

Carmine	2 gm.
Aluminum hydroxide	2 gm.
50% ethyl alcohol	200 ml.
Aluminum chloride, anhydrous	1 gm.

Place the carmine and the dry powdered aluminum hydroxide in a 500 ml. or 1000 ml. pyrex flask. Add the alcohol. Shake the solution and then add the aluminum chloride slowly and carefully. Hydrochloric acid is liberated from the solution at this point. Promptly transfer flask into the boiling water bath and boil the staining solution briskly *for exactly 2½ minutes* with agitation. Allow to cool to room temperature and then filter. The stock solution is stable for several months. Store in the refrigerator.

Mucicarmine Stain (Working Solution)

Stock mucicarmine stain	10 ml.
Distilled water	40 ml.

Do not filter. It is best to make up the working solution shortly prior to use.

Metanil Yellow (Stock Solution)

Metanil yellow	0.25 gm.
Distilled water	100.00 ml.
Glacial acetic acid	0.25 ml. (5 drops)

Note: Dilute 50:50 with distilled water for use.

Staining Procedure

1. Deparaffinize slides and hydrate to water. (Process a control slide with the sections.)
2. Stain nuclei in hematoxylin (Harris's or Weigert's) for *3 to 5 minutes.*
3. Check with microscope. Differentiate, if necessary, and wash again with running water. Leave nuclei slightly overstained.
4. Rinse in distilled water and stain in working solution of metanil yellow for *1 minute.*
5. Rinse in distilled water.
6. Stain in working solution of mucicarmine for *30 to 60 minutes.* Check control slide under the microscope after 30 minutes. Mucin should be deep rose to red.
7. Rinse thoroughly in distilled water, several changes.
8. Dehydrate in two changes of 95% alcohol, three changes of absolute alcohol and clear in three changes of xylene. Mount in Permount or Histoclad.

RESULTS.   Mucin — deep rose to red
Nuclei — blue (if Harris's hematoxylin is used)
black (if Weigert's hematoxylin is used)
Other tissue elements — yellow
Capsule of cryptococcus — deep rose to red

REFERENCES.   Mallory, F. B. *Pathological Technique.* Philadelphia: Saunders, 1938, p. 130.

Southgate, H. W. *J. Path. Bact.* 30:729, 1927.

METHYL GREEN PYRONIN Y STAIN
(After Scudder and Modified from Taft by Dr. Margaret E. Long)

INDICATIONS.   For staining nuclear chromatin, i.e., desoxyribonucleic acid (DNA) and ribonucleic acid (RNA) combinations with protein. Plasma cell stain.

FIXATION.   Absolute methyl alcohol preferred. Carnoy's fluid and 10% alcoholic formalin may be used. *Note:* If tissue has been initially formalin-fixed, a better result will be obtained if tissue is fixed for an additional hour in absolute methyl alcohol and stained for 60 minutes.

TECHNIQUE.   Small pieces of tissue (2–3 mm.) thick, *fixed* in absolute methyl alcohol (two changes) for total of 24 hours. *Dehydrate* in absolute n-butyl alcohol (two changes, each for ½ hour). Tissues are *embedded* in 1:1 n-butyl alcohol/paraffin at 56°C. for *1 hour.* Transfer to pure paraffin (four changes) during a 2-hour interval. Cast block. Cut paraffin sections 4 to 5μ thick. Excessive heat or too long exposure in heated paraffin removes RNA from tissues.

REMARKS.   Samples of methyl green are always mixtures of this dye and methyl violet. Before use as a histochemical reagent, the methyl green should always be freed from the violet component by shaking an aqueous solution with an excess of chloroform, which will dissolve the methyl violet. *Note:* A German dye Chroma-Gesellschaft methyl green GA * is pure methyl green and eliminates chloroform extraction.

* Available from Roboz Surgical Instrument Co., 810 18th St., N.W., Washington, D.C. 20006.

The effect of methyl green is accentuated if used in a solution buffered to pH 4.2 to 4.5.

After the sections are stained, tertiary butyl alcohol is recommended as the dehydrant (stand container in warm water to liquefy).

Solutions

0.2 M ACETIC ACID

Reagent grade glacial acetic acid M.W. 60.05	1.15 ml.
Distilled water	98.85 ml.

0.2 M SODIUM ACETATE

Sodium acetate, reagent grade, M.W. 136.09	2.72 gm.
Distilled water	100.00 ml.

ACETATE BUFFER SOLUTION pH 4.2

0.2 M acetic acid solution	75 ml.
0.2 M sodium acetate solution	25 ml.

Adjust pH to 4.2 with sodium hydroxide or acetic acid.

PREPARATION AND PURIFICATION OF METHYL GREEN STAINING SOLUTION

Dissolve 1 gm. of methyl green in 200 ml. of the acetate buffer solution. Pour mixture into a separatory funnel and add a small amount of chloroform. Shake carefully, releasing the stopper occasionally to reduce pressure. Allow layers of methyl green and chloroform (with methyl violet dissolved in it) to separate. Drain off heavier layer of chloroform. Repeat this process until the chloroform is clear and all traces of methyl violet have disappeared.

This procedure will require the use of a considerable quantity of chloroform (as much as 15 pounds of chloroform may be necessary). Purification will take 2 to 3 hours or more. Let the purified solution stand in an open flask until residual chloroform has evaporated — approximately overnight. Bottle and store in refrigerator.

Note: Use Commission Certified methyl green.

METHYL GREEN-PYRONIN Y SOLUTION

Combine:

Purified methyl green in pH 4.2 acetate buffer	100.0 ml.
Pyronin Y (Commission Certified)	0.1 gm.

Store in refrigerator in brown glass-stoppered bottle. Solution may be reused for months. Bring to room temperature before using.

ALCOHOL DEHYDRATING MIXTURE

Tertiary butyl alcohol	3 parts
Absolute ethyl alcohol	1 part

Staining Procedure

1. Deparaffinize with xylene, absolute ethyl alcohol, 95% alcohol, and two quick rinses in distilled water. Let stand if necessary in 50% alcohol, not distilled water.

2. Stain in methyl green-pyronin Y solution for **5 minutes** (handle each slide individually).

3. Dip **quickly** into distilled water and blot gently but **quickly** with No. 1 filter paper.

4. Place immediately into alcohol dehydrating mixture with **continuous agitation** for ½ **minute**.

5. Rinse quickly in xylene.

6. Transfer to two changes of xylene for **5 minutes each**.

7. Mount in neutral Canada balsam mounting media. Synthetic mountants appear to cause fading of stains.

Note: Handle each slide individually. Wipe forceps dry before carrying another slide through the procedure, so that staining solutions will not be contaminated by the xylene.

RESULTS. Nuclear chromatin (DNA-protein) — blue-green
Cytoplasmic basophilic material (RNA-protein) — rose-pink
Nucleoli — rose pink

Ribonuclease Testing

To confirm the RNA content of the cells, a control is used. A double set of slides on the same material is made. One section is immersed in a ribonuclease (enzyme) solution while the additional section is immersed in plain water. After the prescribed period of time both the treated and the untreated sections are stained.

1. Deparaffinize sections according to step 1 of staining procedure.

2. Immerse one section in a solution of 0.01% ribonuclease in distilled water at room temperature for *1 hour.*

3. Immerse test section in distilled water at room temperature for *1 hour.*

4. Remove both sections and wash together with running tap water for *5 to 10 minutes.*

5. Stain with Methyl Green Pyronin technique, steps 2 through 7.

Note: The material stained in the section which was treated with water only and absent from the section treated with ribonuclease is presumably ribonucleic acid.

REFERENCES.   Long, M. E., and Taylor, H. C.   Nuclear variability in human neoplastic cells. *Ann. N.Y. Acad. Sci.* 63:1095–1106, 1956.

Taft, E. B.   *Stain Techn.* 26:205–212, 1951. Modification by Dr. Margaret E. Long, Lenox Hill Hospital, New York, N.Y. 10021.

MOWRY'S COLLOIDAL-IRON STAIN

This staining technique (after Hale) is based on an affinity of acid mucopolysaccharides for colloidal iron which is subsequently rendered blue by treatment with potassium ferrocyanide and hydrochloric acid (Prussian blue reaction). The colloidal-iron staining method permits counterstaining of nuclei, collagen fibers, and basement membranes. The following technique may be used in combination with the Feulgen test or the periodic acid-Schiff technique.

A duplicate of every section tested should be taken through the treatment in hydrochloric acid and potassium ferrocyanide *without* previous exposure to colloidal iron. In this way, naturally occurring ferric iron will be detected and not mistaken for acidic carbohydrates.

INDICATIONS.   Stain for acid mucopolysaccharides.

Will stain glomerular structures.

Will stain some fungi.

Will show skin changes in collagen disease.

FIXATION. Neutral formalin (10%) or 10% neutral formalin in 90% alcohol preferred. Others may be used.

TECHNIQUE. Paraffin

Solutions

12% ACETIC ACID SOLUTION

Glacial acetic acid	48 ml.
Distilled water	352 ml.

MÜLLER'S COLLOIDAL-IRON OXIDE REAGENT (STOCK SOLUTION)

Bring 250 ml. of distilled water to a boil. While the water is still boiling, pour in 4.4 ml. of (U.S.P. XI) 29% ferric chloride solution and stir. (An equivalent amount of ferric chloride in any other form can be substituted as long as the total volume remains about the same.) If the water is not kept boiling during ferric chloride addition, the conversion to colloidal (hydrous) ferric oxide will be incomplete and the results of its use will be faulty. When the solution has turned dark red, remove from heat and allow to cool. Label "Stock Colloidal Iron." This reagent is dark red, clear, and stable for many months.

COLLOIDAL IRON (WORKING SOLUTION)

Just before use, combine as follows:

Glacial acetic acid	5 ml.
Distilled water	15 ml.
Stock colloidal-iron solution	20 ml.

2% HYDROCHLORIC ACID SOLUTION

Hydrochloric acid, concentrated	2 ml.
Distilled water	98 ml.

2% POTASSIUM FERROCYANIDE SOLUTION

Potassium ferrocyanide	2 gm.
Distilled water	100 ml.

Staining Procedure

1. Deparaffinize sections as usual. Remove mercuric deposits with iodine and hypo, if necessary. Wash sections and place in distilled

water. Reserve control slide in distilled water (until step 5) and process test slide.

2. Rinse section briefly (*30 seconds*) in 12% acetic acid solution. (This prevents watery dilution of reagent used in step 3.)

3. Place slide into freshly prepared working colloidal-iron solution for *1 hour.*

4. Rinse section in four changes of 12% acetic acid for *3 minutes each.*

5. Treat the test section and its control (a duplicate section unexposed to colloidal iron) in a freshly prepared mixture of equal parts of 2% hydrochloric acid solution and 2% potassium ferrocyanide solution for *20 minutes.*

6. Wash gently in tap water for *5 minutes.*

7. If desired, stain nuclei in Harris's hematoxylin (page 227) for *5 minutes.* Wash in running tap water for *2 minutes.* Differentiate the hematoxylin stain in acid alcohol if necessary. Blue in tap water.

8. *Optional.* Dip in a saturated aqueous picric acid solution for *1 minute.* Cytoplasm and red blood cells will stain yellow. Wash in water for a few seconds.

9. Dehydrate in two changes of 95% alcohol, followed by two or three changes of absolute alcohol.

10. Clear in two or three changes of xylene, and mount in Permount.

RESULTS.   Acid polysaccharides will be colored Prussian blue after the complete colloidal iron treatment, but will be unstained in the control section that was subjected to the acid rinses and the hydrochloric acid–potassium ferrocyanide without antecedent colloidal iron. Staining seen in the control section is due to naturally occurring ferric iron and must not be interpreted as indicating acid polysaccharides.

REFERENCE.   Müller, G.   *Acta Histochem.* (Jena) 2:68, 1955.

COLLOIDAL IRON-PERIODIC ACID-SCHIFF STAIN

Solutions

COLLOIDAL-IRON SOLUTIONS (See page 363.)

PERIODIC ACID 0.5%

Periodic acid	0.5 gm.
Distilled water	100.0 ml.

SCHIFF'S REAGENT

(Modification of Lillie's "Cold Schiff")

Combine in order:

Distilled water	192 ml.
Hydrochloric acid, concentrated	2 ml.
Sodium sulfite	5 gm.
Basic fuchsin	2 gm.

Combine the above in a suitable bottle with *50 to 60 ml. of free air space* above the fluid. Shake at 20-minute to 30-minute intervals until the mixture is clear brown to brown-red with no residue. Add *1 gm. of fresh active charcoal.* Shake for 2 minutes and filter. The filtrate should be clear and colorless. The solution is ready for immediate use. Store in refrigerator.

REDUCING RINSE (STOCK MOLAR SOLUTION)

Sodium acid sulfite	10.4 gm.
Distilled water	100.0 ml.

REDUCING RINSE (WORKING SOLUTION)

Stock reducing rinse solution	1 part
Distilled water	19 parts

Prepare fresh just before use.

Staining Procedure

1. Perform steps 1 through 6 as given in the preceding directions for the colloidal-iron stain (page 363). As indicated before, include

a control duplicate section treated only with the hydrochloric acid-potassium ferrocyanide (unexposed to colloidal iron).

2. Oxidize sections in 0.5% aqueous periodic acid for *10 minutes.*

3. Wash in running tap water for *5 minutes.* Rinse in distilled water.

4. Treat in Schiff's reagent for *10 minutes.*

5. Rinse in two changes of the working reducing rinse for *2 minutes each.*

6. Wash in running tap water for *2 minutes.*

7. If desired, counterstain nuclei in Harris's hematoxylin (page 227) for *1 to 5 minutes.* Wash in tap water for *2 minutes.* If indicated, differentiate hematoxylin in acid alcohol. Blue in water.

8. *Optional.* Dip in saturated aqueous picric acid for *1 minute.* (This colors cytoplasm and red blood cells yellow.) Rinse for *a few seconds* in tap water.

9. Dehydrate in 95% alcohol, followed by two or three changes of absolute alcohol.

10. Clear in several changes of xylene and mount in Permount.

RESULTS.   Exclusively acid substances (e.g., mucins of soft connective tissue) — blue

Neutral polysaccharides — magenta

Certain substances (e.g., most epithelial mucins) are colored by both colloidal iron and the periodic acid-Schiff, resulting in varying shades of purple to very deep blue.

Other features appear about the same as after the customary periodic acid-Schiff method.

REFERENCE.   Mowry, R. W. *Lab. Invest.* 7:566, 1958.

PEARSE TRICHROME PAS
(Periodic Acid-Schiff Technique — Pearse After Hotchkiss)

INDICATIONS.   Differential stain for cells of the pituitary
Stain for basement membranes, glycogen, and fungi

FIXATION.   Formalin (10%), Zenker's fluid, or Helly's fluid

TECHNIQUE.   Paraffin

Solutions

Periodic Acid Solution

Periodic acid	0.4 gm.
95% ethyl alcohol	35.0 ml.
M/5 sodium acetate *	5.0 ml.
Distilled water	10.0 ml.

*M/5 sodium acetate

6.8 gm. (M.W. 136.09)	sodium acetate
250.0 ml.	distilled water

The periodic acid solution should be kept in the dark at room temperature and used at this temperature. Discard solution when orange color appears, and remake. Solution usually lasts 2 or 3 weeks. May be reused.

Hotchkiss Reducing Rinse

Potassium iodide	1.0 gm.
Sodium thiosulfate	1.0 gm.
95% ethyl alcohol	30.0 ml.
Distilled water	20.0 ml.
2N hydrochloric acid *	0.5 ml.

*2N hydrochloric acid

Hydrochloric acid, conc., s.g. 1.19	83.5 ml.
Distilled water	416.5 ml.

Dissolve the potassium iodide and sodium thiosulfate in the alcohol and water. Add 0.5 ml. of 2N hydrochloric acid. A deposit of sulfur forms which can be ignored. The solution lasts for about 14 days but no longer. Keep solution at room temperature. Solution may be reused.

Schiff's Reagent
(Double strength)

Distilled water	200 ml.
Basic fuchsin	2 gm.
Sodium metabisulfite	4 gm.
1N hydrochloric acid *	40 ml.

*1N hydrochloric acid

Hydrochloric acid, conc., s.g. 1.19	83.5 ml.
Distilled water	916.5 ml.

Bring water to boiling point. Remove from flame and at once dissolve basic fuchsin in water, adding the dye slowly. Cool to 60°C. and filter. Add 4 gm. sodium metabisulfite; shake solution. Add 40 ml. of 1N hydrochloric acid, shake solution. Solution should be deep amber color. Leave overnight in the dark at room temperature for 18 to 24 hours. In the morning the solution should be light amber color. *Add 600 mg. activated charcoal* and shake for 1 minute. Filter through filter paper and store solution in dark bottle in refrigerator. The solution after filtering should be clear water-white. Repeat filtration until clear. Allow reagent to reach room temperature before use. Discard solution if precipitate forms or if pink tint appears.

CELESTIN BLUE SOLUTION

Ferric ammonium sulfate	2.50 gm.
Distilled water	50.00 ml.
Celestin blue R	0.25 gm.
Glycerol	7.00 ml.

Dissolve the iron alum in water by letting stand overnight at room temperature. Add 0.25 gm. celestin blue and boil for 3 minutes. Filter when cool and add 7 ml. of glycerol. Save stain and reuse.

ORANGE G SOLUTION

Orange G	2 gm.
5% aqueous phosphotungstic acid	100 ml.

Dissolve the orange G in the 5% phosphotungstic acid solution. Let stand for 48 hours and use the supernatant. Save stain and reuse. The staining solution may appear cloudy, but this turbidity will not interfere with its staining qualities.

Staining Procedure

1. Bring sections down to water. Remove mercuric deposits if necessary.
2. Rinse in 70% alcohol.
3. Immerse in periodic acid solution for *5 minutes* to oxidize.
4. Rinse in 70% alcohol.
5. Immerse in the reducing bath (Hotchkiss) for *1 minute.*
6. Rinse in 70% alcohol.
7. Place in Schiff's reagent for *7 to 10 minutes.*
8. Wash in running water for *10 minutes.*

9. Stain nuclei with celestin blue for ½ *minute to 3 minutes.*

10. Rinse quickly in water.

11. Stain nuclei in hematoxylin for *1 to 3 minutes* (one used in H and E series will do).

12. Rinse in tap water and decolorize in 0.5% or 1.0% acid alcohol. Rinse in water. Check the nuclei with microscope. Decolorize or restain if necessary.

13. Counterstain with orange G (dip slides in and out few times). Wash off orange G in water and check with microscope. If orange G is too heavy and is masking other stains, water will remove the excess.

14. Dehydrate in several changes of 95% alcohol and absolute alcohol.

15. Clear in several changes of xylene and mount.

RESULTS.   Nuclei — blue to brown
Basement membranes, glycogen, fungi — purple-red
Differential staining of cells of the pituitary:
    Acidophils — orange-yellow
    Basophils — deep purple-red
    Amphophils — pale pink

REFERENCE.   Pearse, A. G. E.   *Histochemistry: Theoretical and Applied* (2d ed.). Boston: Little, Brown, 1960, p. 431.

MODIFIED SCHMORL'S METHOD FOR ADRENOCHROME
(After McManus and Mowry)

DISCUSSION.   Adrenochrome after strong chromic oxidation shows an affinity for the eosin and methyl violet components of Giemsa's stain.

INDICATIONS.   For staining adrenal medullary cells.

FIXATION.   Fix fresh material for 24 hours in potassium dichromate-formalin fixative (see below).

TECHNIQUE.   Paraffin

Solutions

POTASSIUM DICHROMATE FIXATIVE

3% potassium dichromate	8 parts
Full-strength formalin (37–40%)	2 parts

Prepare just before use.

DILUTE GIEMSA STAIN

Giemsa stain	5 ml.
Distilled water	100 ml.

OR

Add 1 drop Giemsa stain to each milliliter of distilled water. There are approximately 20 drops in 1 ml. of fluid.

Staining Procedure

1. Fix tissue block in potassium dichromate fixative for *24 hours.*
2. Wash *1 hour* or more in running tap water.
3. Dehydrate and embed in paraffin. Bring paraffin sections to water as usual.
4. Stain sections for *15 to 24 hours* in dilute Giemsa stain (or for *2 to 6 hours* in a paraffin oven at 58°C.).
5. Rinse in tap and distilled waters.
6. Blot dry.
7. Dehydrate rapidly with acetone followed by equal parts of acetone and xylene.
8. Clear in several changes of xylene and mount in Permount.

RESULTS.   Adrenal medullary cells – bright red to violet
Cortical cells – blue
Erythrocytes – pink
Eosinophil granules – red

REFERENCES.   Schmorl, G.   Method for Chromaffin Cells. *Die pathologischhistologischen Untersuchungsmethoden* (7th ed.). Leipzig: F. C. W. Vogel, 1914, p. 293.
McManus, J. F. A., and Mowry, R. W. *Staining Methods, Histologic and Histochemical.* New York: Hoeber Med. Div., Harper & Row, 1960, p. 321.

SCHMORL REACTION

INDICATIONS. Valuable for the identification of pigments in tissue sections.

FIXATION. 10% buffered neutral formalin.

TECHNIQUE. Paraffin sections cut 6μ thick.

DISCUSSION. Components of some pigments (melanins, argentaffin granules, lipofuscins, and tissue components containing sulfhydryl groups) will reduce ferric ferricyanide to ferric ferrocyanide, which is then seen as a blue precipitate (Prussian blue). The reaction generally occurs within 1 to 5 minutes. To prevent overstaining, it is best to check section periodically with the microscope and remove it from the solution when the reaction has occurred.

Solutions

1% FERRIC CHLORIDE (STOCK SOLUTION)

Ferric chloride lumps	1 gm.
Distilled water	100 gm.

1% POTASSIUM FERRICYANIDE (STOCK SOLUTION)

Potassium ferricyanide	1 gm.
Distilled water	100 ml.

FERRIC CHLORIDE-POTASSIUM FERRICYANIDE WORKING SOLUTION

Ferric chloride stock solution	150 ml.
Potassium ferricyanide	50 ml.

Prepare fresh just before use.

Staining Procedure

Use chemically clean glassware throughout.

1. Deparaffinize sections through to water.
2. Immerse in ferric chloride-potassium ferricyanide working solution for *5 minutes* (see DISCUSSION).

3. Wash in running water.

4. Counterstain nuclei in 0.1% nuclear fast red (page 378) for 5 *minutes.* This step optional.

5. Dehydrate rapidly in alcohols, clear in xylene, and mount in Permount.

RESUTS. Melanin — dark blue

Argentaffin granules — dark blue

Lipofuscin — dark blue

Components containing active sulfhydryl groups — dark blue

Nuclei — pink, if counterstain is used

REFERENCE. Pearse, A. G. E. *Histochemistry: Theoretical and Applied.* Boston: Little, Brown, 1960, p. 925.

SHORR S3 AND HEMATOXYLIN STAIN

INDICATIONS. Stain for inclusion bodies

FIXATION. Any well-fixed tissue

TECHNIQUE. Paraffin sections; smears; membrane filters

Solutions

1% ACID ALCOHOL

Hydrochloric acid, concentrated	1 ml.
Ethyl alcohol, 70%	99 ml.

SHORR'S STAINING SOLUTION

Ethyl alcohol, 50%	100.000 ml.
Biebrich scarlet, water-soluble	0.500 gm.
Orange G	0.250 gm.
Fast green, FCF	0.075 gm.
Phosphotungstic acid, C.P.	0.500 gm.
Phosphomolybdic acid, C.P.	0.500 gm.
Glacial acetic acid	1.000 ml.

Combine and do not use until all the ingredients have completely dissolved.

HARRIS'S HEMATOXYLIN
(See page 227.)

AMMONIA WATER
(See page 26.)

Staining Procedure

1. Deparaffinize sections as usual and bring to water.
2. Stain in Harris's hematoxylin for *3 to 5 minutes.*
3. Rinse in water and differentiate in 1% acid alcohol until there is no hematoxylin in the cytoplasm of the cells. Check with microscope. (Leave nuclei slightly darker than usual.)
4. Wash in water and blue sections in ammonia water.
5. Wash in running tap water *10 minutes.*
6. Place sections in Shorr's staining solution for *1 minute.*
7. Wash in 95% alcohol. Check with microscope. Connective tissue will be a clear light green when differentiation is complete.
8. Rinse several times in absolute alcohol, clear in two or three changes of xylene, and mount in Permount or Clarite.

RESULTS. Inclusion bodies – bright red
Connective tissue – light green
Elastic tissue – purple-red
Muscle – red
Nuclei – blue
Keratin – orange
Erythrocytes – orange-red

REFERENCES. Page, W. G., and Green, R. G. *Cornell Vet.* 32:265–268, 1942.
Shorr, E. *Science* 94:545–546, 1941.

SCHULTZ CHOLESTEROL TEST

DISCUSSION. This is an impermanent "wet mount" procedure and must be examined by the pathologist *immediately* after step 5.

INDICATIONS.   To demonstrate the presence of cholesterol.

FIXATION.   Formalin (10%)

TECHNIQUE.   Frozen sections. A section of adrenal cortex may be used as a control.

Solutions

2.5% IRON ALUM

Ferric ammonium sulfate	2.5 gm.
Distilled water	100.0 ml.

CONCENTRATED SULFURIC-GLACIAL ACETIC ACID MIXTURE

Place *2 to 5 ml. of glacial acetic acid* in a small test tube and immerse tube in ice water. Then add gradually the *same volume of concentrated sulfuric acid* while the tube is still held in the ice water. Prepare fresh just before use.

Staining Procedure

1. Cut thin (10 to 15μ) frozen sections of formalin-fixed tissue.

2. Mordant sections in a closely stoppered bottle for *3 days* at 37°C. in 2.5% iron alum solution. (Lillie gives this alternate method of mordanting: 1 to 3 minutes in 3% hydrogen peroxide solution or 1% sodium iodate.)

3. Rinse in distilled water, float onto slides, and blot dry with filter paper.

4. Treat with a few drops of the freshly prepared acetic-sulfuric mixture dropped on with a glass rod.

5. Cover section with a coverglass and examine the wet mount at once.

RESULTS.   A positive test for cholesterol or its esters is indicated by the appearance of a blue-green color within a few seconds which reaches its maximum intensity within a few minutes. The stain is not permanent and within 30 minutes the sections may acquire a brown discoloration. At least two or more sections of the material under test should be treated with the acetic-sulfuric mixture and examined before considering the test negative.

REFERENCE. Lillie, R. D. *Histopathologic Technic and Practical Histochemistry* (2d ed.). New York: McGraw-Hill, 1954, p. 317.

SUDAN BLACK B STAIN

Propylene glycol is recommended as a solvent for Sudan black B to replace commonly employed alcohol-acetone mixtures for general lipid staining in tissue sections. The solution is easily prepared, and there is excellent control of differentiation without loss of dye from lipid particles.

INDICATIONS. For staining fat in sections.

FIXATION. Formalin (10%). Fat cuts more easily when fixed.

TECHNIQUE. Frozen sections

Solutions

SUDAN BLACK B SOLUTION

Dissolve *0.7 gm. of Sudan black B in 100 ml. of absolute propylene glycol* by heating to 100° to 110°C., stirring thoroughly for a few minutes. Do not exceed 110°C., since a useless gelatinous suspension will result. Filter hot through Whatman No. 2 paper to remove excess dye. After cooling to room temperature, filter through a fritted glass filter of medium porosity with the aid of suction. This is a stable solution.

85% PROPYLENE GLYCOL SOLUTION

Propylene gylcol	85 ml.
Distilled water	15 ml.

Staining Procedure

1. Cut frozen sections. Collect in distilled water and allow to remain for *2 to 5 minutes* to remove excess formalin.

2. Dehydrate sections in absolute propylene glycol for *5 to 10 minutes.* Occasional movement of sections is desirable because of the viscosity of the glycol.

3. Stain for *10 to 30 minutes* in Sudan black B solution. Agitate sections occasionally.

4. Transfer sections to 85% propylene glycol solution for *2 to 3 minutes.* Agitate gently.

5. Wash in distilled water for *3 to 5 minutes.*

6. Counterstain, if desired, in nuclear fast red (page 378) for a few minutes.

7. Wash well.

8. Transfer sections to slides. Drain off excess water and mount in glycerin jelly or any commercial aqueous mountant.

RESULTS.   Fat — black, blue, or blue-black
Nuclei — red if counterstain is used

REFERENCE.   Chifelle, T. L., and Putt, F. A. *Stain Techn.* 26:51, 1951.

UNNA-PAPPENHEIM METHYL GREEN-PYRONINE STAIN

This is the simplest of the methyl green-pyronine stains and one of the oldest. All methyl green-pyronine stains are capricious. Since this is the simplest, it is worth trying before turning to the more complex techniques.

INDICATIONS.   Stain for plasma cells

FIXATION.   Carnoy's fluid, absolute alcohol, 10% formalin, or Helly's solution

TECHNIQUE.   Paraffin

Solutions

PAPPENHEIM STAIN
(Ready to use from supplier *)

Staining Procedure

1. Deparaffinize as usual and bring to water.
2. Stain sections in Pappenheim stain for *20 to 30 minutes.*
3. Rinse rapidly in water. Blot gently and quickly with smooth filter paper.
4. Differentiate and dehydrate rapidly in absolute ethyl alcohol. *Note:* Acetone may be used in place of the alcohol to dehydrate because it has less tendency to extract the pyronine from the cytoplasm of the cells.
5. Clear in xylene and mount in Permount.

RESULTS.   Nuclei — green

Cytoplasm — rose to red

REFERENCE.   Mallory, F. B. *Pathological Technique.* Philadelphia: Saunders, 1938, p. 176.

VON KOSSA'S METHOD FOR DEMONSTRATING CALCIUM

Von Kossa has shown that calcium phosphate can be demonstrated by means of silver nitrate, which forms silver phosphate on the surface of the granules and blackens in the presence of light.

FIXATION.   Alcohols or 10% neutral formalin. Alcohols preferred.

TECHNIQUE.   Paraffin

* Pappenheim stain #VS27860. Aloe Scientific, 1831 Olive St., St. Louis, Mo. 63103.

Solutions

5% SILVER NITRATE SOLUTION

Silver nitrate	5 gm.
Distilled water	100 ml.

5% SODIUM THIOSULFATE

Sodium thiosulfate	5 gm.
Distilled water	100 ml.

KERNECHTROT* NUCLEAR FAST RED STAIN

Dissolve *0.1 gm. of nuclear fast red powder in 100 ml. of 5% aqueous aluminum sulfate solution* with the aid of heat. Cool and filter. Add a *crystal of thymol* as a preservative. Keeps well at room temperature. Can be reused.

Staining Procedure

1. Deparaffinize sections through two changes of xylene, absolute and 95% alcohols down to distilled water.

2. Place in 5% silver nitrate solution for *30 to 60 minutes* exposed to direct sunlight or a 100-watt desk-lamp light. *Use chemically clean container.*

3. Rinse in distilled water.

4. Reduce in 5% sodium thiosulfate for *2 to 3 minutes* to remove excess silver nitrate.

5. Wash well in distilled water.

6. Counterstain in nuclear fast red for *5 minutes.*

7. Wash in distilled water.

8. Dehydrate in two changes of 95% alcohol, two changes of absolute alcohol, and clear with two or three changes of xylene.

9. Mount in Permount or balsam.

RESULTS. Calcium salts — black
Nuclei — red
Cytoplasm — pink to rose

* May be procured from Roboz Surgical Instrument Co., 810 18th St., N.W., Washington, D.C. 20006.

REFERENCE. Mallory, F. B. *Pathological Technique.* Philadelphia: Saunders, 1938, p. 144.

WEIGERT'S STAIN FOR FIBRIN

FIXATION.   Carnoy's fluid or alcohol-formalin. Zenker's or Helly's fluid may also be used.

TECHNIQUE.   Paraffin

Solutions

LITHIUM CARMINE SOLUTION

Carmine	4 gm.
Lithium carbonate, saturated aqueous solution (1.25%)	100 ml.
Thymol	1 gm.

Dissolve the carmine in the lithium carbonate solution. Boil for 10 to 15 minutes. When cool, add *thymol* to prevent growth of molds. Always filter this stain just before use.

CRYSTAL VIOLET (SOLUTION A)

Absolute alcohol	33 ml.
Aniline	9 ml.
Crystal violet to saturate (approx. 5 gm.)	in excess

CRYSTAL VIOLET (SOLUTION B)

Crystal violet	2 gm.
Distilled water	100 ml.

CRYSTAL VIOLET WORKING SOLUTION

Solution A	3 ml.
Solution B	27 ml.

The stock solutions will keep indefinitely, the combined stain for only 1 to 2 weeks.

Staining Procedure

1. Deparaffinize in xylene, absolute alcohol, and 95% alcohol to water.

2. Stain nuclei with freshly filtered lithium carmine for *2 to 5 minutes.*

3. Transfer sections directly to 1% acid alcohol for *a few seconds* to fix the dye in the nuclei and differentiate the section.

4. Wash thoroughly with tap water.

5. Stain sections for *6 to 10 minutes* in the working solution of crystal violet.

6. Drain and blot with filter paper.

7. Pour Gram's iodine (page 29) over the sections. Allow it to act for *5 to 10 minutes.*

8. Drain off solution and blot with filter paper.

9. Differentiate in a mixture of equal parts of aniline oil and xylene (two changes) until the section is well differentiated and no more purple washes out. Check slides with microscope to control differentiation. Reticulum, elastica, and basement membranes should be colorless.

10. Blot. Rinse in xylene, several changes, to remove aniline.

11. Mount in Permount.

Note: Avoid inhaling the aniline.

RESULTS.   Fibrin — blue to blue-black
Gram-positive bacteria — blue to blue-black
Nuclei — red

REFERENCE.   Mallory, F. B. *Pathological Technique.* Philadelphia: Saunders, 1938, p. 193.

APPENDIX II

Glossary

absorption   A soaking up throughout the mass.

achromatic   Without color. Not staining readily.

acid   A compound containing hydrogen, which in water solution forms no positive ions but hydrogen ions.

acid-fast   Most bacteria when placed in carbol-fuchsin for sufficient time will stain deeply. However, all bacteria except tuberculosis and leprosy bacilli lose their color when treated immediately thereafter with an acid. *Mycobacteria tuberculosis* and *B. leprae* are thus often termed "acid-fast."

acidophilic   Readily stained with acid dyes.

adsorption   A soaking up only on the surface.

aldehyde   An organic compound containing the CHO group.

ameba   One-celled protozoan animal. One type parasitic to man causes amebic dysentery.

amorphous   Without a definite shape.

amphoteric   Referring to a compound which may ionize as a base in the presence of a strong acid, and as an acid in the presence of a strong base.

amyloid   A starchlike *protein* complex which is an abnormal extra-cellular product. In disease it is usually found in the spleen, liver, and kidneys.

anaplasia   A condition in tumor cells in which there is loss of normal differentiation or organization.

anhydrous   Material from which the water has been removed.

anode   The positive terminal of an electric cell.

anthracosis   Black carbon pigment found in the lungs and mediastinal lymph nodes. It resists all reactions, bleaches, and solvents.

aqua regia   A mixture of concentrated nitric and hydrochloric acids.

argentaffin   Having an affinity for silver or other metallic salts; staining with silver solutions. The difference between the "argentaffin reaction" and silver impregnation methods is that the argentaffin cells have the property (capacity of the tissue component itself) of reducing ammoniacal silver solutions to metallic silver. See also *argyrophil*.

argyrophil   Having an affinity for silver or other metallic salts; staining with silver solutions. Argyrophilic tissue can be impregnated by silver solutions when an artificial reducer is employed.

artefact   Something produced artificially. A modification of the appearance or structure of tissue caused by a chemical or some other exterior agent.

aspiration   Withdrawal, by suction, of fluid or soft tissue from the body; e.g., needle aspirates of liver, kidney, or sternal marrow.

autogenous pigment   Natural pigment, made by the cell inside the body (e.g., melanin).

autolysis   Tissue decomposition unconnected with bacterial decay. Dead cells liberate enzymes that digest the tissue. Highly specialized organs such as brain, spinal cord, and glands autolyze more rapidly than, for example, connective tissue. The adrenal gland autolyzes very rapidly.

autopsy   Examination of the body or tissues removed from the body after death.

Autotechnicon   Commercial name of a tissue-processing machine which automatically fixes, washes, dehydrates, clears, and infiltrates tissue. Also employed by some laboratories to stain tissue.

base   A compound containing the hydroxyl group which, when dissolved in water, forms no negative ions but hydroxyl ions.

basophilic   Having an affinity for or staining readily with basic dyes.

benign   Favorable for recovery. Not malignant.

biopsy   Excision of a small piece of living tissue for microscopic examination.

birefringent   Doubly refractive.

blocking   See *embedding.*

cancer   See *carcinoma.*

carbohydrates   Compounds containing carbon, hydrogen, and oxygen, usually with the hydrogen and oxygen present in the ratio of two to one.

carcinoma   A malignant new growth (cancer). It differs from benign tumors in its ability to metastasize (spread beyond its site of origin). This is accomplished either by direct invasion of adjacent structures or by dissemination through the lymphatic system or blood stream. Cancer may arise from any type of cell and is classified according to the tissue and type of cell origin. Hundreds of classifications exist which fall under three major types: *Carcinoma,* arising from epithelial cells (very cellular tumor); *Sarcoma,* those cancers arising from connective and supporting tissue; and the *lymphomas* and *leukemias* that involve blood-forming tissue.

casting   See *embedding.*

catalyst   A substance that promotes or retards a reaction.

cathode   The negative electrode or terminal.

cell block   The closely packed cellular sediment ("button") obtained when samples of body fluids are centrifuged, and the supernatant fluid decanted. The cell block is removed from the tube and processed exactly like a tissue section.

celloidin   Purified form of collodion or nitrocellulose used for impregnating tissue.

centigrade temperature   Temperature on the Centigrade scale which has $0°$ for the freezing point of water and $100°$ for the boiling point at a pressure of 760 mm.

chelate   (from the Greek "chēlē" claw) Chemically it means to combine with a metal in weakly dissociated complexes in which the metal is part of a ring.

chromatin   The more readily stainable portion of the cell nucleus (DNA). It is the carrier of the genes of inheritance. Portion of nucleus readily stained by basic dyes such as hematoxlyin.

chromophors   Certain groups whose presence results in compounds having a color.

clearing   A process serving two functions. Clearing dealcoholizes in both embedding and mounting procedures. Clearing renders the tissue transparent.

colloid   A particle in an extremely fine state of subdivision.

colloidal   Existing in the form of extremely small-sized particles.

crystallization   The process of forming crystals from a solution.

crystals   Solids separated from solutions having a definite shape or structure.

cytogenics   Microscopic study of human chromosomes.

cytology   The study of cells: their origin, structure, and function.

cytoplasm   Protoplasm of a cell, excluding the nucleus. It is made up of complexes of fats, carbohydrates, and proteins.

decalcification   Removal of lime salts from bone or other calcified specimens so that thin sections can be cut.

decolorization   Removal of stain or excess stain from tissue sections.

decomposition   Decay of tissue produced by bacterial invasion. Decomposition may be retarded by cold.

dehydration   Removal of free water from tissue.

dichroism   The quality of presenting one color in reflected and another in transmitted light (i.e. with polarizing lens Congo red will change from red to green).

differentiation   Removal of excess stain from tissue until color is retained only by the tissue elements to be studied, usually visually controlled with the microscope.

diffusion   The intermingling of liquids and gases.

diluent   A diluting agent, such as water in a solution.

embedding   Enclosing tissue in a solid block of the medium used for infiltration. Also called "casting" or "blocking."

embedding process   Complete method of processing tissue, including fixation, dehydration, infiltration, and casting.

endogenous pigment   Pigment made inside the body (e.g., bile pigment).

enzyme   Complex chemical substance acting upon other substances and causing them to split up into simpler substances. Capable of accelerating greatly the course of specific cellular chemical reactions.

ester   A compound formed by the reaction between an acid and an alcohol.

exfoliation   The shedding of sheets or layers of cells.

exogenous pigment   Various substances which enter the body and are deposited there as pigments (e.g., carotin, carbon, silver).

fahrenheit temperature   Temperature on the Fahrenheit scale with 32° as the freezing point of water and 212° as the boiling point at a pressure of 760 mm.

fixation   A process of hardening and preserving pathologic specimens.

friable   Easily crumbled.

fungi   A group of living organisms resembling yeasts or molds, some of which are pathogenic to man.

gel   A jelly-like solid.

glycogen   A colorless carbohydrate cell product related to starch and dextrin, commonly found in liver. It is water-soluble.

Golgi apparatus   A delicate intracellular network of fibers within the nerve cell. It is seen only after special staining.

ground substance   Reticulum, collagen, and elastin are connective tissue elements embedded in a cementing substance known as ground substance.

hematein The active coloring agent in hematoxylin solutions. It is the product of oxidation (ripening) of the solution.

hematogenous Produced in or derived from the blood.

hemofuscin Hematogenous pigment occurring as light yellow granules. It will *not* react to iron-staining reaction.

hemosiderin Hematogenous pigment occurring as bright yellowish-brown granules and masses. It *will* react to iron-staining reaction (e.g., Prussian blue).

histology The microscopic study of structure, composition, and function of tissues and organs.

honing The first step of knife sharpening. Honing removes nicks and sets the bevel of the knife.

homogeneous The same throughout.

homologous Having a similar general structure.

hydrolysis The reaction of water with a salt to form the acid and the base of which the salt was a product; it opposes neutralization reactions.

hygroscopic Having a tendency to pick up water vapor.

hypo Sodium thiosulfate, in common use in photographic developing.

inert substance One which does not react at all with other substances under the usual conditions of chemical reactions.

infiltration Impregnation of tissue with a substance that will support cells so that they may be cut into thin sections.

inorganic Pertaining to mineral matter, or matter not connected with living material.

ion An atom or group of atoms which carries an electric charge.

ion-exchange resins Granules of resins that absorb either positive or negative ions.

ionization The formation of ions from polar compounds by action of a solvent.

irradiation   Exposure to light, especially ultraviolet light.

keratin   A scleroprotein found in epidermis, hair, nails, and horny tissues.

level   See *step sections.*

lipoid   Substance resembling fat in appearance and solubility.

lysis   Dissolution of cells.

malignant   Virulent, tending to go from bad to worse. Unfavorable for recovery.

mast cells   Large cells containing basophil granules believed to contain heparin.

melanin   A dark-brown natural pigment that is found in cells (e.g., skin) as brown or black granules.

metachromasia   Change of color — a tissue color reaction different from that of the stain used, such as a violet color after toluidine blue staining.

microtome   Machine designed to cut thin sections of human, animal, or plant tissue.

miscible   Capable of being mixed.

mitochondria   Small granules or rod-shaped structures found, after differential staining, in the cytoplasm of cells.

mitoses   Indirect cell division.

molar solution   One gram-molecular weight of a substance dissolved in enough solvent to make one liter of solution.

mole   That number of grams of a substance which is exactly equal to its molecular weight.

molecular weight   The sum of the weights of the atoms in a molecule.

monomer   A substance composed of a single part.

mordant   Substance that unites with a dye linking it with the object to be dyed. In histologic techniques tissues are "mordanted." When we mordant tissue, the substance is picked up by the tissue; the mordant, now absorbed by the tissue, takes up the dye, making possible a staining reaction. While not all dyes demand a mordant, many require one in order to stain tissues at all. Mordants are also used to ensure specific staining reactions.

morphology The science of form and structure. Morphology deals with size, shape, appearance, and interrelationships.

mount The word has several applications: (1) To attach tissue blocks to the block holder. (2) To place tissue sections on slides for staining and observation. (3) To place coverglasses over tissue sections which have been stained.

mucin A highly viscous mucopolysaccharide or glycoprotein.

neoplasm A new and abnormal growth, such as a tumor. May be either benign or malignant.

nitrocellulose Embedding medium derived from gun cotton. Used in the same manner as celloidin, especially for eye embedding.

osmosis The passage of liquids and gases through porous membranes.

oxidation Chemical reactions in which oxygen is taken up, giving rise to the formation of oxides. Chemically it consists in the increase of positive charges on an atom or the loss of negative charges.

pH A numerical scale that indicates the concentration of hydrogen ions in a solution; 7 is neutral, less than 7 is acid, and greater than 7 is basic.

polychrome Multicolor.

polymers Substances made up of many parts.

polymerization The process by which many monomers join together to form polymers.

postmordanting Immersing tissue in a mordant (i.e. ferric chloride, potassium bichromate, picric acid solutions, etc.) usually after initial fixation in formalin.

precipitation Separation of a solid substance from a solution by action of a reagent. The substance separated is the precipitate.

properties   The characteristics by which we identify materials.

pyknotic   A condition in which the nucleus shrinks in size and chromatin condenses to a solid structureless mass or masses. Nucleus stains densely and appears shriveled.

radical   A group of atoms which acts like a single atom in forming compounds.

reagent   A substance of known chemical composition used to produce a chemical reaction with another substance.

reducing agent   An agent that removes oxygen from a material.

reduction   A chemical reaction in which hydrogen is taken up by a compound or oxygen is removed.

resins   Gum from trees. Hard substances, usually amber in color. Used in histologic techniques to aid differentiation (e.g., colophonium or cherry resin); also used as a base for mounting media (e.g., Canada balsam, gum dammar). Both natural and synthetic resins are used.

rosin   See *resins.*

sarcoma   See *carcinoma.*

sclerosis   Hardening or induration.

serial sections   Unbroken sequence of sections throughout the tissue block. All sections are saved. It is necessary to avoid losing any of the sections cut. Ribbons are cut and placed conveniently on a sheet of cardboard in proper order.

smear   Fluid or semifluid tissue spread in a film upon a glass slide.

step sections (*levels*)   Tissue sections taken from different parts of the block; e.g., section taken from the top, center, and bottom of block.

stropping   Second step in knife sharpening. Stropping removes wire edge caused by honing and sharpens knife.

supernatant   The liquid floating over the solid particles of a substance separated by precipitation or centrifugation.

synthetic resins   Plastics produced by chemical synthesis.

titration   Determination of the concentration of a solution by comparing it with a standard solution, usually employing burettes for the operation.

touch preparation   Tissue material left on a clean glass slide when freshly cut tissue (especially bone marrow) is placed against it.

ultraviolet rays   Invisible radiations having a shorter wave length than violet light.

valence   The number of electrons gained, lost, or shared in forming a chemical bond.

volatile   Easily vaporized.

wetting agents   Materials that reduce the surface tension of a liquid, causing it to spread out better.

Prefixes and Suffixes

The Registry of Medical Technologists requires the knowledge of prefixes, suffixes, and word stems used in medical terminology.

A hyphen before the affix indicates a suffix.

A hyphen after indicates a prefix.

A hyphen before and after indicates use both as a prefix and as a suffix.

a-, an-	negative (not)
aer-	air
-algia	pain
apo-	from, opposed
-ase	enzyme
auto-	self
bi-, bis-	twice, double
-cele	tumor, cyst, hernia
cent-	hundred
-chrom-, chromo-	color
circum-	around
cyst-	bag, bladder
-cyte	cell
-derma-	skin
di-	double, apart from
dys-	difficult, bad
ecto-	out, on the outside
-ectomy	cutting out
-emia	relating to blood
endo-	within

epi-	upon
-fuge	drive away
gastr-, gastro-	stomach
-gen, -genesis	origin, formation
-gram	tracing, mark
hem-, hemato-	relating to blood
hepa-, hepar-, hepato-	relating to liver
homo-, homeo-	same, similar
hydra-, hydro-	relating to water
hypo-	under, below
hyper-	over, above, excessive
inter-	between
intra-, intro-	within
-itis	inflammation
kerat-	horny
latero-	side
leuco-, leuko-	white
-lite, -lith	stone, calculus
-lysis	setting free, disintegration
macro-	large
mal-	bad
mega-	large, great
micro-	small
mono-	single
multi-	many
my- or myo-	relating to muscle
neur-, neuro-	relating to nerves
-oid	form, resemblance
-oma	tumor
-orchid-	testicle
-otomy	cutting into
pan-	all, entire
para-	alongside of
-path-, -pathy	disease
peri-	around
pneum-	relating to air or lungs
poly-	much, many
post-	after

pre-	before
pseud-, pseudo-	false
py-, pyo-	pus
sclero-	hard
-scopy	to see
trans-	across
-uria	relating to urine
vaso-	vessel

First Aid

1. Keep laboratory well lighted and well ventilated.
2. Exert great care in handling acids and caustic alkalis.
3. Check Bunsen burners regularly for gas leaks. Replace tubing when necessary.
4. Do not light matches or smoke cigarettes while working with volatile reagents (ether, etc.).
5. Dye stains on the hands are to be avoided. When fingers become stained, the prompt local application of acid alcohol followed by running water will usually be effective in removing the dye. Dyes should not be permitted to remain on the skin because they are slowly absorbed and may produce later injurious effects. Avoid dye absorption by wearing disposable plastic gloves when handling slides and solutions. The plastic gloves are dissolved by xylene.

EMERGENCY FIRST AID SUPPLIES

Keep the following handy on a laboratory shelf:

1. Mild antiseptic for cuts and scratches: 1% tincture of iodine, 70% isopropyl alcohol, or a bottle of sterile saline.
2. Adhesive bandages or sterile dressings.
3. 2% solution of acetic acid.
4. Bicarbonate of soda.
5. Petroleum jelly.

FIRST AID TREATMENT

burns, acid   Wash promptly with soap and water. Soak area in bi-carbonate of soda in water or apply paste of bicarbonate of soda.

burns, alkali   Do not use water, as this will spread the alkali. Rinse burn thoroughly with 2% acetic acid.

burns, heat   For a minor burn (skin is reddened but not denuded) apply a thin coating of petroleum jelly to the area. For a serious burn, *do not treat;* see physician.

cuts   For minor cuts and scratches, wash cut. Check to be sure that there are no foreign bodies (glass) in wound. Rinse with sterile saline or 70% alcohol or apply mild antiseptic. Cover with adhesive bandage or loose dressing.

If the edges of the injury gape, or wound is serious enough to warrant suturing, do not apply any antiseptic. See doctor promptly. After treatment it may be necessary to protect cut with a finger cot. Do not leave on longer than absolutely necessary, as it delays healing.

eyes   If formalin or any other liquid is splashed into the eye, do not stop to find suitable neutralizing agent. Wash eye out immediately with copious amounts of running tap water. If irritation persists, see physician.

fainting   If someone feels faint, have her sit with her head between her knees. When someone has fainted, no treatment is necessary other than to place the person flat on the floor. Clothing around the neck may be loosened, or a cold cloth may be applied to the head.

Useful Information

gm.   =   gram
gr.   =   grain
mm.   =   millimeter
cm.   =   centimeter
ml.   =   milliliter
cc.   =   cubic centimeter
μ =   micron
$m\mu$ =   millimicron
A   =   angstrom unit

U.S.P.   Abbreviation for United States Pharmacopoeia, an official book that specifies strengths and degrees of purity.

C.P.   Abbreviation for "chemically pure," generally exceeding U.S.P. requirements.

A.R.   Analytical or reagent grade, unexcelled in purity and uniformity.

M, mole.   Mole is the number of grams of a substance which is exactly equal to its molecular weight.

M.W., molecular weight.   Molar solution is one gram-molecular weight of a substance dissolved in enough solvent to make 1 liter of solution.

N   abbreviation for Normal. A Normal solution is one that contains one gram-equivalent of a substance dissolved in enough solvent to make 1 liter of solution. Normal solutions are made up so that in 1 liter of solution there is either (1) 1 gram of hydrogen which can be replaced; or (2) sufficient quantity of some other substance to replace directly or indirectly 1 gram of hydrogen. For instance, if 1000 ml. of a normal solution of any acid is added to 1000 ml. of a normal solution of any base we have exact neutralization. In other words, normal acid solutions neutralize normal base solutions, milliliter for milliliter. *Equal volumes of solutions of equal normality are equivalent.*

Normal solutions may be two or three times normal, but more often they are diluted until they are 0.1N, 0.01N, or any other fractional normality.

PREPARATION OF MOLAR AND NORMAL SOLUTIONS[*]

Preparation of Molar Solutions

A molar solution contains 1 gram molecular weight (one gram molecule) of the chemical in 1 liter of solution. For example:

Sodium β-glycerophosphate.

Molecular weight of sodium β-glycerophosphate $= 315.13$
Molar solution $(M) = 315.13$ gm. in 1000 ml. distilled water
$0.1\ M = 31.513$ gm. in 1000 ml. distilled water.

The chemical is dissolved in a small quantity of the water and the volume is made up to one liter.

Preparation of Normal Solutions

A normal solution contains one gram molecular weight of the substance, divided by the hydrogen equivalent of the substance. For example:

(a) Sodium hydroxide, NaOH

Molecular weight of sodium hydroxide $= 40.0$.   Valency $= 1$.
Normal solution $= 40.0$ gm. in 1000 ml. distilled water divided by 1
$\qquad = 40.0$ gm. in 100 ml. distilled water.

[*]Source: Bancroft, J. D. *Introduction to Histochemical Technique.* London: Butterworth, 1967, p. 252.

(b) For liquids, the following formula may be used:
ml. of acid per 1000 ml. of distilled water

$$= \frac{\text{mol. wt.}}{\text{valency} \times \text{spec. gravity} \times \text{concn.}}$$

For example: Hydrochloric acid, HCl

Valency 1, spec. gravity 1.18, Concn. 36%, mol. wt. 36.4

$$\frac{36.4}{1 \times 1.18 \times 0.36} = 85.6 \text{ ml.}$$

N HCl = 85.6 ml. HCl + 914.4 ml. distilled water.

For example: Sulphuric acid, H_2SO_4

Valency 2, spec. gravity 1.835, Concn. 98% mol. wt. 98.08

$$\frac{98.08}{2 \times 1.835 \times 0.98} = 29.1 \text{ ml.}$$

N $H_2S_2O_4$ = 29.1 ml. H_2SO_4 + 970.9 ml. distilled water.
0.1 N H_2SO_4 = 2.91 ml. H_2SO_4 + 997.09 ml. distilled water.

MEASUREMENTS

Solids are weighed in **grams.** Length is measured in **centimeters** or **millimeters.** Liquids are measured in **milliliters.** The prefix **centi** = $\frac{1}{100}$. The prefix **milli** = $\frac{1}{1000}$. A centigram is $\frac{1}{100}$ of a gram. A milliliter is $\frac{1}{1000}$ of a liter.

Weight Units

The basic weight unit is a **gram.** There are 454 gm. to a pound.

1 grain	=	0.0648 gm. (nearly)		
1 milligram	=	0.001 gm.		
1 centigram	=	0.01 gm.		
1 gram	=	0.001 kilogram (kg.)	=	(15.4324 grains)
1 ounce	=	28.35 gm.		
1 pound	=	454.00 gm.		
1 kilogram	=	1000.00 gm.		

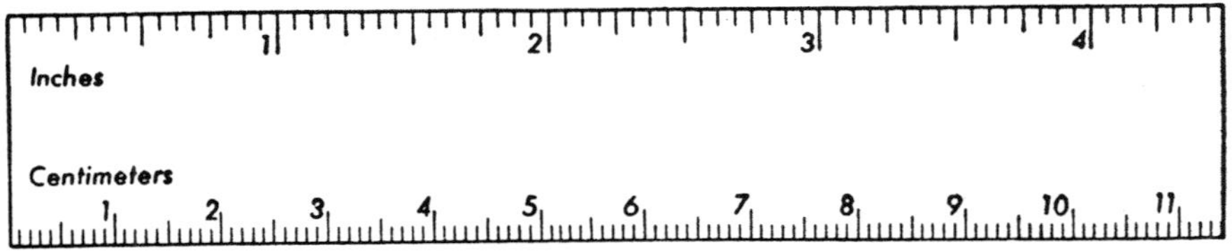

Figure A-1. Centimeter-inch ratio: 1 inch = 2.54, 1 centimeter = 0.394 inch

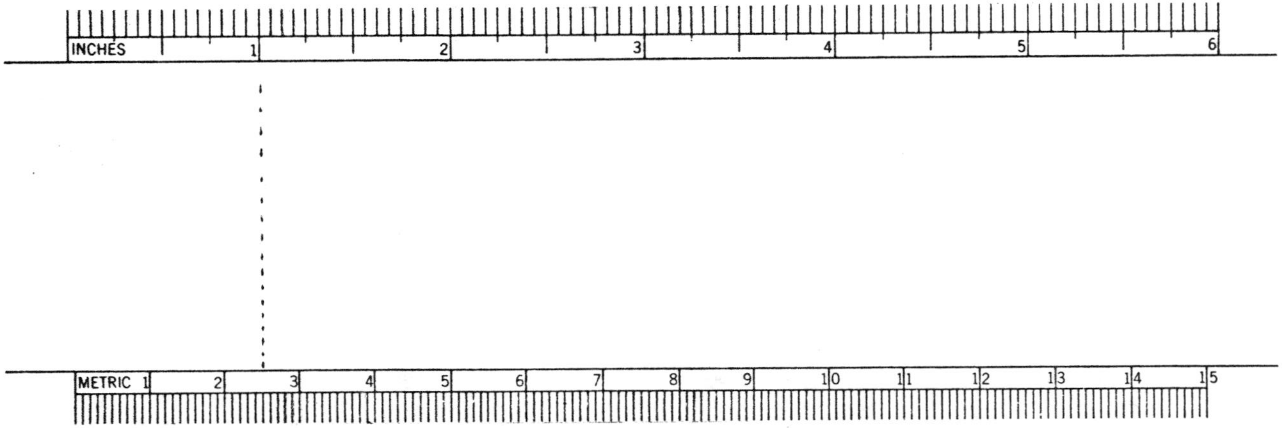

Figure A-2. Millimeter-inch ratio with 25.4 millimeters to an inch; 1.0 millimeter is equal to 0.03937 of an inch

Linear Measurements

The *meter* is the basic unit of length. A meter is equal to slightly more than a yard. It is 39.37 inches (3.281 feet).

1 millimeter	=	0.03937 inch (1000 microns)
1 centimeter	=	0.3937 inch (10 millimeters)
1 inch	=	2.54 centimeters (25.4 millimeters)
1 angstrom (A)	=	0.0000000001 meter
1 millimicron (mμ)	=	0.000000001 meter
1 micron (μ)	=	0.000001 meter
1 millimeter (mm.)	=	0.001 meter
1 centimeter (cm.)	=	0.01 meter
1 micron	=	0.001 millimeters (mm.)
1 angstrom unit	=	0.1 millimicrons (mμ.)
1 angstrom unit	=	0.0001 microns (μ.)
1 micron	=	1000 millimicrons or 10,000 angstrom units

Liquid Measurements

The *liter* is the basic unit of volume in the metric system. One liter is nearly equivalent to 1 liquid quart measure (1.06 quart).

1 liter	=	1000 milliliters
1 gallon	=	3785 milliliters
4 liters	=	4000 milliliters

1 milliliter (1.0 ml.)	=	0.001 liter
1 cubic centimeter (1.0 cc.)	=	0.001 liter
(in practice 1 cc. = 1 ml.)		

1 milliliter = approximately 20 drops

TEMPERATURES

A change of 1°C. = a change of 1.8°F.
A change of 1°F. = a change of 0.54°C.

Body temperature = 37°C. (98.6°F.)
Room temperature = 22°C. (70°F.)
Refrigerator temperature = 5° to 10°C.
Freezer temperature = —20 to —30°C.
Dry ice temperature = approximately —70° to —75°C.

Conversion Table for Temperature

°F.	°C.	°C.	°F.
0	—17.7	0	32.0
95	35.0	35.0	95.0
96	35.5	35.5	95.9
97	36.1	36.0	96.8
98	36.6	36.5	97.7
99	37.2	37.0	98.6
100	37.7	37.5	99.5
101	38.3	38.0	100.4
102	38.8	38.5	101.3
103	39.4	39.0	102.2
104	40.0	39.5	103.1
105	40.5	40.0	104.0
106	41.1	40.5	104.9
107	41.6	41.0	105.8
108	42.2	41.5	106.6
109	42.7	42.0	107.6
110	43.3	100.0	212.0

$$°C. = (°F. - 32) \times \tfrac{5}{9} \qquad °F. = (°C. \times \tfrac{9}{5}) + 32$$

CONVERSION TABLE FOR METRIC SYSTEM

To Convert From:	To:	Multiply By:
milligrams	grains	0.01543
angstrom units	centimeters	1×10^{-8}
angstrom units	microns	0.0001
centimeters	inches (U.S.)	0.3937
grams	grains	15.4324
inches (U.S.)	centimeters	2.5400
inches (U.S.)	millimeters	25.4001

LIST OF COMMON ELEMENTS

Name	Symbol	Approximate Atomic Weight	Name	Symbol	Approximate Atomic Weight
Aluminum	Al	27	Magnesium	Mg	24
Antimony	Sb	121.8	Manganese	Mn	55
Arsenic	As	75	Mercury	Hg	200.6
Barium	Ba	137	Molybdenum	Mo	96
Bismuth	Bi	209	Nickel	Ni	58.7
Bromine	Br	80	Nitrogen	N	14
Calcium	Ca	40	Oxygen	O	16
Carbon	C	12	Phosphorus	P	31
Chlorine	Cl	35.5	Platinum	Pt	195
Chromium	Cr	52	Potassium	K	39
Cobalt	Co	59	Silicon	Si	28
Copper	Cu	63.5	Silver	Ag	108
Fluorine	F	19	Sodium	Na	23
Gold	Au	197	Strontium	Sr	87.6
Hydrogen	H	1	Sulfur	S	32
Iodine	I	127	Tin	Sn	118.7
Iron	Fe	56	Titanium	Ti	48
Lead	Pb	207	Tungsten	W	184
Lithium	Li	7	Zinc	Zn	65

VALENCES SHOWN BY COMMON ELEMENTS AND RADICALS

Name	Symbol	Valence	Name	Symbol	Valence
Aluminum	Al	+3	Lead	Pb	+2
Ammonium	NH_4	+1	Lithium	Li	+1
Barium	Ba	+2	Magnesium	Mg	+2
Calcium	Ca	+2	Mercuric	Hg	+2
Chromium	Cr	+3	Mercurous	Hg	+1
Cobalt	Co	+2	Molybdenum	Mo	+2, +3
Cupric	Cu	+2	Nickel	Ni	+2
Cuprous	Cu	+1	Potassium	K	+1
Ferric	Fe	+3	Silver	Ag	+1
Ferrous	Fe	+2	Sodium	Na	+1
Hydrogen	H	+1	Zinc	Zn	+2
Acetate	$C_2H_3O_2$	−1	Hypochlorite	ClO	−1
Bicarbonate	HCO_3	−1	Iodide	I	−1
Bisulfate	HSO_4	−1	Nitrate	NO_3	−1
Bromide	Br	−1	Nitrite	NO_2	−1
Carbonate	CO_3	−2	Oxide	O	−2
Chlorate	ClO_3	−1	Permanganate	MnO_4	−1
Chloride	Cl	−1	Phosphate	PO_4	−3

Name	Symbol	Valence	Name	Symbol	Valence
Chromate	CrO_4	−2	Sulfate	SO_4	−2
Ferricyanide	$Fe(CN)_6$	−3	Sulfide	S	−2
Ferrocyanide	$Fe(CN)_6$	−4	Sulfite	SO_3	−2
Hydroxide	OH	−1	Tartrate	$C_4H_4O_6$	−2

NOTE: Metalic ions may exist in several valence states. (See *Handbook of Chemistry and Physics*. Published by the Chemical Rubber Publishing Co., 2310 Superior Ave., N.E., Cleveland, Ohio.)

Buffer Tables *

pH 0.65 to 5.20

50 ml. 1N sodium acetate + x ml. 1N HCl, made up to 250 ml. (Walpole, 1914.)

pH	x ml. HCl	pH	x ml. HCl	pH	x ml. HCl
0.65	100	1.99	52.5	3.79	42.5
0.75	90	2.32	51.0	3.95	40.0
0.91	80	2.64	50.0	4.19	35.0
1.09	70	2.72	49.75	4.39	30.0
1.24	65	3.09	48.5	4.58	25.0
1.42	60	3.29	47.5	4.76	20.0
1.71	55	3.49	46.25	4.92	15.0
1.85	53.5	3.61	45.0	5.20	10.0

pH 2.2 to 8.0

200 ml. mixtures of x ml. 0.2M $Na_2 HPO_4$ with y ml. 0.1M citric acid. (McIlvaine, 1921.)

x ml. $Na_2 HPO_4$	y ml. citric acid	pH	x ml. $Na_2 HPO_4$	y ml. citric acid	pH
4.0	196	2.2	107.2	92.8	5.2
12.4	187.6	2.4	111.5	88.6	5.4
21.8	178.2	2.6	116.0	84.0	5.6
31.7	168.3	2.8	120.9	79.1	5.8
41.1	158.9	3.0	126.3	73.7	6.0
49.4	150.6	3.2	132.2	67.8	6.2
57.0	143.0	3.4	138.5	61.5	6.4

* From Pearse, A. G. E. *Histochemistry: Theoretical and Applied* (2d ed.). Boston: Little, Brown, 1960, pp. 779–781.

pH 2.2 to 8.0 — Continued

x ml. Na₂ HPO₄	y ml. citric acid	pH	x ml. Na₂ HPO₄	y ml. citric acid	pH
64.4	135.6	3.6	145.5	54.5	6.6
71.0	129.0	3.8	154.5	45.5	6.8
77.1	122.9	4.0	164.7	35.3	7.0
82.8	117.2	4.2	173.9	26.1	7.2
88.2	111.8	4.4	181.7	18.3	7.4
93.5	106.5	4.6	187.3	12.7	7.6
98.6	101.4	4.8	191.5	8.5	7.8
103.0	97.0	5.0	194.5	5.5	8.0

pH 3.6 to 5.6

200 ml. mixtures of 0.1N acetic acid and 0.1N sodium acetate. (Walpole, 1914.)

pH	0.1N acetic acid (ml.)	0.1N sodium acetate (ml.)	pH	0.1N acetic acid (ml.)	0.1N sodium acetate (ml.)
3.6	185	15	4.8	80	120
3.8	176	24	5.0	59	141
4.0	164	36	5.2	42	158
4.2	147	53	5.4	29	171
4.4	126	74	5.6	19	181
4.6	102	98			

pH 5.29 to 8.04

100 ml. mixtures of M/15 Na₂ HPO₄ and M/15 KH₂ PO₄. (Sörensen, 1909–12.)

pH	M/15 Na₂ HPO₄ (ml.)	M/15 KH₂ PO₄ (ml.)	pH	M/15 Na₂ HPO₄ (ml.)	M/15 KH₂ PO₄ (ml.)
5.29	2.5	97.5	6.81	50	50
5.59	5	95	6.98	60	40
5.91	10	90	7.17	70	30
6.24	20	80	7.38	80	20
6.47	30	70	7.73	90	10
6.64	40	60	8.04	95	5

pH 7.8 to 10.0

50 ml. 0.2M H_3BO_3 + 0.2M KCl + x ml. 0.2M NaOH, diluted to 200 ml. (Clark and Lubs, 1916.)

pH	x ml. 0.2M NaOH	pH	x ml. 0.2M NaOH
7.8	2.65	9.0	21.40
8.0	4.00	9.2	26.70
8.2	5.90	9.4	32.00
8.4	8.55	9.6	36.85
8.6	12.00	9.8	40.80
8.8	16.40	10.0	43.90

pH 8.45 to 12.77

100 ml. mixtures of 0.1M glycine and 0.1M NaCl with 0.1M NaOH. (Sörensen-Walbum, 1920.)

pH	x ml. glycine-NaCl	y ml. NaOH	pH	x ml. glycine-NaCl	y ml. NaOH
8.45	95	5	11.14	50	50
8.79	90	10	11.39	49	51
9.22	80	20	11.92	45	55
9.56	70	30	12.21	40	60
9.98	60	40	12.48	30	70
10.32	55	45	12.66	20	80
10.90	51	49	12.77	10	90

pH 2.62 to 9.16

Stock solution: 9.174 gm. sodium acetate $3H_2O$ + 14.714 gm. sodium barbiturate in CO_2-free distilled water, made up to 500 ml. 5 ml. of this solution + 2 ml. of 8.5% NaCl (may be omitted) treated with x ml. of 0.1N HCl and $(18 - x)$ ml. water. (Michaelis, 1931.)

x ml. 0.1N HCl	pH	x ml. 0.1N HCl	pH	x ml. 0.1N HCl	pH
16.0	2.62	9.0	4.93	4.0	7.66
15.0	3.20	8.0	5.32	3.0	7.90
14.0	3.62	7.0	6.12	2.0	8.18
13.0	3.88	6.5	6.75	1.0	8.55
12.0	4.13	6.0	6.99	0.75	8.68
11.0	4.33	5.5	7.25	0.5	8.9
10.0	4.66	5.0	7.42	0.25	9.16

pH 7.4 to 9.0

Mixtures of M/5 boric acid with M/20 sodium tetraborate. (Holmes.)

pH	M/5 H_3BO_3 (ml.)	M/20 $Na_2B_4O_7$ 10 H_2O (ml.)	pH	M/5 H_3BO_3 (ml.)	M/20 $Na_2B_4O_7$ 10 H_2O (ml.)
7.4	18	2	8.2	13	7
7.6	17	3	8.4	11	9
7.8	16	4	8.7	8	12
8.0	14	6	9.0	4	16

pH 7.19 to 9.10

25 ml. of 0.2M tris (hydroxymethyl) aminomethane; Eastman-Kodak (M.W. 121.14), + x ml. 0.1N HCl and distilled water up to 100 ml. (Gomori.)

pH	x ml. 0.1N HCl	pH	x ml. 0.1N HCl
7.19	45.0	8.23	22.5
7.36	42.5	8.32	20.0
7.54	40.0	8.41	17.5
7.66	37.5	8.51	15.0
7.77	35.0	8.62	12.5
7.87	32.5	8.74	10.0
7.96	30.0	8.92	7.5
8.05	27.5	9.10	5.0
8.14	25.0		

INDEX

Index

STAINS FOR:

Notes

Notes

Notes

Notes